A. J.

OXFORD MEDICAL PUBLICATIONS

THE ESSENTIALS OF PERIMETRY

STATIC AND KINETIC

THE ESSENTIALS OF PERIMETRY
STATIC AND KINETIC

SECOND EDITION

HOWARD REED

M.B., M.S.(Lond.), F.R.C.S.(Eng.), F.R.C.S.(C), F.A.C.S.

*Assistant Professor, Department of Ophthalmology,
University of Manitoba*

*Ophthalmologist to Winnipeg Clinic, Winnipeg
General Hospital, Children's Hospital, and
Misericordia Hospital, Winnipeg*

and

STEPHEN M. DRANCE

M.B., Ch.B.(Edin.), M.D.(Sask.), F.R.C.S.(Eng.), C.R.C.S.(C)

Professor of Ophthalmology, University of British Columbia

*Ophthalmologist to Vancouver General and Shaughnessy
Hospitals, Vancouver*

OXFORD
OXFORD UNIVERSITY PRESS
LONDON NEW YORK TORONTO

Oxford University Press, Walton Street, Oxford OX2 6DP

OXFORD LONDON GLASGOW
NEW YORK TORONTO MELBOURNE WELLINGTON
KUALA LUMPUR SINGAPORE JAKARTA HONG KONG TOKYO
DELHI BOMBAY CALCUTTA MADRAS KARACHI
IBADAN NAIROBI DAR ES SALAAM CAPE TOWN

ISBN 0 19 265403 9

© Oxford University Press 1960, 1972

First edition 1960
Second edition 1972
Reprinted 1978

All rights reserved. No part of this publication may be reproduced, stored in a retrieval system, or transmitted, in any form or by any means, electronic, mechanical, photocopying, recording, or otherwise, without the prior permission of Oxford University Press

Printed in Great Britain by
Hazell Watson & Viney Ltd, Aylesbury, Bucks

CONTENTS

PREFACE TO THE FIRST EDITION ... vii
PREFACE TO THE SECOND EDITION ... ix
INTRODUCTION ... xi

PART I
THE APPLIED ANATOMY OF THE VISUAL PATHWAY

1. THE RETINA AND THE OPTIC NERVE ... 3
2. THE OPTIC CHIASMA, THE OPTIC TRACTS, AND THE LATERAL GENICULATE BODIES ... 9
3. THE OPTIC RADIATIONS AND THE VISUAL CORTEX ... 16

PART II
THE VISUAL FIELD AND ITS ASSESSMENT

4. THE VISUAL FIELD ... 25
5. APPARATUS FOR THE MEASUREMENT OF VISUAL FIELDS ... 33
6. VISUAL FIELD EXAMINATION ... 42
7. STATIC PERIMETRY ... 54
8. TYPES OF FIELD DEFECTS ... 61

PART III
FIELD DEFECTS AND THEIR INTERPRETATION

9. GLAUCOMA ... 66
10. RETINAL LESIONS ... 90
11. THE TOXIC AMBLYOPIAS ... 95
12. OPTIC NERVE LESIONS ... 108
13. CHIASMAL LESIONS ... 124
14. RETROCHIASMAL LESIONS ... 141
15. OTHER LESIONS CAUSING FIELD DEFECTS ... 160
    INDEX ... 173

PREFACE TO THE FIRST EDITION

The opinion persists among some ophthalmologists that examination of the visual fields is not only a complicated, time-consuming procedure, but that it is frequently unrewarding. It is the aim of this book to present a simple account of the field defects, and to show that field examination may be both rapid and of great diagnostic value.

During recent years many elaborate perimeters have been put on the market. These have tended to complicate a simple examination, and make perimetry less popular. A hatpin with a small white head and a Bjerrum screen with suitable targets are usually adequate for making the diagnosis.

It is hoped that this book will serve as an introduction to perimetry for students of ophthalmology, and as an aid to revision for both anxious examinees and busy practitioners. Physicians and neurologists sometimes seek a simple statement of the principles of perimetry. I trust this book will meet their needs.

Some of the more important principles of perimetry have been repeated in different parts of the book. This has been done for two reasons. Firstly, repetition is an accepted maxim of good teaching and, secondly, it is irritating to be constantly referred to other sections of a book for important related information.

The anatomy drawings of the visual pathway are simple line drawings. In the diagrams of field defects only one or two isopters are given in order to illustrate the shape of the essential defect. Miss Nancy Joy, medical artist in the Department of Surgery, University of Manitoba*, gave unstintingly of her thought and time to the illustration of this book. To Dr. I. Maclaren Thompson, Professor of Anatomy in the University of Manitoba, my thanks are due for careful editing of the opening chapters on anatomy and for many sections of brain from which the drawings were made. Many friends have made suggestions which have contributed much to any merit which may be found in this book. In particular I wish to thank Dr. Rankin K. Hay, neurosurgeon to the Winnipeg Clinic, and Mr. Ian W. Payne, ophthalmic surgeon to the Royal Eye Infirmary, Plymouth, England, for so carefully reading the typescript and helping to eliminate errors and ambiguity. Finally I must express my gratitude to Professor Arnold Sorsby. He taught me more ophthalmology than did anyone else and without his encouragement this book would never have been completed.

Winnipeg, Manitoba, Canada H. R.
  April 1959

* Now Head of the Department of Art as Applied to Medicine, University of Toronto.

PREFACE TO THE SECOND EDITION

Eleven years have passed since the first edition of this book was published. It has been out of print for some time and it has proved a challenge to attempt to bring it up to date. During the past eleven years great strides have been made in ophthalmology. Whilst the basic concepts and principles of perimetry remain largely unchanged there is now much additional information to be added to that contained in the 1960 edition.

The whole book has been carefully read and edited. Some changes have been made in the text on most pages, many sections have been rewritten, and new sections have been added.

Whilst it is still true that for practical purposes almost all diagnoses may be made with a few coloured pins using the confrontation test, followed by analysis on a Bjerrum screen, many newer sophisticated instruments have been introduced which are essential for the detailed analysis necessary in research. These newer pieces of equipment are described and a chapter on static perimetry has been added. The chapter dealing with glaucoma has been rewritten.

Static perimetry has revealed much new knowledge concerning the development of field defects, particularly in glaucoma. In the chapter on glaucoma this new information is amply illustrated by static perimetric studies of patients. However, most of the original illustrations of the field defects found by using the tangent screen have been retained in this edition because the book has been written particularly for practising ophthalmologists. Most eye specialists in practice rely on the tangent screen and are likely to continue to use it for many years to come.

The preface to the first edition clearly states the purpose of this book. However, social and economic changes are occurring throughout the world which will alter the pattern of practice not only of ophthalmology but of the whole of medicine. Following the European example there is a great increase in the medical coverage of the general population by prepaid insurance. This factor, plus the dissemination of medical information by popular press, radio and television, has so increased the demand for medical service that the practice of medicine is becoming a race to cope with the volume of work, much of it of a technical nature. In the previous edition it was emphasized that all field examinations should be carried out by the ophthalmologist personally. However, ophthalmologists must change with the times and this no longer seems to be a reasonable opinion. Whilst it is true that the ophthalmologist must understand the principles of perimetry thoroughly, it is not right to insist that he should do all field examinations personally. A well-trained ophthalmic assistant or orthoptist can relieve the busy ophthalmologist of much of this technical work, particularly in such procedures as the routine examination of visual fields of known glaucoma subjects, or the recording of the extent of the defect in a patient whose diagnosis is established. The static perimetry fields in this book were in fact charted by Miss C. Wheeler, Mrs. M. Fairclough and Miss J. Bryett to whom we wish to express our thanks. When doubt arises the ophthalmologist must be prepared to investigate the visual field himself. It is hoped that this book will be of value not only to ophthalmologists but also to technicians who wish to learn the principles of perimetry.

H. R.
S. M. D.

July 1971

INTRODUCTION

Although the principles of perimetry have been known for a generation, patients are still seen with advanced disease which has been overlooked because these principles have not been applied. This occurs particularly in cases of glaucoma and of cerebral tumours compressing the optic nerves, chiasma, or radiations.

The expectation of life is increasing; hence there is a corresponding increase in the incidence of glaucoma. It has been shown by many observers that 2 per cent of the general population above the age of forty have ocular hypertension. This proportion increases with age, and above the age of sixty-five about 4·6 per cent are affected. If all those who examine eyes were more familiar with the methods of simple and rapid examination of the visual fields, more cases would be diagnosed before the field loss is severe.

When light falls upon the retina, nervous impulses arise in the rod and cone layer and pass along the optic nerves. These impulses then travel via the optic chiasma, optic tracts, and optic radiations to the visual cortex at the occipital poles. The visual pathway therefore passes from the front to the back of the brain. Interference with the conduction of nerve impulses by injury, tumour, inflammation, or vascular lesions at any site along this extensive pathway causes field defects. From these the site of a lesion can often be deduced. Hence the great value of perimetry.

Symptoms suggestive of visual field loss such as bumping into objects, difficulty in keeping to the line when reading, or pallor of the optic disc all indicate the need for field examination.

A distinction should be made between an examination to determine the presence of a field defect and the analysis of one that is known to be present. If a defect is suspected, no more than 5 minutes are required to detect and plot its form with one or two targets. From the simple chart thus produced, a diagnosis may often be confirmed. For the sake of clarity, most of the illustrations show no more than one or two isopters. This is not intended to imply that analysis of a known defect is unnecessary. Every defect should be analysed. As many targets as are necessary should be used for this analysis which may be either by dynamic or static techniques. This may take 30 or more minutes. For this reason it is often advisable to do the locating and the analysis at separate sittings. The more complicated field chart resulting from the analysis of a defect may be compared with a similar analysis at a later date and give much information about the advance or recovery of a disease.

In order to examine a visual field efficiently yet quickly the diagnostic features of a suspected disease must be known. A knowledge of these features is sound only when based upon the anatomy of the visual pathway.

PART I

THE APPLIED ANATOMY OF THE VISUAL PATHWAY

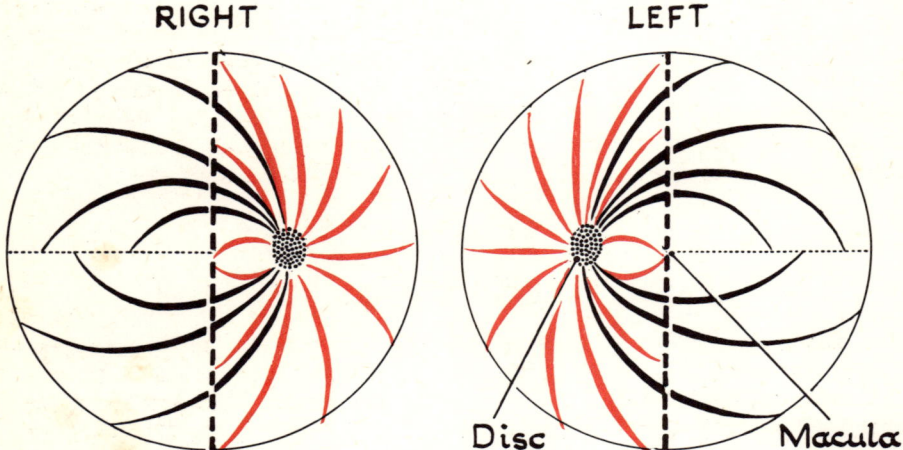

FIG. 3. The nasal and temporal halves of the retinae.

1
THE RETINA AND THE OPTIC NERVE

The anatomy of the visual pathway is known fairly well, but there is still some doubt about several minor details. A simple account of the generally accepted concepts will be given. These have been worked out by the following methods:
1. Correlation of clinical features and findings at operation in cases of tumours and injuries.
2. Correlation of ante-mortem and post-mortem findings in patients with visual defects.
3. Dissection of the nerve fibres of the visual pathway in the anatomy dissecting room.
4. Studies of degeneration resulting from experimental lesions in anthropoids.
5. Studies of field defects resulting from photocoagulation of different sites in the retinae of eyes about to be removed because of intraocular tumours.

THE RETINA

The retina may be considered as comprising three sets of neurones [FIG. 1]:
1. The rod and cone neurones.
2. The intermediate neurones.
3. The ganglion cell neurones.

The outer neurone is the receptor neurone, and it is dependent upon the choriocapillaris for its nutrition. The inner two neurones are supplied by the retinal blood vessels. After exit from the scleral canal, the third neurone is supplied by the blood vessels supplying the optic nerve, chiasma, and optic tracts.

A nerve fibre or axon arises from each ganglion cell and passes in the nerve fibre layer of the retina to the optic disc. It traverses the optic nerve, the optic chiasma, and an optic tract, to end in the appropriate lateral geniculate body. Between the ganglion cell in the retina and the lateral geniculate body there is no synapse, and field defects due to lesions of these nerve fibres are called conduction defects.

A lesion of any part of the visual pathway anterior to the lateral geniculate bodies causes optic atrophy in addition to a field defect. The nearer the lesion to the eyeball, the earlier the atrophy occurs. Pallor of the optic disc is seen about four weeks after a retrobulbar neuritis or injury to the optic nerve, but it may take months to appear in a tract lesion. When one optic nerve is damaged the related optic disc becomes paler than the other, but when one optic tract is damaged both optic discs become pale and it is more difficult to determine that optic atrophy is present. Visual field studies are essential in tract lesions.

It should be borne in mind that developmentally the retina is part of the brain. Therefore the optic nerves, chiasma, and tracts correspond to medullated tracts of the brain rather than to peripheral nerves. Peripheral nerves possess sheaths of Schwann which are essential for regeneration. But the cerebral tracts and the optic nerves lack them and therefore lack the faculty of regeneration.

ARRANGEMENT OF RETINAL NERVE FIBRES

The retinal nerve fibres arising from ganglion cells nasal to the disc pass directly to it, but on the temporal side they are arranged differently [FIG. 2].

The fibres passing from the macular area form a spindle-shaped bundle known as the maculopapillary fibres. This bundle comprises one-third of all the retinal fibres. Its situation corresponds to a spindle shaped area of the visual field known as the centrocaecal area which lies between the fixation point and the blind spot.

A horizontal raphe extends from the fovea to the temporal periphery. This raphe is the anatomical boundary between the functional superior and inferior halves of the retina. The arrangements of the nerve fibres may be likened to a feather which points from the macula to the temporal periphery. The raphe resembles the shaft, and the nerve fibres diverge from it like barbs from the shaft of the feather.

The retinal fibres which diverge from the raphe arch around the macular area and are known as the arcuate fibres [FIG. 2]. Damage to them causes arcuate defects in the visual field. These are characteristic of glaucoma and other conditions listed on page 66.

The horizontal raphe is represented in the

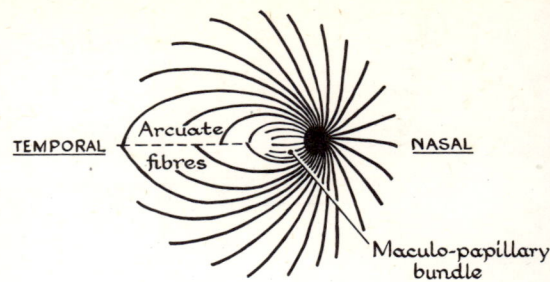

FIG. 2. The course of the retinal nerve fibres.

occipital lobes of the brain in the depths of the calcarine and post-calcarine fissures.

An imaginary vertical line drawn through the fovea divides the retina into nasal and temporal halves [FIG. 3]. All nerve fibres arising from ganglion cells to the temporal side of this vertical line pass, without crossing, into the optic tract on the same side. Those arising from the nasal side of this line cross at the chiasma into the optic tract of the opposite side. The most commonly accepted view is that with the exception of the arcuate fibres all axons of ganglion cells pass directly to the optic disc. Those physiological nasal fibres arising between the optic disc and a vertical line through the fovea actually cross the temporal edge of the disc. *It follows that a chiasmal lesion involving only the decussating nasal fibres causes atrophy and pallor of the whole of the optic disc.*

The fovea forms the physiological centre of the retina. Damage to the visual pathway behind the optic disc causes field defects based upon the fovea.

The disc forms the anatomical centre of the retina because the retinal arteries diverge from it, and the veins and retinal nerve fibres converge to it. Lesions of the retinal vessels or nerve fibres in the region of the optic disc, therefore, cause field defects based upon the optic disc [see FIGS. 72 and 73, p. 61].

Wolff's experiments upon rabbits and monkeys and observations in human cases of choroiditis [see p. 160] suggest that the peripheral and central nerve fibres have a definite arrangement in the retina [FIG. 4]. In the nerve fibre layer, fibres from peripheral areas of the retina lie to the outer side of those arising more centrally. The latter are therefore closest to the vitreous. At the optic disc they maintain their

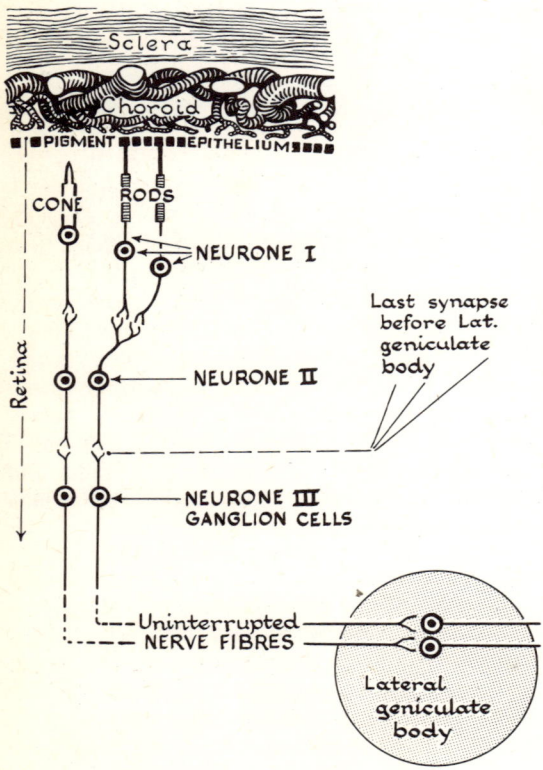

FIG. 1. The three groups of neurones of the retina.

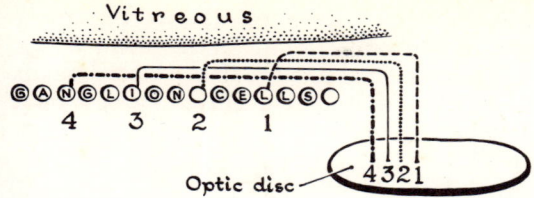

FIG. 4. The relationship of the peripheral to the central nerve fibres in the retina and at the optic disc.

central position, entering and traversing the optic nerve surrounded by the peripheral fibres.

This simple arrangement is modified by the macular group of fibres. It has already been pointed out that these fibres form a spindle-shaped group known as the maculopapillary bundle. This maculopapillary bundle enters the optic nerve through the temporal region of the disc. The nerve fibres from the temporal areas of the retina arch around this maculopapillary bundle and cross the upper and lower margins of the optic disc to enter the upper and lower segments of the optic nerve. The fibres from the retina nasal to the disc take the shortest route and pass straight to the optic disc across its nasal margin [FIGS. 2 and 3].

Hoyt and Tudor photocoagulated the centrocaecal area in a monkey and showed that the degenerating fibres occupied the temporal sector of the optic nerve immediately behind the optic disc. This supports the classical view that no fibres from ganglion cells in the temporal area of the retina cross the nasal border of the optic disc.

THE BLOOD SUPPLY OF THE RETINA

The outer neurones of the retina are supplied by the choriocapillaris of the choroid. No choroidal blood vessels penetrate the retina but its oxygenation is maintained by diffusion.

The retinal vessels supply the two inner neurones of the retina. The retinal artery divides into an upper and lower branch, each of which immediately divides again into nasal and temporal branches. The pattern varies from individual to individual, but four main branches are usually present. These follow the general direction of the nerve fibres. Like the nerve fibres the superior and inferior temporal vessels do not cross the temporal horizontal raphe. Occlusion of either of these arteries therefore causes a field defect with a horizontal edge.

Occasionally a cilioretinal artery supplies the macular area [FIGS. 109 and 110, p. 92]. A network of radial peripapillary capillaries has been described in the superficial nerve fibre layer surrounding the disc. Superiorly and inferiorly capillaries arise from this network, assume an arcuate course and follow the nerve fibre bundles. These capillaries form few anastomoses with adjacent vessels. It has been postulated that glaucoma field changes may occur as a result of circulatory embarrassment in these capillaries.

THE OPTIC NERVE

The nerve fibres of the maculopapillary bundle occupy the temporal quadrant of the optic nerve as far as the entrance of the central retinal artery [FIG. 5]. This occurs about 1 cm. behind the eyeball and here the maculopapillary bundle sinks into the centre of the optic nerve. From this point on the peripheral retinal fibres are situated peripherally in the nerve and the central fibres are central.

The classical teaching was that just before the optic nerve joins the chiasma a nasal rotation of the nerve fibres begins [FIG. 6]. It was considered that this nasal rotation of fibres continued through the optic chiasma and the optic tracts until at the lateral geniculate bodies the superior fibres of the retina were medial and the inferior fibres of the retina were lateral in situation.

Hoyt and Luis have reported experiments which cast doubt upon the orthodox view [see Chapter 2]. They photocoagulated small areas in the retina of monkeys and then followed the path of the degenerating fibres in the visual pathway. Their experiments indicated that no nasal rotation occurs in the monkey optic nerve. The rotation commences in the chiasma and is not significant until the nerve fibres enter the optic tract, where the superior fibres

THE RETINA AND THE OPTIC NERVE

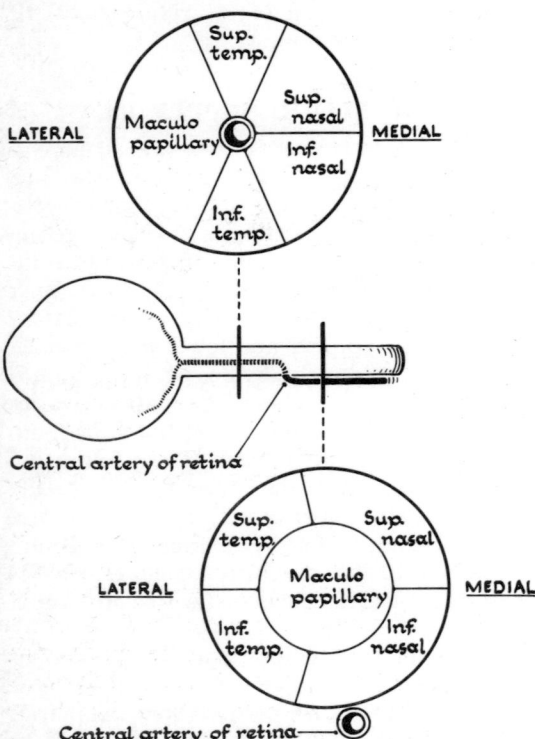

FIG. 5. The arrangement of the nerve fibres in the optic nerve.

are superomedial in position and the inferior fibres are inferolateral.

Another finding which contradicts the standard view is that whilst the peripheral retinal fibres are orderly and peripheral in situation in the optic nerve, the macular fibres are distributed diffusely throughout the nerve and are found peripherally as well as centrally.

A fibrous septum is present in the optic nerve close to its junction with the chiasma. This septum separates the nasal from the temporal fibres of the retina. Damage to the medial aspect of the optic nerve at this site, e.g. an aneurysm of the anterior communicating artery, may cause a temporal defect in the visual field. A lesion of the lateral aspect of the optic nerve close to the chiasma may cause a nasal field defect.

RELATIONS OF THE OPTIC NERVE

The optic nerve passes from the orbit through the optic foramen of the sphenoid bone into the middle cranial fossa. Its intraorbital portion is about 3 cm. long, the intraforaminal part is 0·6 cm. and the intracranial course varies from 1 cm. to more than 2 cm. in length. Its relations are best considered in these three situations.

ORBITAL RELATIONS

The nerve lies within the rectus muscle cone, and at the apex of the cone the medial and superior rectus muscles actually arise in part from the optic nerve sheath [FIG. 7]. This attachment is thought to cause the sickening pain on extreme rotation of the eyes in retrobulbar neuritis. Four nerves enter the apex of the muscle cone through the superior orbital fissure. At the apex they lie between the optic nerve and the origin of the lateral rectus muscle. They are:

1. The upper and lower divisions of the oculomotor nerve (III).
2. The nasociliary nerve (V).
3. The abducens nerve (VI).
4. The sympathetic root to the ciliary ganglion.

INTRAFORAMINAL RELATIONS

The optic nerve is surrounded by the three meninges, dura, arachnoid, and pia. At the

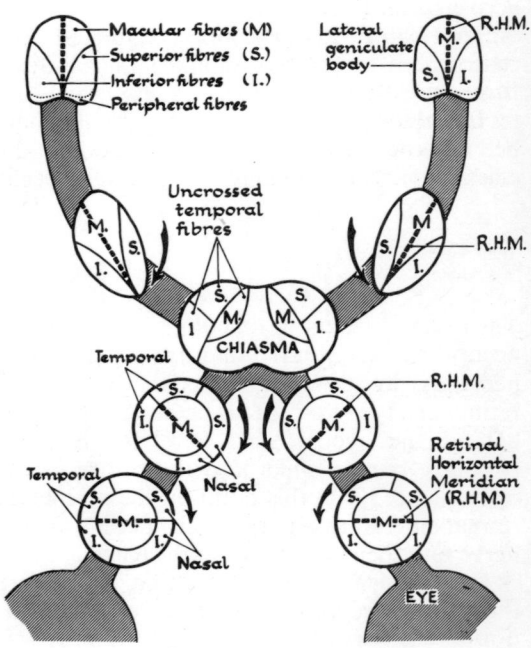

FIG. 6. The nasal rotation of nerve fibres (after Henschen).

optic foramen the dura of the optic nerve joins the periorbita to line the optic canal. Elsewhere these three membranes, dura, arachnoid, and pia, are not adherent, but in the foramen they are attached superiorly to each other and to the nerve. The nerve is therefore tethered, so that a piston-like movement of the nerve in the foramen is prevented during rotation of the eyeball. The most common result of an injury to the optic nerve is a defect in the inferior half of the visual field. It is believed that blood vessels entering the nerve are torn in the region of this superior fixation and this results in atrophy of the nerve fibres in the upper part of the nerve [FIG. 144, p. 121].

Below the nerve and within the dural sheath is the ophthalmic artery.

Medially the nerve is related to the sphenoidal sinus. A large posterior ethmoid cell may sometimes be a medial relation. Occasionally either the sphenoid sinus or a posterior ethmoid cell may spread into the roots of the lesser wing of the sphenoid and even completely surround the optic nerve. If such a sinus becomes infected retrobulbar neuritis may occur, but this is a rare clinical event.

RELATIONS IN THE MIDDLE CRANIAL FOSSA

On emerging from the optic foramen of the sphenoid bone the optic nerve at once becomes closely related to important anatomical structures in the middle fossa.

Laterally are the anterior clinoid process and the internal carotid artery as it emerges from the roof of the cavernous sinus. Just above the

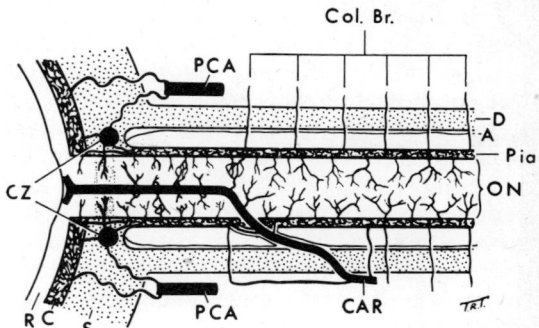

FIG. 8. Blood supply of the optic nerve.
A = arachnoid; C = choroid; CAR = central artery of retina; Col. Br. = collateral branch; CZ = circle of Zinn; ON = optic nerve; PCA = posterior ciliary artery; R = retina; S = sclera.
[Hayreh (1963) *Brit. J. Ophthal.*, by permission of the Author and Editor.]

level of the anterior clinoid process are the anterior perforated substance and the medial root of the olfactory tract. The anterior cerebral artery crosses the upper surface of the optic nerve from the lateral to the medial side.

Inferiorly, the optic nerve lies first upon the ophthalmic artery at its origin from the internal carotid and then upon the anterior end of the cavernous sinus. Below the level of the angle formed by the two optic nerves is the anterior part of the pituitary gland which is roofed by the diaphragma sellae.

These anatomical relationships are of great importance in cases of tumours and inflammation in this region. Accurate diagnosis depends upon the correlation of the field defects, cranial nerve palsies, and other clinical signs.

BLOOD SUPPLY OF THE OPTIC NERVE

The blood supply of the optic nerve is arranged in two different systems, the axial and the peripheral.

AXIAL SYSTEM

François and Neetens maintained that the central or axial part of the optic nerve is supplied by the central optic nerve artery which is derived from the ophthalmic artery and divides into an anterior and a posterior branch. François believed that it supplies the macular nerve fibres, that it probably does not anastomose with the peripheral system, and that this may have some bearing on the pathogenesis of central scotomata.

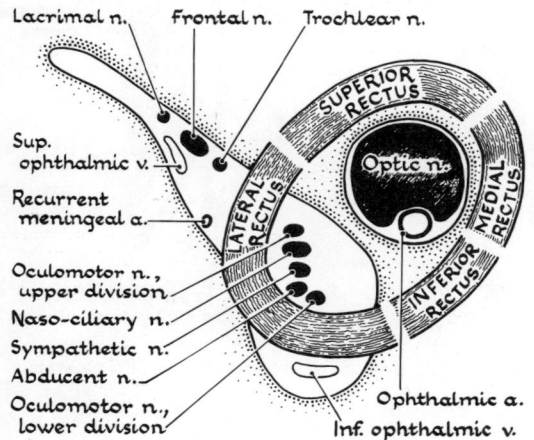

FIG. 7. Anatomical relations at the apex of the right orbit.

Hayreh, however, after extensive investigations by latex injection, disagreed with the description of the anatomy by François and Neetens in the following respects [FIG. 8]:

1. In the majority of cases the central retinal artery gives off numerous branches to the optic nerve and contributes to both the axial and peripheral systems. It plays a major role in the blood supply of the anterior part of the optic nerve but is less important in supplying blood to the posterior part, though sometimes it supplies blood as far as the optic canal.

2. No typical anterior and posterior central optic nerve arteries were seen by Hayreh in 100 specimens, but in a few cases rudimentary arteries 3–4 mm. long were observed.

However, Hayreh emphasized that there was extreme variation in the pattern of branches and anastomosis of the central retinal artery so that it cannot be said that any one arrangement is usual.

A knowledge of the blood supply in the region of the disc may aid considerably in the understanding of the changes occurring in glaucoma and other manifestations associated with ischaemia. The posterior aspect of the lamina cribrosa is supplied by short branches from the intraneural portion of the central retinal artery. The anterior aspect of the lamina receives its blood supply from the ciliary system via the choriocapillaris. The circumferential areas of the lamina are supplied by the short posterior ciliary arteries plus a pial component from the outer layers of the optic nerve. The venous drainage is through the central retinal vein and the vortex system. Fluorescein angiographic studies suggest that the vascular territories of the individual ciliary vessels remain separate in their areas of supply to the nerve head. This could explain some of the changes seen clinically in which there appears to be an insufficient supply of blood to discrete sectors of the optic disc.

PERIPHERAL SYSTEM

The outer fibres of the optic nerve are nourished by blood vessels from the pial sheath. Small pial branches are given off by larger arteries in the neighbourhood of the optic nerve throughout its course.

In the orbit the nerve receives branches from the ophthalmic and lacrimal arteries. Near the eye small branches from the long and short posterior ciliary branches supply the optic nerve sheath and form the intrascleral anastomosis of Zinn and Haller.

Within the cranium the outer fibres of the optic nerve are supplied by minute branches from the internal carotid, anterior cerebral, and anterior communicating arteries.

REFERENCES AND FURTHER READING

FRANÇOIS, J., and NEETENS, A. (1954) Vascularization of the optic pathway. I. Lamina cribrosa and optic nerve, *Brit. J. Ophthal.*, **38**, 472.

FRANÇOIS, J., and NEETENS, A. (1956) Vascularization of the optic pathway; study of intraorbital and intracranial optic nerve by serial sections, *Brit. J. Ophthal.*, **40**, 45, 341, 730.

FRANÇOIS, J., NEETENS, A., and COLLETTE, J. M. (1955) Vascular supply of the optic pathway. II. Further studies by micro-arteriography of the optic nerve, *Brit. J. Ophthal.*, **39**, 220.

HAYREH, S. S. (1963) The central artery of the retina. Its role in the blood supply of the optic nerve, *Brit. J. Ophthal.*, **47**, 651.

HENKIND, P. (1967) New observations on the radial peripapillary capillaries, *Invest. Ophthal.*, **6**, 103.

HOYT, W. F., and TUDOR, R. C. (1963) The course of parapapillary temporal retinal axons through the anterior optic nerve, *Arch. Ophthal.*, **69**, 503.

WOLFF, E., and PENMAN, G. G., *XVI Concil. Ophthalmologicum 1950*. The position occupied by the peripheral retinal fibres in the nerve-fibre layer and at the nerve head, p. 625, British Medical Association.

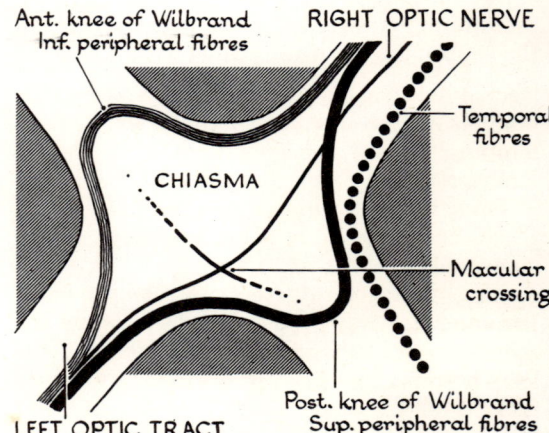

FIG. 9. The crossing of the nasal fibres in the chiasma.

2

THE OPTIC CHIASMA, THE OPTIC TRACTS, AND THE LATERAL GENICULATE BODIES

THE OPTIC CHIASMA

The chiasma is a tablet-like mass of nerve fibres. It is about 12 mm. from side to side and 8 mm. from front to back. The two optic nerves join its anterior horns and the two optic tracts leave its posterior horns.

It is situated in a subarachnoid basal cistern in the middle cranial fossa, where it is bathed in cerebrospinal fluid. It lies at the junction of the anterior wall and the floor of the third ventricle and forms a ridge on the inside of the third ventricle.

Objects in the nasal field set up impulses in the retina on the temporal side of the fovea. Fibres carrying these impulses pass through the chiasma without decussation. They pass along the lateral border of the chiasma to the optic tract of the same side.

Objects in the temporal field set up impulses in the retina on the nasal side of the fovea. All these nasal fibres cross to the opposite optic tract at the chiasma. In man, there are approximately 50 per cent more nasal fibres than temporal fibres corresponding to the larger temporal field.

There are three points to remember about these nasal fibres which decussate at the chiasma [FIG. 9]:
1. The inferior peripheral nasal fibres cross in the anterior part of the chiasma and enter the opposite optic nerve for a short distance. This loop is sometimes known as the anterior knee of Wilbrand.
2. The superior peripheral nasal fibres cross in the posterior part of the chiasma and pass a short distance into the optic tract of the same side. This loop is known as the posterior knee of Wilbrand.
3. The fibres arising from the nasal half of the macular area of each retina fan out into a broad band as they cross in the posterior part of the chiasma.

The anterior knees of Wilbrand and the posterior macular crossing are fairly constant in situation, but the posterior knees of Wilbrand are less so. The four knees are formed by peripheral fibres, and between these the remainder of the nasal fibres from both retinae spread out and form a mesh of nerve fibres.

The detailed internal structure of the chiasma is not known with accuracy. At the termination of the tracts and in the lateral geniculate bodies the nerve fibres which started in a superior position in the optic nerves are medial in situation, and the lower fibres in the optic nerves become lateral in the tracts and bodies. This rotation results in the superior temporal retinal fibres being more medial than the inferior temporal fibres [FIG. 6, p. 6]. It was always believed that the nasal rotation of nerve fibres started in the optic nerves and continued throughout the chiasma and optic tracts. It was accepted that this nasal rotation explained the fact that midline compression of the chiasma damages the superior temporal retinal fibres before the inferior temporal ones, and thus usually results in the lower nasal quadrants of the two visual fields being lost before the upper nasal quadrants. However, Hoyt and Luis found no evidence of nasal rotation in the optic nerves and chiasma in their monkey experiments.

Previous workers have reported that the fibres of the nasal macular areas cross in the posterior portion of the chiasma. But Hoyt and Luis found in their experiments with monkeys that the macular fibres were widely diffused throughout the chiasma, a thin layer of the anterior and posterior parts of the floor of the chiasma being the only portions free of macular fibres. In fact, the degeneration which occurred when the macula was photocoagulated was so diffuse throughout the chiasma that they consider that the chiasma must be regarded as primarily a macular structure.

Another interesting finding by Hoyt and Luis, not previously emphasized, was that the macular fibres were principally of small calibre in contrast with the larger calibre of fibres arising from more peripheral areas of the retina. They confirmed the findings of earlier workers that the small macular fibres pass from the central portion of the optic nerve through the chiasma to the superior segments of the optic tracts.

ANATOMICAL RELATIONS OF THE OPTIC CHIASMA

The optic nerves emerge from the optic foramina in the middle cranial fossa and pass upwards and backwards to the chiasma at a variable angle which is usually about 35 degrees. The length of the optic nerves also varies, so that the height of the optic chiasma above the diaphragma sellae is by no means constant. It is usually about 1 cm. A pituitary tumour must therefore rise at least 2 cm. above the level of the clinoid processes before pressure on the chiasma is severe enough to interfere with conduction of nerve impulses and cause field defects.

The chiasma is tilted at an angle, which follows the direction of the optic nerves, and from each posterior corner arises an optic tract. At this situation in the middle cranial fossa the whole of the visual pathway is encircled by the arterial circle of Willis [FIG. 10]. The posterior communicating arteries are approximately horizontal so that the anterior cerebral arteries lie above and in front of the optic chiasma at its junction with the optic nerves, and the posterior cerebral arteries lie below the optic tracts. Aneurysms commonly arise from this arterial circle and cause field defects by compressing the optic nerves, optic chiasma, or optic tracts.

In front and above the chiasma are the anterior cerebral and anterior communicating arteries.

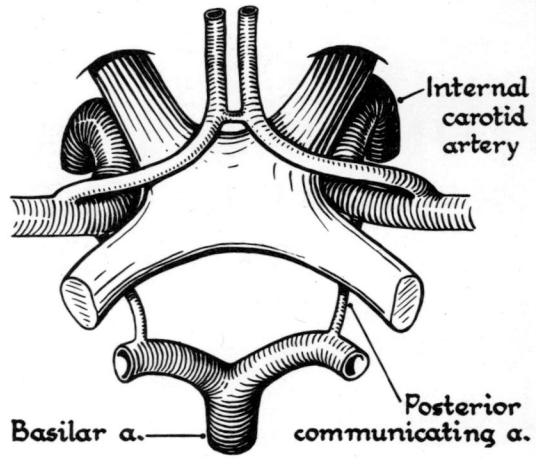

FIG. 10. The circle of Willis.

Behind is the third ventricle with the infundibulum descending to the pituitary body.

On each side the internal carotid artery passes upwards in the angle between the optic nerve and the optic tract after having pierced the roof of the cavernous sinus.

Above the chiasma are the third ventricle and the hypothalamus.

Below it are the optic groove of the sphenoid in front, and the pituitary body behind. The outer border of the chiasma is related below to the cavernous sinus and its contents [FIG. 11].

The inconstancy of the relationship of the chiasma to the pituitary gland was demonstrated by de Schweinitz [FIG. 12]. He dissected 125 heads and found that in 5 per cent the optic nerves were so short that the chiasma occupied the optic groove of the sphenoid bone. This is known as the pre-fixed chiasma. In 12 per cent the optic nerves were longer, so that the chiasma was above the middle of the sella turcica. The commonest relationship was that in which the chiasma was above the posterior two-thirds of the sella. This occurred in 79 per cent of cases. In 4 per cent the chiasma was post-fixed. In these the optic nerves were long and the major portion of the chiasma was behind the sella.

Not only does the optic chiasma vary in its relationship to the pituitary and to its surrounding structures, but space-occupying lesions seldom grow symmetrically. For example, a pituitary tumour once out of its fossa may expand predominantly to one side. The

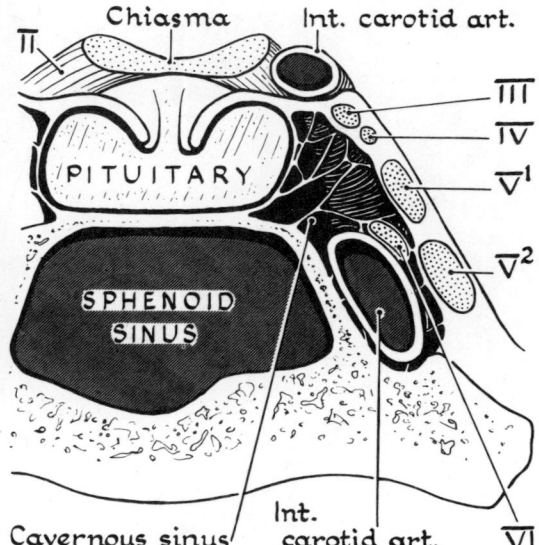

FIG. 11. The cavernous sinus from behind.

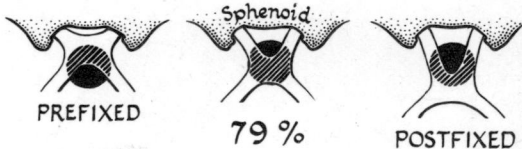

FIG. 12. Pre-fixation and post-fixation of the chiasma.

valuable guide to the site of compression, they occasionally seem unreliable.

BLOOD SUPPLY OF THE OPTIC CHIASMA

The optic chiasma lies within the circle of Willis and derives its blood supply from arteries forming the circle. It is supplied chiefly by the internal carotid, the anterior cerebral, and the anterior communicating arteries. The middle cerebral, the posterior communicating, and the anterior choroidal arteries also contribute to its nourishment [FIG. 10].

CLINICAL APPLICATIONS

The field defects will be discussed in more detail later [see Chapter 13], but since they are so important in the diagnosis of chiasmal compression a few commonly observed clinical patterns will be mentioned here. The correlation of the anatomy and the field defects will aid an understanding of both.

It has already been mentioned that a chiasma may be stretched in one situation and compressed against a fixed or relatively resistant structure elsewhere. A tumour may cause relative ischaemia by squeezing small nutrient arteries, or oedema and congestion by constricting veins. Thus nerve fibres some distance away may be more severely affected than those adjacent to the tumour. Consequently, although in most cases the field defects are a

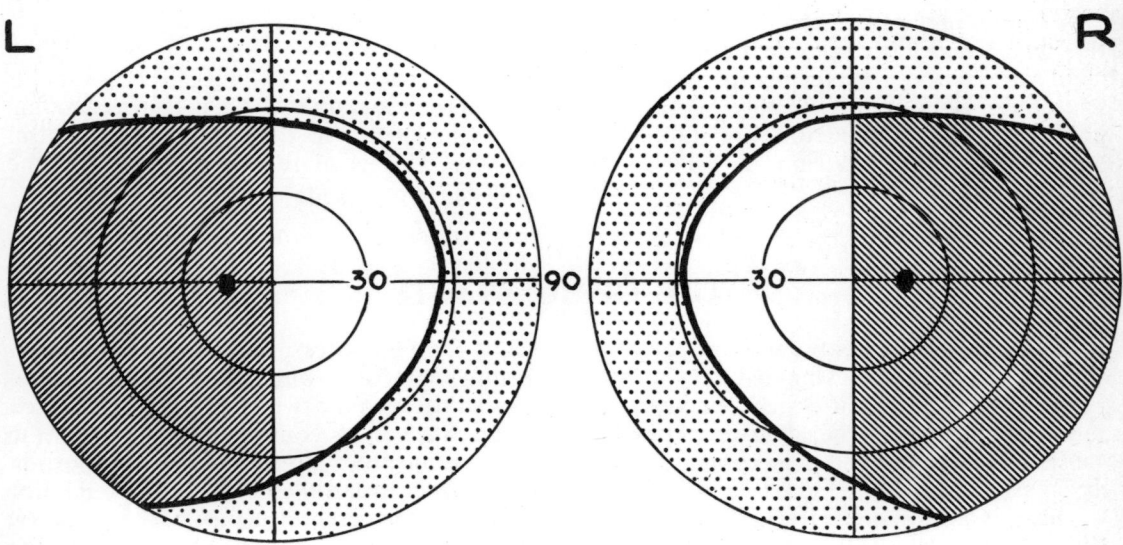

FIG. 13. Bitemporal hemianopia.

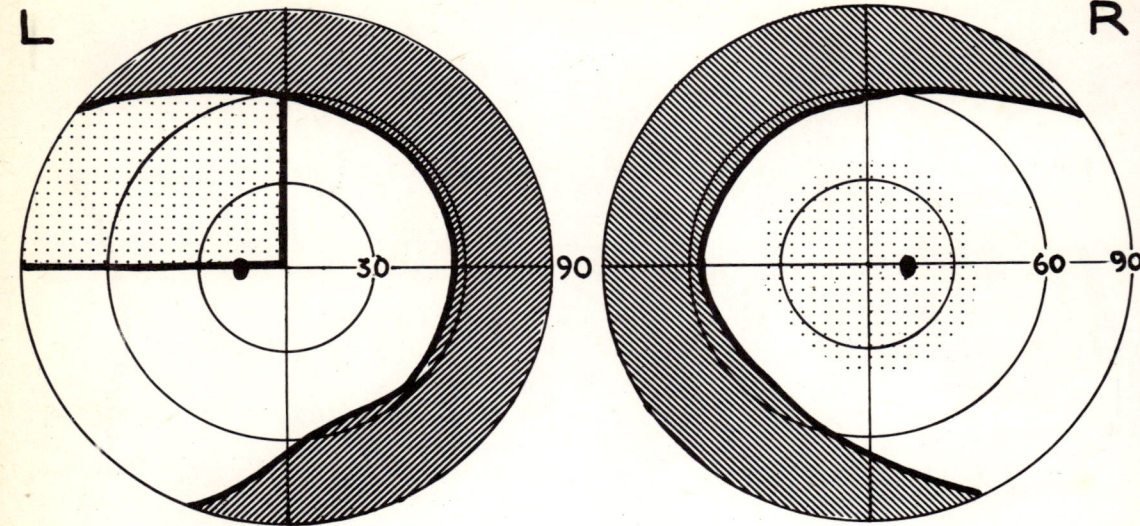

Fig. 14. Field defects resulting from damage to the right optic nerve and the right anterior knee of Wilbrand.

pituitary tumour must rise some 2 cm. above the level of the posterior clinoid processes before serious stretching of the chiasma occurs. If the enlargement is in the midline the nasal decussating fibres are affected first, giving rise to bitemporal defects [FIG. 13].

With progressive enlargement the crossed fibres degenerate and form a thin fibrous sheet on the upper aspect of the tumour. The uncrossed temporal fibres lie more laterally and may remain undamaged for a long period. At this stage the field defects often appear to remain stationary despite further increase in the size of the tumour, presumably because the uncrossed fibres are able to move still farther up and out before stretching is sufficient to interfere with conduction.

Pressure upon an optic nerve at its junction with the chiasma interferes with the anterior knee of Wilbrand. Conduction in the inferior peripheral nasal fibres from the other eye may be impaired and result in an upper temporal quadrantic defect in the visual field [FIG. 14]. This is seen especially in meningiomata of the inner one-third of the sphenoidal ridge.

An inferior temporal quadrantic defect from interference with the posterior knee of Wilbrand is less commonly seen.

Stretching of the chiasma in the midline posteriorly by an expanding pituitary tumour hinders conduction in the macular decussating fibres and tends to cause bitemporal central defects. This is more likely to occur if the chiasma is pre-fixed.

THE OPTIC TRACTS

From each posterolateral corner of the optic chiasma, an optic tract, rounded like the optic nerve, passes lateroposteriorly, between the tuber cinereum and the anterior perforated substance. Here the posterior communicating artery crosses below it [FIGS. 10 and 15].

The next portion of the tract is flattened, and winds around the junction of the basis pedunculi of the midbrain and the internal capsule.

Thus the two bases pedunculi and the interpeduncular fossa with its contents are embraced between the two optic tracts. Here each optic tract is in contact medially with the descending motor fibres [FIG. 16]. This portion of the tract is partly embedded in the inferior aspect of the cerebral hemisphere just below the lentiform nucleus. It passes above the uncus, immediately medial to the choroidal

THE OPTIC TRACTS

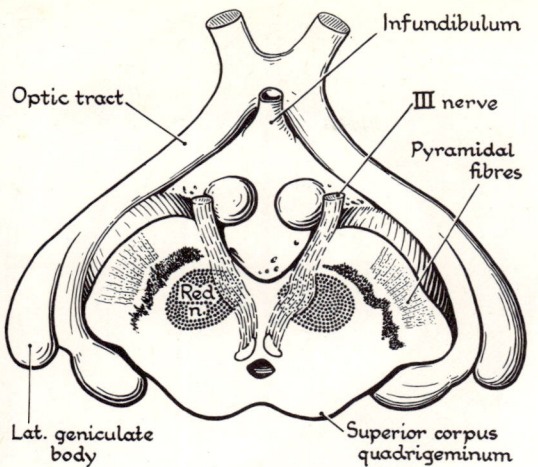

Fig. 15. The optic tracts viewed from below at the level of the superior corpus quadrigeminum.

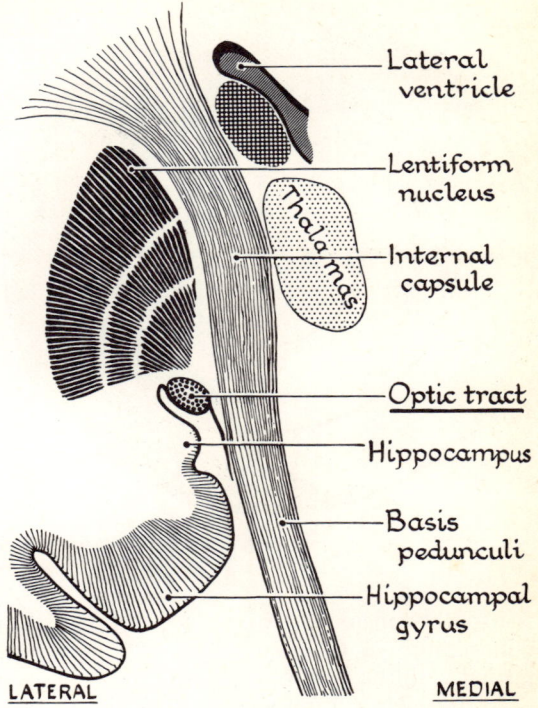

Fig. 16. Coronal section showing the anatomical relations of the optic tract.

fissure of the inferior horn of the lateral ventricle.

It ends by dividing into two roots. The longer lateral root goes to the lateral geniculate body and the smaller medial root goes to the medial geniculate body. Each optic tract is about one inch in length.

All the fibres concerned with vision (about 90 per cent of those in the optic tract) end in the lateral geniculate body.

There is some uncertainty about the constitution of the medial root of the optic tract. It

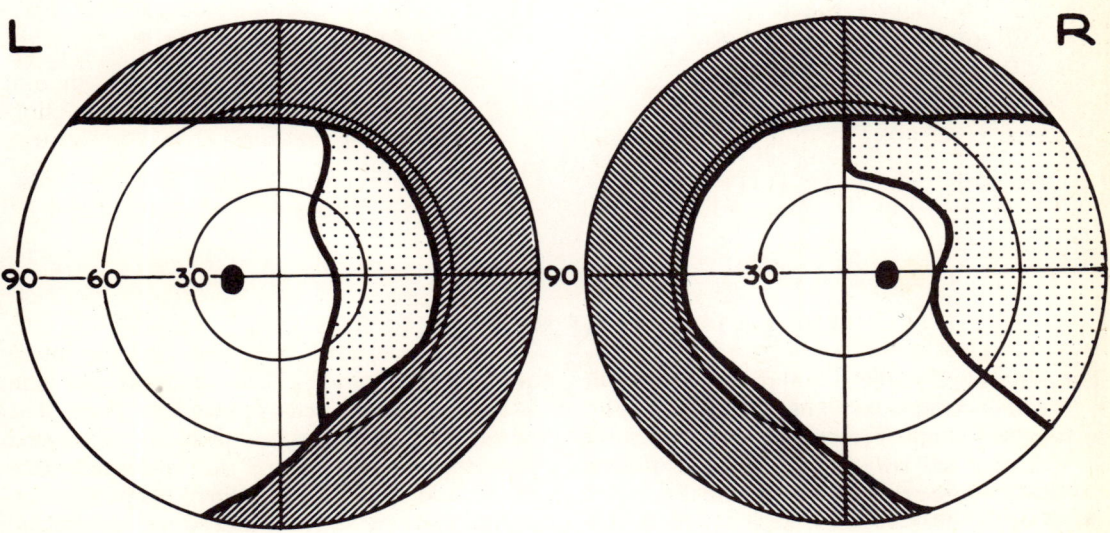

Fig. 17. Homonymous hemianopia showing incongruity due to a lesion of the left optic tract.

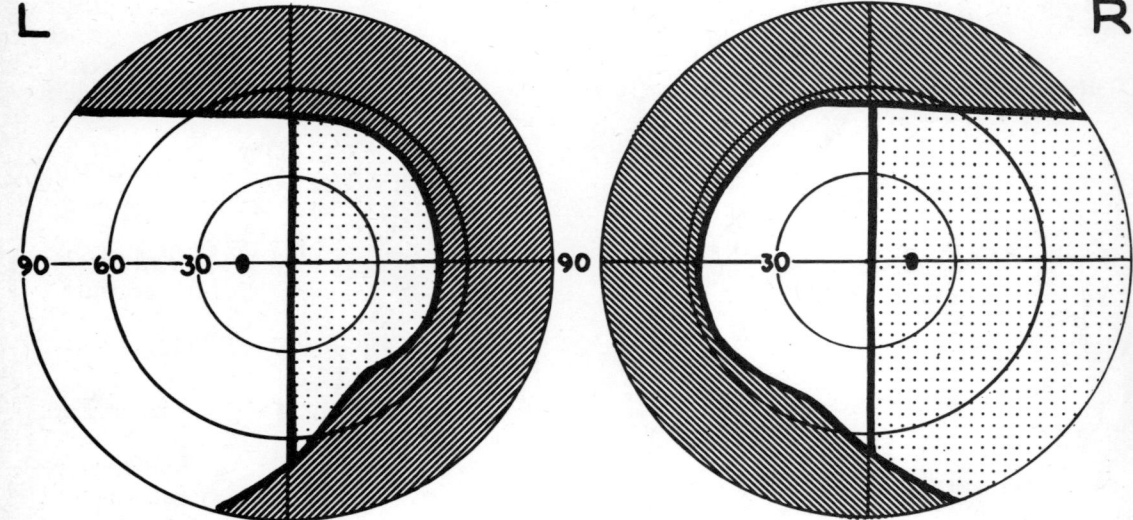

Fig. 18. Homonymous hemianopia with splitting of the macula due to destruction of the left optic tract.

is usually considered to contain fibres of the commissure of Gudden which may be connected with the auditory system.

As the nerve fibres pass backwards in the optic tracts, those from corresponding areas in the two retinae become more closely associated, until in the lateral geniculate bodies an accurate relationship is established. The clinical evidence for this is that a lesion of the anterior end of an optic tract is likely to cause bilateral field defects which are not exactly alike, an important feature known as incongruity [Fig. 17].

Another feature which may occur in tract lesions is splitting of the macula, in which the field defect bisects the macular area [Fig. 18]. Lesions posterior to the lateral geniculate bodies, i.e. those of the optic radiations and visual cortex, usually spare the macula by 3 degrees or more.

Although there is some uncertainty about an orderly nasal rotation commencing in the optic nerves and continuing through the chiasma, there is no doubt about the 90 degree rotation in the optic tracts. The fibres from the corresponding upper quadrant of each retina are medial, and those from the lower quadrants are lateral. On coronal section the macular fibres occupy a wedge-like area near the upper part of the tract [Fig. 6, p. 6].

BLOOD SUPPLY OF THE OPTIC TRACTS

The anterior choroidal and posterior communicating arteries supply the optic tracts.

THE LATERAL GENICULATE BODIES

The nerve fibres in the lateral root of each optic tract end in synapses with nerve cells in the corresponding lateral geniculate body. Since the 90 degree nasal rotation of fibres is already complete, those arising from the corresponding upper quadrants of each retina end in the medial portion of the body. Those arising from the lower quadrants of each retina are represented laterally. The macular fibres end in a large wedge-shaped area between them. The fibres from the nasal periphery of each retina carrying impulses from the crescentic temporal field end inferiorly [Fig. 6, p. 6].

On coronal section the lateral geniculate body is seen to be composed of six layers of cells [Fig. 19], each layer being separated from

THE LATERAL GENICULATE BODIES

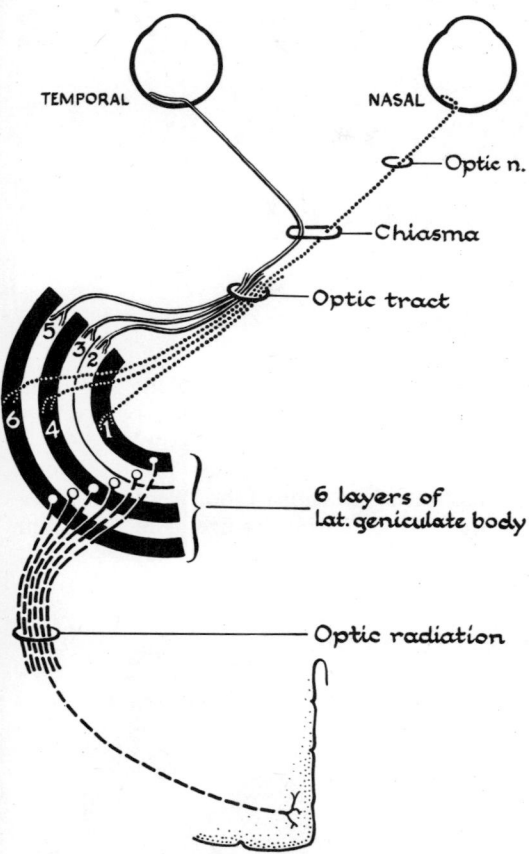

FIG. 19. The six layers of the lateral geniculate body.

the next by a lamina of nerve fibres. The nerve cell layers have been numbered from 1 to 6 from within outwards. The uncrossed retinal fibres end in layers 2, 3, and 5, and the crossed fibres terminate in layers 1, 4, and 6. The nerve fibres of the optic radiation arise from all six cell layers.

A small lesion in the temporal region of the retina of one eye causes patches of atrophy in layers 2, 3, and 5 of the lateral geniculate body of the same side. Damage to the nasal half of the retina causes atrophy in layers 1, 4, and 6 of the opposite lateral geniculate body. A lesion in the visual cortex, however, causes an area of atrophy in all six layers of the lateral geniculate body of the same side. It is usually considered, therefore, that in the lateral geniculate body there is accurate localization of corresponding retinal points, just as there is in the visual cortex. However, there is growing evidence that correlation of corresponding points is not completely accurate until the posterior areas of the radiations are reached, because the more meticulous the study of lesions of the anterior parts of the radiations, the more often incongruity is demonstrated.

BLOOD SUPPLY OF THE LATERAL GENICULATE BODY

The posterior cerebral artery and the anterior choroidal artery form an anastomotic network on the surface of the lateral geniculate body. Branches arise from this network and penetrate the body.

CLINICAL APPLICATIONS

Gliomata of the temporal lobe are the tumours which most frequently affect this area. By the time they are large enough to damage the visual pathway they distort the adjacent structures so much that it is often difficult to be sure whether the interference is in the posterior end of the optic tract, the lateral geniculate body, or the beginning of the optic radiation. All three structures may be involved. The clinical evidence for the detailed internal anatomy of the optic tracts and lateral geniculate bodies is somewhat scanty.

REFERENCES AND FURTHER READING

BULL, J. (1956) The normal variations in the position of the optic recess of the third ventricle, *Acta radiol. (Stockh.)*, **46**, 72.

DE SCHWEINITZ, G. E. (1923) Concerning certain ocular aspects of pituitary body disorders mainly exclusive of the usual central and peripheral hemianopic field defects, Bowman Lecture, *Trans. ophthal. Soc. U.K.*, **43**, 12.

HOYT, W. F., and LUIS, O. (1962) Visual fibre anatomy in the infrageniculate pathway of the primate, *Arch. Ophthal.*, **68**, 94.

HOYT, W. F., and LUIS, O. (1963) The primate chiasma, *Arch. Ophthal.*, **70**, 69.

SCHAEFFER, J. P. (1924) Some points in the regional anatomy of the optic pathway, with especial reference to tumours of the hypophysis cerebri and resulting ocular changes, *Anat. Rec.*, **28**, 243.

3

THE OPTIC RADIATIONS AND THE VISUAL CORTEX

THE OPTIC RADIATIONS

It should be noted that both geniculate bodies are parts of the thalamus. The thalamus is a mass of nerve cells and from these arise nerve fibres which radiate to the cortex. Each optic radiation is the posterior portion of this thalamocortical projection system in each hemisphere. It is composed of nerve fibres which arise from cells in each lateral geniculate body and carry impulses to the striate area in the corresponding occipital lobe.

After leaving the lateral geniculate body, the optic radiation ascends for a very short distance in the retrolentiform portion of the posterior limb of the internal capsule [FIG. 20]. In this situation it passes immediately behind the main ascending sensory pathway. This is a most important relation, because a vascular lesion of the internal capsule may involve the optic radiation. If this occurs the hemiplegia is accompanied by homonymous hemianopia.

The optic radiation then sweeps laterally and posteriorly around the outer side of the inferior and posterior horns and the adjacent part of the body of the lateral ventricle [FIGS. 21 and 22]. In this situation the radiation is deep to the superior and the middle temporal convolutions.

The horizontal portion of the optic radiation is composed of three bundles. The superior bundle carries impulses from the medial group of cells in the lateral geniculate body to the visual cortex above the calcarine fissure and the anterior end of the post-calcarine fissure. This bundle, therefore, conveys impulses from the extramacular area of the corresponding upper quadrant of each retina.

The middle bundle, which constitutes nearly half the total number of radiation fibres, conveys macular impulses. The fibres begin in the cells in the wedge-like area in the lateral geniculate body. They pass to the posterior pole of the occipital lobe and end both above and below the post-calcarine fissure.

The inferior bundle arises in the lateral group of cells and ends in the visual cortex below the post-calcarine fissure. The uniocular

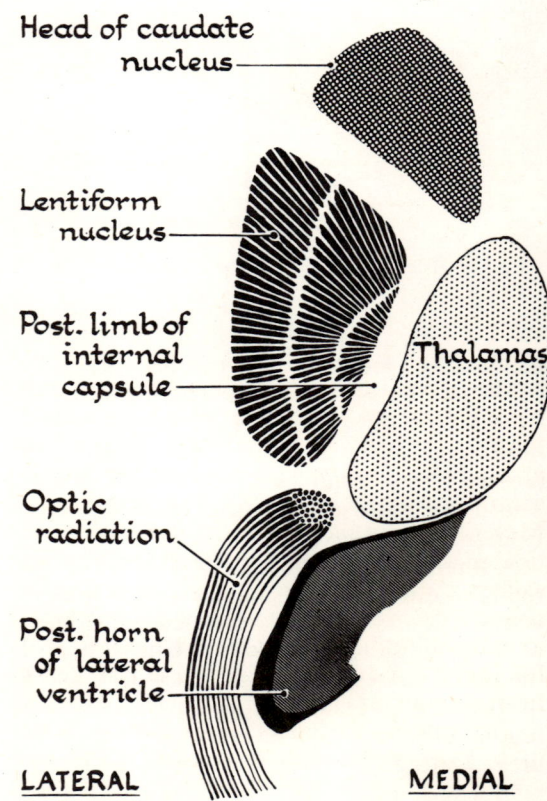

FIG. 20. Horizontal section showing the relation of the optic radiation to the internal capsule and to the lateral ventricle.

THE OPTIC RADIATIONS

field is believed to be represented by the most medial fibres in the inferior and superior bundles.

Temporal rotation therefore occurs in each optic radiation. In the visual cortex the corresponding superior quadrant of each retina is represented above the post-calcarine fissure and the appropriate inferior quadrant of each retina is represented below it. It will be recalled that in the lateral geniculate body the superior fibres are represented medially and the lower fibres are represented laterally. Thus the nasal rotation of fibres which occurs between the eyes

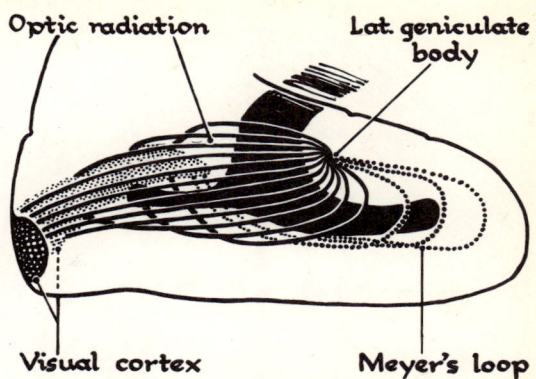

Fig. 22. The optic radiation and its relation to the lateral ventricle.

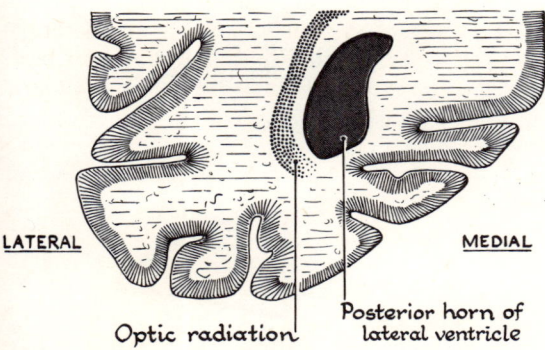

Fig. 21. Coronal section showing the relation of the optic radiation to the posterior horn of the lateral ventricle.

and the lateral geniculate bodies is corrected by a temporal rotation in the optic radiations.

Meyer first demonstrated by dissection that the inferior bundle of fibres swings anteriorly towards the pole of the temporal lobe while arching over the inferior horn of the lateral ventricle [FIGS. 22 and 23]. The presence of Meyer's loop has been denied by some authorities but the weight of evidence is in favour of its existence. It is probable, however, that there is considerable variation in the degree of anterior looping of the fibres, just as the depth and folding of the cerebral convolutions differ from person to person.

The anterior extremity of the inferior horn of the lateral ventricle is 4 cm. behind the temporal pole. When excising a part of the temporal lobe for temporal epilepsy Penfield measured the extent of the excision backwards from the pole. He found that if more than 4 cm.

was excised, the inferior horn was opened and a homonymous upper quadrantopia usually occurred [FIG. 24]. But if 8 cm. was amputated homonymous hemianopia was produced. There was, however, no precise correlation between the size of the amputation and the extent of the field defect.

These findings have been confirmed and amplified by French and others. French reported that following temporal pole amputations involving Meyer's loop the defect was always adjacent to the vertical meridian. This indicates that the fibres from the most superior retinal areas are most anterior in the loop. He found that, whilst there was no close correlation, the larger the amputation the greater the field defect, which enlarged towards the horizontal meridian. The smaller defects did not reach fixation [FIG. 25]. In fact some were outside the 30 degree isopter. The defects were always congruous and the vertical edge was always sharp. As the amputations increased in

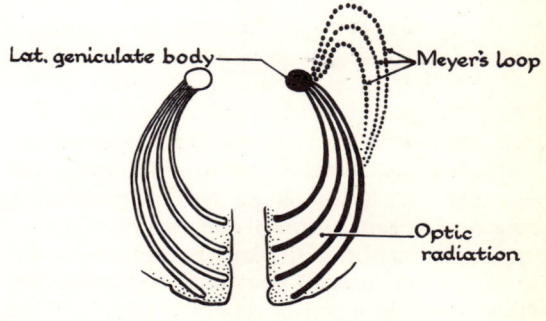

Fig. 23. Meyer's loop.

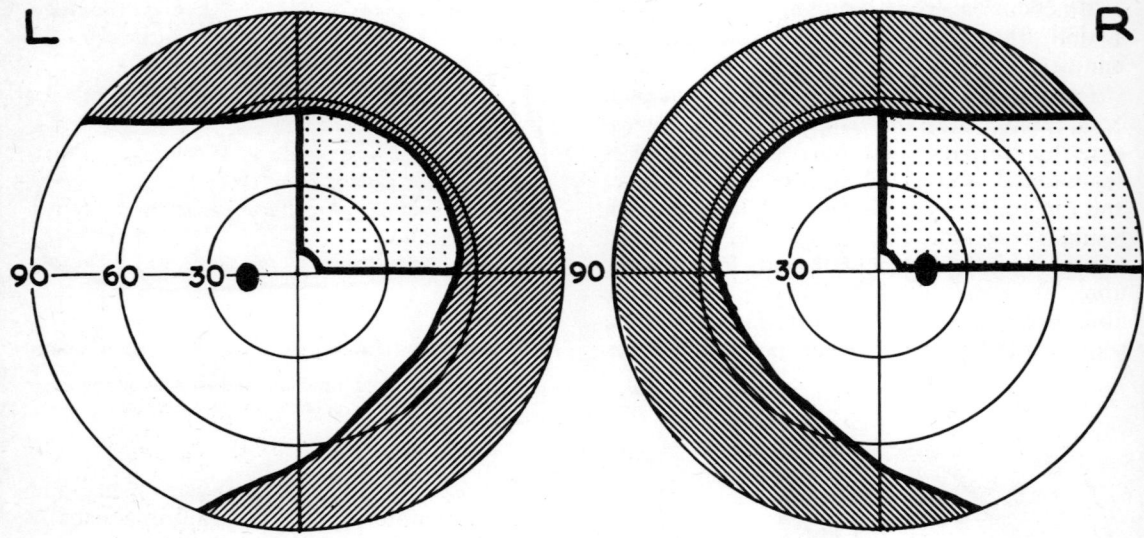

FIG. 24. Congruous homonymous quadrantopia with macular sparing, characteristic of a left temporal lobe lesion.

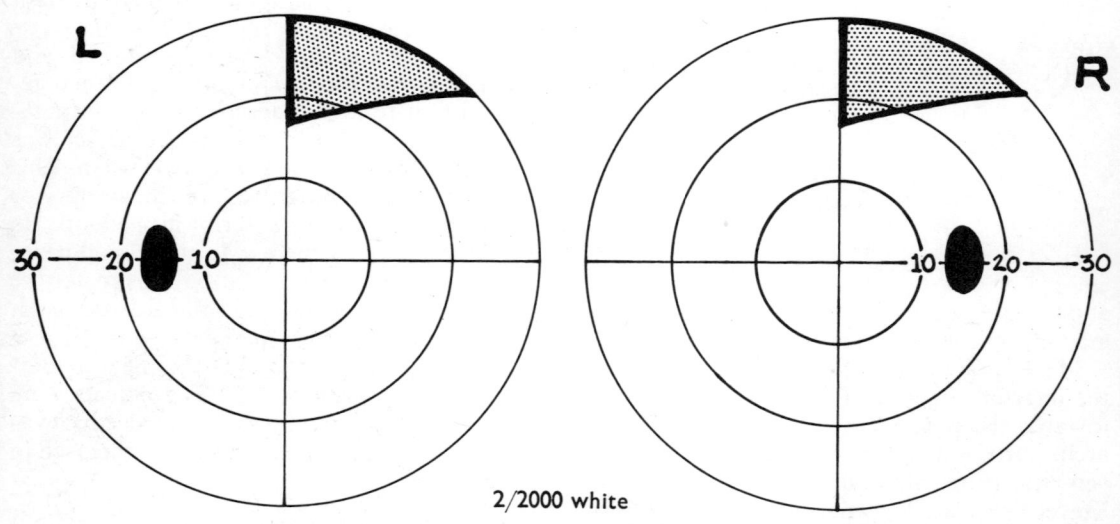

2/2000 white

FIG. 25. Field defect following a small amputation of the left temporal lobe.

size the defects invaded the fixation area [FIG. 26] and tended to produce a complete quadrantopia [FIG. 27]. This suggests that there is an anatomical separation of the superior and inferior retinal fibres. Still larger amputations led to complete hemianopia, indicating that the fibres from the superior retinal quadrants form a compact bundle.

The characteristic field defect of a lesion situated further back in the optic radiations is a congruous homonymous hemianopia with macular sparing [FIG. 28]. Depending upon its site, the lesion may involve only the upper or lower fibres of the radiation and thus cause a lower or upper quadrantopia in the opposite fields.

THE OPTIC RADIATIONS

Much has been written about the cause of the phenomenon of macular sparing in lesions of the optic radiations. It probably occurs because the macula has such a large area of representation. Destruction of all the fibres and cells associated with the macular area is therefore uncommon. There is no anatomical basis for the old belief that each point in the macular area is represented in the visual cortex of both occipital lobes [see p. 157].

BLOOD SUPPLY OF THE OPTIC RADIATION

The blood supply of the optic radiation may be divided into three areas:
1. Its anterior end is supplied by the perforating branches of the anterior choroidal artery.
2. In the middle of its course, where it is lateral to the descending horn of the lateral ventricle, it is supplied mainly by the deep optic branch

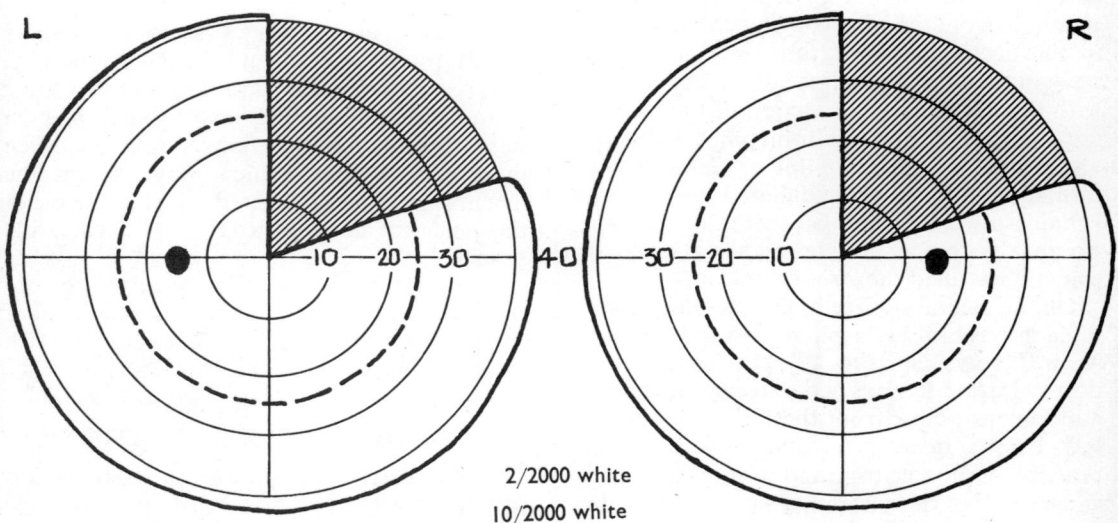

FIG. 26. Larger amputation of temporal lobe resulting in defect invading fixation.

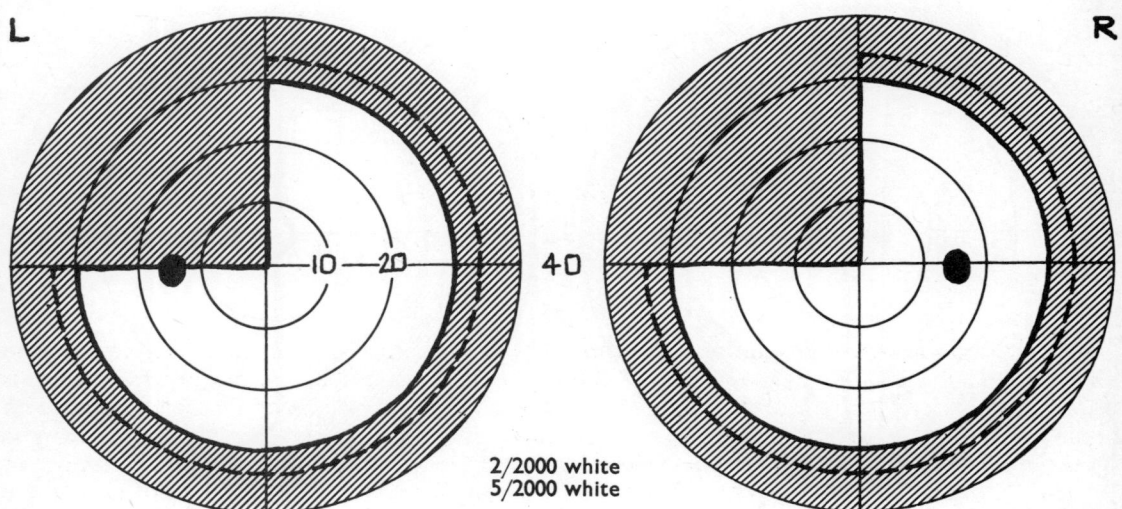

FIG. 27. Defect caused by larger amputation.

of the middle cerebral artery which penetrates the anterior perforated substance. The lower fibres of the radiation receive an additional supply from the posterior cerebral artery.

3. The posterior part of the radiation, where the fibres are fanning out to end in the striate area, is supplied by perforating cortical branches from the calcarine branch of the posterior cerebral artery and from the middle cerebral artery.

THE VISUAL CORTEX

The shape and depth of the convolutions and fissures of the brain vary from individual to individual, but the situation of the visual cortex in the occipital lobe is fairly constant. It is recognized by a white line which can be seen with the naked eye in a section of the cortical grey matter. This line is sometimes called the visual stria, or the white line of Gennari. It is formed of a layer of medullated nerve fibres running just below and parallel to the surface. Because of this white line the visual cortex is sometimes called the striate area.

On the medial surface of the occipital region of each cerebral hemisphere two well-marked fissures can be seen [FIG. 29]. The calcarine and post-calcarine fissures separate the precuneus and cuneus above from the lingual gyrus below. Passing downwards and forwards to the junction of the calcarine and post-calcarine fissures is the parieto-occipital fissure. It divides the precuneus in front from the cuneus behind.

BLOOD SUPPLY OF THE VISUAL CORTEX

The striate area receives its blood supply chiefly from the calcarine branch of the posterior cerebral artery and to a lesser degree from the middle cerebral artery. Near the posterior pole there is an anastomosis between these two arteries, which may explain the macular sparing associated with occlusion of the posterior cerebral artery or its calcarine branch.

Occlusion of the calcarine artery is not uncommon, and causes an abrupt development of congruous homonymous hemianopia with macular sparing [FIG. 28].

CORTICAL REPRESENTATION

The pear-shaped visual cortex or striate area is situated both above and below the calcarine and post-calcarine fissures. Opinions differ

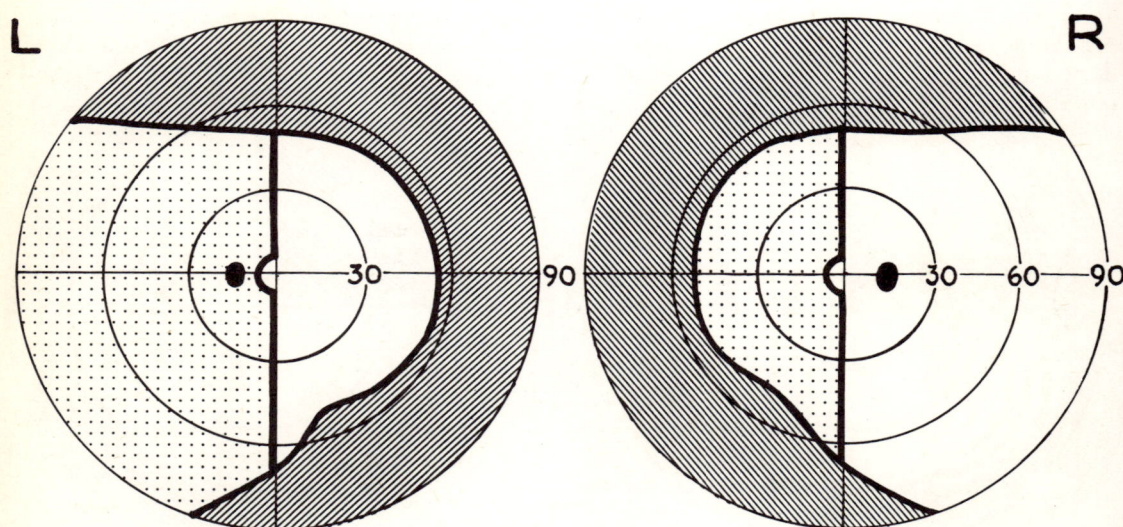

FIG. 28. Congruous homonymous hemianopia with macular sparing due to a lesion of the right optic radiation.

THE VISUAL CORTEX

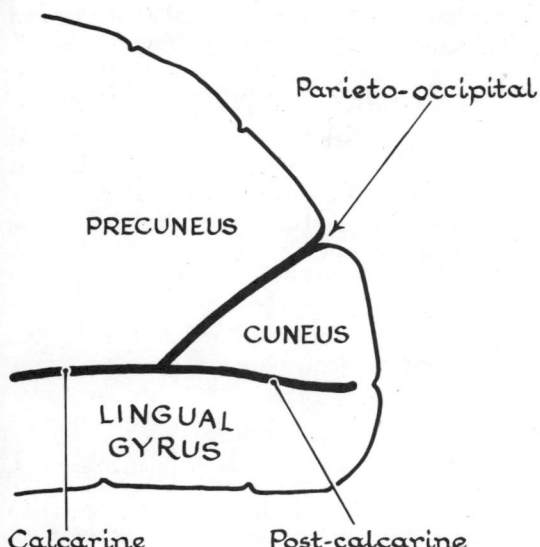

FIG. 29. Medial surface of the right occipital lobe.

concerning the representation in the region of the calcarine fissure. Most believe that the uniocular field is represented both above and below it. Since the retinal horizon is represented by the calcarine and post-calcarine fissures it seems likely that this is correct. Some authorities consider that the uniocular field is represented only below the calcarine fissure. Others hold that the visual area does not extend anterior to the parieto-occipital fissure. The probability is that considerable variation exists from person to person, depending upon the development of the gyri.

The following points should be remembered concerning the representation of the binocular visual field in the visual cortex [FIG. 30].

1. The calcarine and post-calcarine fissures represent the junction between the upper and lower halves of the visual fields. The upper lip of the fissure receives impulses from the corresponding upper quadrants of both retinae, which are associated with the lower quadrant of the binocular field on the opposite side. The inferior lip is related to the superior quadrant of the binocular field on the opposite side.

2. The macula is represented posteriorly by an extensive area of the visual cortex. In a large number of human brains the post-calcarine fissure extends slightly onto the posterolateral aspect of the occipital lobe. This is important when considering bullet wounds and similar injuries of the occipital lobe.

3. The periphery of the retina is represented anteriorly.

4. The uniocular field is represented most anteriorly and is probably in front of the junction of the parieto-occipital and calcarine fissures.

5. There is accurate localization in the occipital cortex, i.e. each pair of corresponding points in the retinae is represented by a specific area in the visual cortex of the appropriate cerebral hemisphere.

Dr. I. Maclaren Thompson, Professor of Anatomy in the University of Manitoba, has made an interesting calculation. If the eye is regarded as approximately a sphere of 12 mm. radius, its area ($4\pi r^2$) is about 1,810 mm². The radius of the macula is about 1 mm., so that its area is 3 mm².

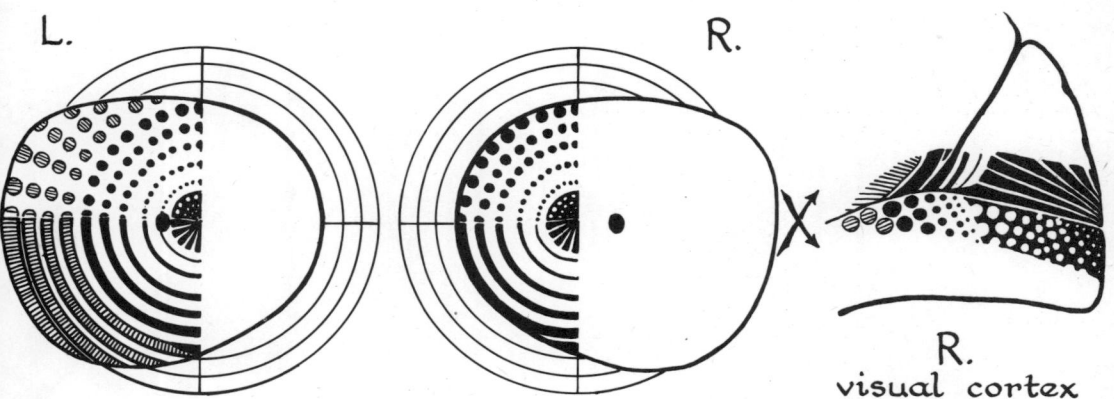

FIG. 30. Scheme to show the cortical representation of the visual field.

The striate area of the cerebral cortex has been estimated by Elliot Smith (quoted by Whitnall) to cover about 3,000 mm^2. At least one half of this area is concerned with macular vision, i.e. 1,500 mm^2. The following ratios are of interest:

RETINO-CORTICAL RATIOS

	Retinal Area	Cortical Area	Ratio
Extramacular retina	900 mm.^{2}	1,500 mm.^{2}	1 : 1·7
Macula	3 mm.^{2}	1,500 mm.^{2}	1 : 500

These figures are of course approximate but they emphasize the relatively large area of cortex concerned with macular function compared with that associated with extramacular function. They also indicate that whilst a point-to-area relationship may exist between the extramacular retina and the visual cortex, such a relationship certainly does exist between the macula and its cortical area.

CLINICAL APPLICATION

It will be noted that there is no fundamental difference between the field defect caused by a lesion of the optic radiation and that caused by damage to the visual cortex. Both are of course homonymous, both usually show congruity, and both usually exhibit macular sparing. The field defects alone give no reliable guide to the exact site of a lesion in the visual pathway behind the lateral geniculate body.

REFERENCES

FRENCH, L. A. (1962) Studies on the optic radiations, *J. Neurosurg.*, **29**, 552.

PENFIELD, W., and PAINE, K. (1955) Results of surgical therapy for focal epileptic seizures, *Canad. med. Ass. J.*, **73**, 515.

PART II

THE VISUAL FIELD AND ITS ASSESSMENT

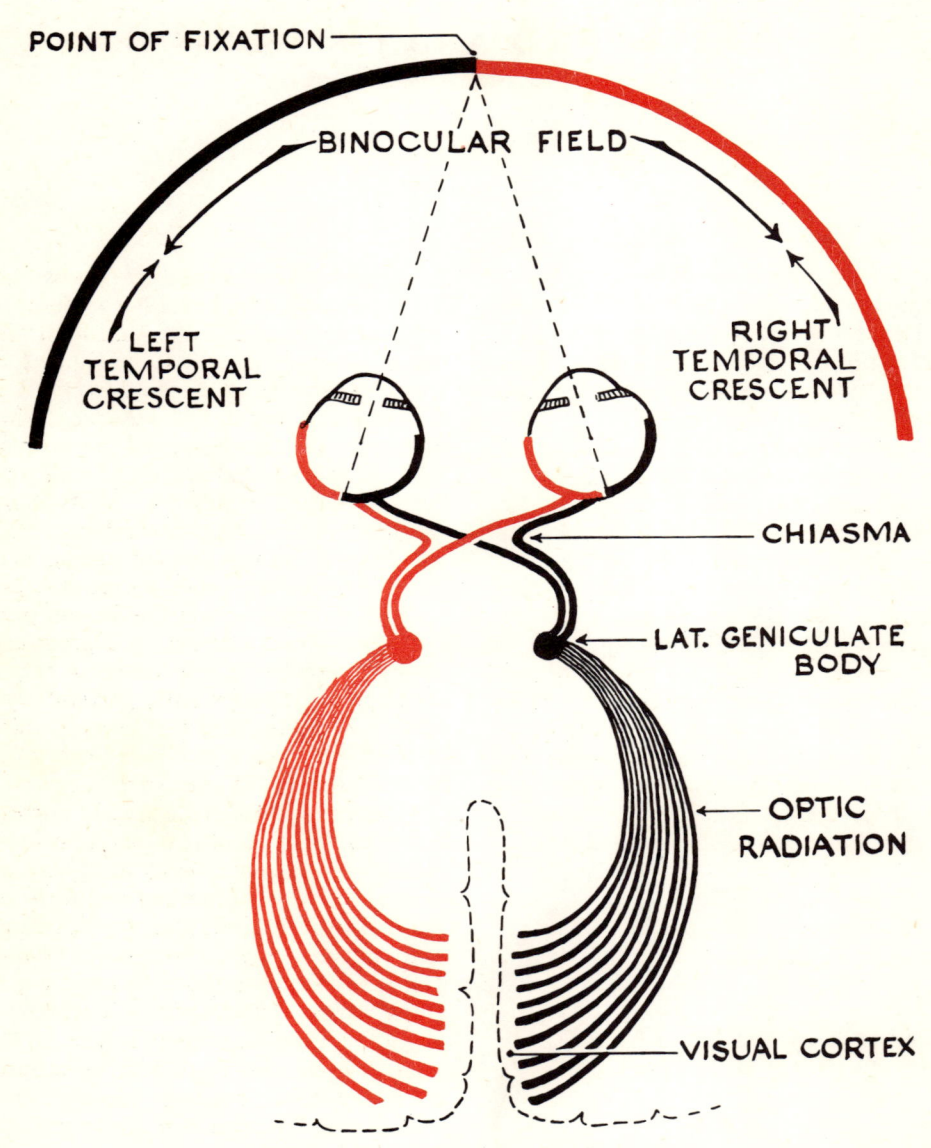

FIG. 31. The pathway from visual field to cortex.

4
THE VISUAL FIELD

The visual field is that area of one's surroundings which is visible at one time. It is limited by the facial contours and the size of the sentient retina. Only those rays of light which pass through the lens and reach the sentient retina result in a visual sensation [FIG. 31].

If the eye is considered to be situated at the centre of a sphere, then the visual axis is that radius which joins the fovea of the eye and the point on the inner surface of the sphere to which the eye is directed.

The normal monocular visual field extends approximately 100 degrees laterally, 60 degrees medially, 60 degrees upwards, and 75 degrees downwards [FIG. 32]. These values are approximate since they vary slightly from patient to patient. The centre of the blind spot is situated about 15 degrees temporally and 1·5 degrees below the horizontal meridian. In hypermetropic eyes it is farther out, and in myopic eyes it is closer to the fixation point.

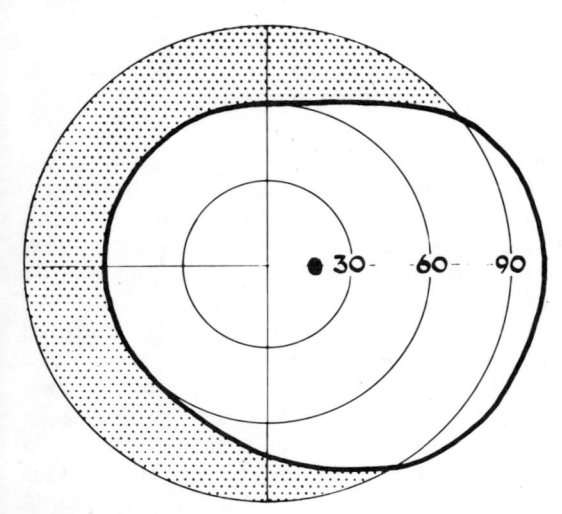

FIG. 32. A normal monocular visual field.

The normal blind spot has two components. There is a central absolute scotoma corresponding to the scleral canal through which the nerve fibres pass and a peripheral relative scotoma the size of which depends upon the diameter and brightness of the target. In earlier literature the dimensions of the normal blind spot are given as being about 7·5 degrees in its vertical and 5·5 degrees in its horizontal meridian. Armaly has shown that with a 1/1000 white target, using a tangent screen, 10 degrees and 7 degrees are more accurate sizes whilst the 1–2–e target, with a Goldmann perimeter, gives diameters of about 14 degrees and 9–10 degrees. Smaller or less luminous targets give still larger measurements, particularly in the vertical meridian, and may even exhibit baring of the blind spot which was once thought to be characteristic of glaucoma.

Uncorrected or inadequately corrected refractive errors result in the diffusion of the retinal image over a wider area with a reduction in intensity of illumination. Early cataracts and other conditions causing clouding of the media have the same effect. Any of these conditions may therefore result in apparent enlargement of the blind spot, particularly in the vertical meridian, and in baring of the blind spot. It must also be remembered that ageing itself leads to gradual contraction of all isopters, enlargement of the blind spot and baring of the blind spot when standard targets become threshold stimuli for the blind spot area [see p. 49].

VISUAL FIELD CHART

The centre of a field of vision chart represents the point of fixation, i.e. the point on the internal surface of the sphere to which the eye is directed. Circles are arranged concentrically around this point of fixation and represent the angles made with the visual axis at the nodal point.

The problem of charting spherical features on a flat chart is familiar to makers of maps. A true estimate of the size and shape of countries in the far north or south can be appreciated better by looking at a sphere than at a map. This same problem confronts perimetrists. A record on a spherical surface would be more accurate, but it would be difficult to store. Charts are therefore used. The standard perimeter chart is composed of concentric circles, but this rather schematic form of chart gives a distorted representation of the visual field. Various improved charts are available and they will be described in the section dealing with the recording of visual field defects.

The size of the visual field may be reduced slightly if the patient has a prominent nose, bushy projecting eyebrows, high cheek-bones, or drooping eyelids.

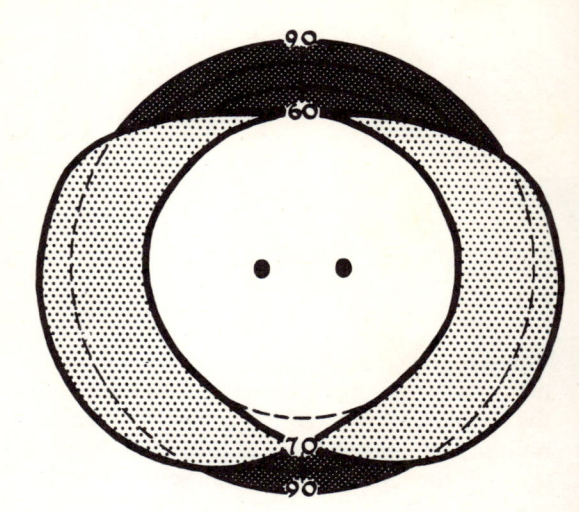

FIG. 33. The binocular visual field.

RELATIVE FIELD

The relative field is the visual field measured without moving the head to remove these obstacles.

ABSOLUTE FIELD

The absolute field is recorded by moving the head so as to remove each restricting factor when measuring the appropriate meridian, e.g. the nose, prominent eyebrows, etc. It is found that the absolute field is normally very little larger than the relative field—not usually more than 10 degrees in each meridian. This may be thought somewhat surprising at first, but it will be remembered that the periphery of the sentient retina extends farther forwards nasally than temporally and slightly more anteriorly above than below.

When examining a visual field the facial characteristics such as nose, eyebrows, cheek-bones, and drooping lids should be noted at the beginning. If none of these features is unusually prominent the relative field may be taken. But if an eyebrow or eyelid is obviously restricting the field in a region which is important for diagnosis then it is wise to measure the absolute field and record this fact on the chart.

BINOCULAR FIELD

The binocular field is the total visual field as seen with both eyes directed to a distant fixation point [FIG. 33]. The measurement of this field is of little clinical value, except perhaps as part of the driving test, because a field defect in one eye only would not be revealed by plotting the binocular field. It is sometimes measured roughly by confrontation in cases of homonymous hemianopia. But such a test is merely a preliminary to an examination of each field separately.

TEMPORAL CRESCENT OR MONOCULAR FIELD

The temporal crescent is that part of the binocular field which is always monocular, i.e. the crescentic area situated temporally beyond 60 degrees [FIG. 33]. It will be remembered that visual impulses from this area in each eye are represented in the antero-inferior portion of the lateral geniculate body, in the most medial fibres of the optic radiation, and in the most anterior area of the visual cortex of the same side. The temporal crescent may on occasions be lost, whilst the binocular field is intact, and sometimes it may remain whilst a homonymous hemianopia involves the rest of the associated binocular field.

VISUAL FIELD CHART

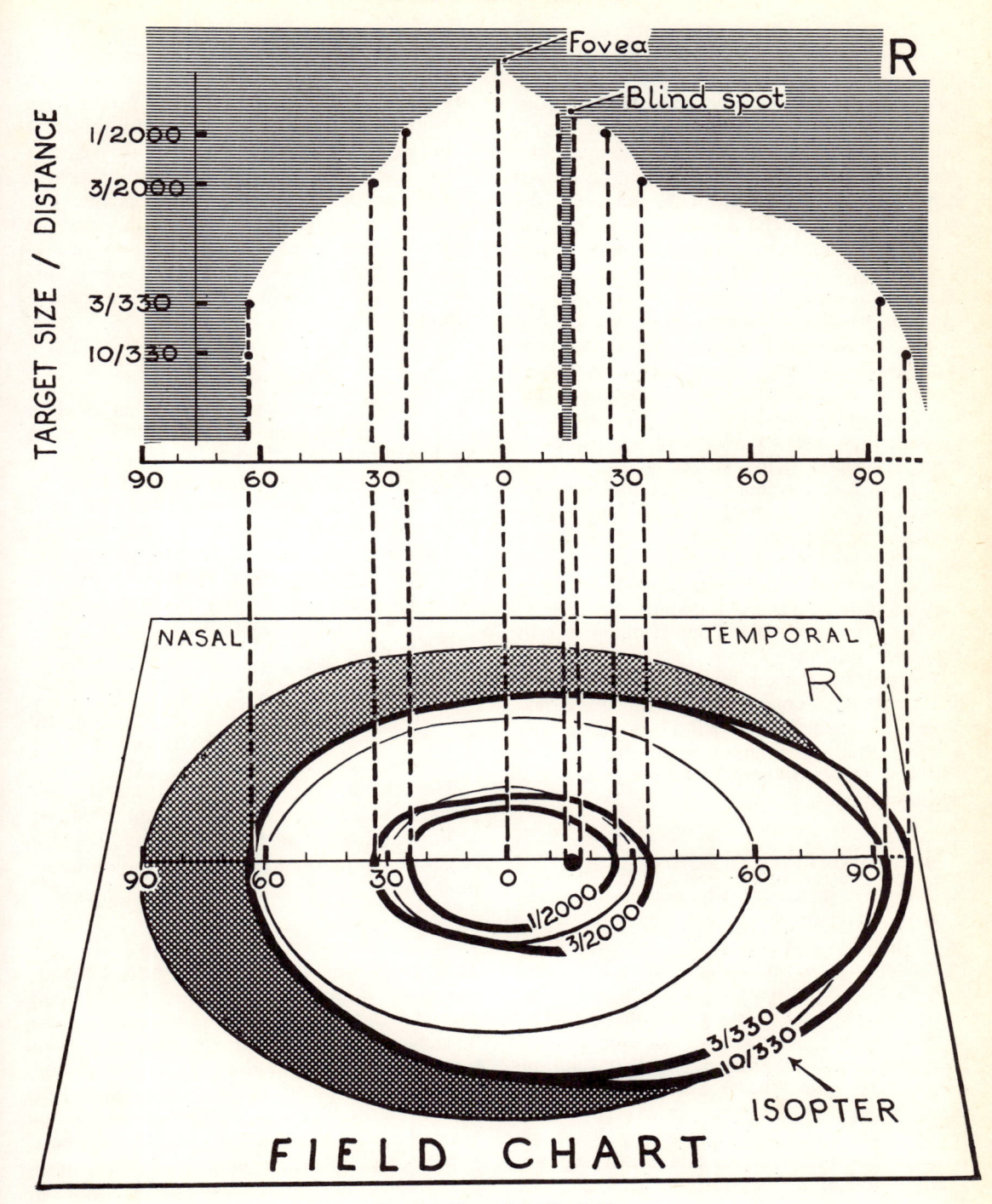

FIG. 34. Traquair's hill of vision.

TRAQUAIR'S CONCEPTION OF HILL OF VISION

Traquair likened the visual field to a hill or an island and the visual field chart to a contour map [FIG. 34]. Large white targets are visible out to the periphery with the normal eye, but a small target can be seen only when it is moved near to the point of fixation. As the size of the target is reduced, the area within which it is visible becomes smaller, so that a series of ever diminishing circles is formed. These are known as isopters and they resemble the contour lines of a map which enclose an area above a certain height. An isopter therefore encloses an area within which a target of a given size is visible. Each isopter is plotted by moving the target from an area of the field where it is not seen to an area in which it is seen and recording the point at which it is just visible.

If depression or general reduction in vision occurs it is as if the 'hill of vision' had partly sunk below the surface of the sea. When plotted with standard targets it appears as a contraction of the field, but considerable contraction may occur before the visual acuity falls below 20/30. This type of visual defect may occur in syphilitic optic atrophy.

To continue the simile, a defect of the periphery resembles coast erosion with subsidence of the cliff. In such a case all the isopters show a corresponding indentation in the area. A scotoma may be likened to a pool or lake excavating the hill.

THE IMPORTANCE OF VISUAL ACUITY

Reduced visual acuity, whether due to a refractive error or to medial opacities, blurs small targets and makes the findings of a field examination unreliable. The target is not seen by an eye with reduced vision until it is moved closer to the fixation point than the isopter for the normal eye. All isopters are therefore contracted, the degree of contraction depending upon the reduction in visual acuity. If a patient has a refractive error which reduces his uncorrected vision to 20/40 or less, he should wear spectacles during an examination of the central field. Bifocals are obviously unsuitable for this purpose unless the segment is placed low and the patient is intelligent enough to co-operate by tilting the head downwards slightly to prevent the segment confusing the findings in the lower field.

The peripheral field has a low visual acuity but it is sensitive to movement. Large targets are therefore used and refractive errors have less effect upon the findings. For this reason it is not necessary for the patient to wear glasses when the peripheral field is being examined. Moreover, the rim or side of the glasses may obscure the target. Small abnormalities of the field which may have important clinical significance should always be checked with different correcting lenses to exclude refractive artefacts.

COLOURED TARGETS

A coloured target stimulates the retina less than a white target of the same size, but given a sufficient intensity almost all colours can be recognized even at the periphery of the retina. The intensity of the stimulus produced by a coloured target is really the product of its size and luminosity. Thus, in perimetry, coloured targets in use are larger than white targets. Their purpose is to stimulate a larger area of the retina with a reduced intensity.

If a coloured target is moved from the periphery of the screen towards the centre, it is always seen some time before its hue can be recognized. It is the actual site at which the hue is recognized that should be recorded when charting a colour isopter.

The recognition of colour is largely dependent upon the intensity of illumination. Yellow and blue targets usually give slightly larger fields than red targets, depending upon their hue.

DISPROPORTION

With the illumination found in most consulting rooms, which is about 10 foot candles, and at 2 metres from the screen, the colour of the 15 mm. and 30 mm. diameter red targets will normally be recognized at about the 15 and 25 degree circles respectively. A 2 mm. white target can usually be seen about 25–30 degrees from the fixation point on the screen. These values vary with the illumination and hue of the targets. Each ophthalmologist will quickly become accustomed to the lighting and values obtained in his own office.

When a field charted with a red target, e.g. 30/2000, is found to be much smaller than that

VISUAL FIELD CHART

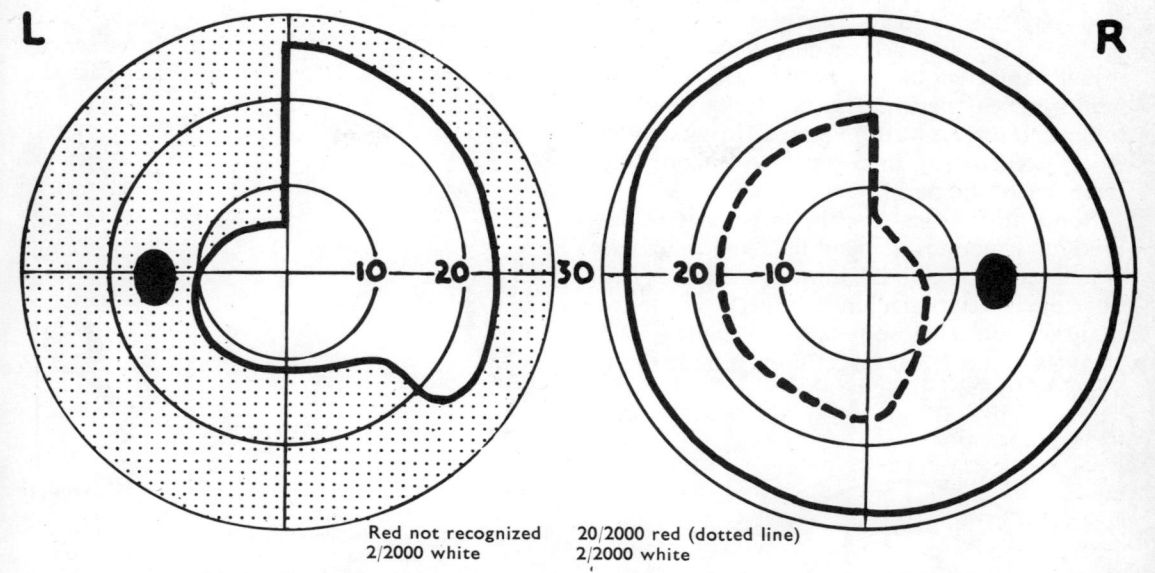

L   **R**

Red not recognized
2/2000 white   20/2000 red (dotted line)
2/2000 white

FIG. 35. Chiasmal compression resulting in disproportion in the right visual field.

demonstrated with a corresponding white target, e.g. 2/2000, disproportion is said to be present. When this is found, it suggests that a disease process is either progressing or retrogressing. For example, a pituitary tumour which is beginning to compress the chiasma will cause a defect which may be more easily defined when plotted with a red target than with a comparable white target [FIG. 35]. A retrobulbar neuritis will also cause disproportion which results in a larger central defect for red than for a corresponding white target [FIG. 36].

USE OF ULTRA-VIOLET ILLUMINATION

Harrington has suggested coating both the target and the fixation point on the screen with luminous blue paint. The screen and the test object are illuminated with a dull ultra-violet lamp, the intensity of which is not enough to endanger the eye of the patient or the observer. The ultra-violet radiation is absorbed by the screen, so that the fixation spot and the target glimmer upon a black background. Such targets emit a narrow spectral band and have an almost pure hue, so that it is not necessary for the patient to recognize the colour. He need say only when it is visible. Harrington has found that patients are able to be more definite in their answers when this form of blue luminous test object is used. This facilitates the accurate plotting of minute scotomata due to early macular lesions and to early damage to the optic nerve, which are difficult to detect with small white targets.

RECORDS

The visual fields are recorded schematically upon charts. On all charts the right visual field is charted on the right and the left field on the left [FIG. 37]. It is important to remember that the optical system of the eye produces an inverted retinal image of the visual field. Thus a retinal lesion above and nasal to the fovea in the right eye will produce a defect below and temporal to the fixation point on the chart [FIG. 38].

When recording the results of a visual field examination it is important to state the diameter of the target used, its colour, the distance of the patient's eye from the target and the diameter of the pupil. This is recorded in the following manner:

$$\frac{\text{Diameter of target in mm.}}{\text{Distance of patient's eye from screen in mm.}} \text{ colour,}$$

e.g. $\dfrac{2}{2000}$ white

Pupil diameter =   mm.

The date on which the examination is made

must be recorded to aid assessment of the progress of a lesion at a later date. The corrected visual acuity should be noted, and with the hemispherical perimeters the background illumination must also be stated. In glaucoma it is particularly important to record the diameter of the pupil.

Some authorities give the target size in degrees and minutes, depending upon the angle it subtends at the nodal point of the eye. It can be remembered that a 1 mm. target at a distance of 1,000 mm. corresponds to an angle of 3·5 minutes and a 1/330 target corresponds to an angle of 10·5 minutes.

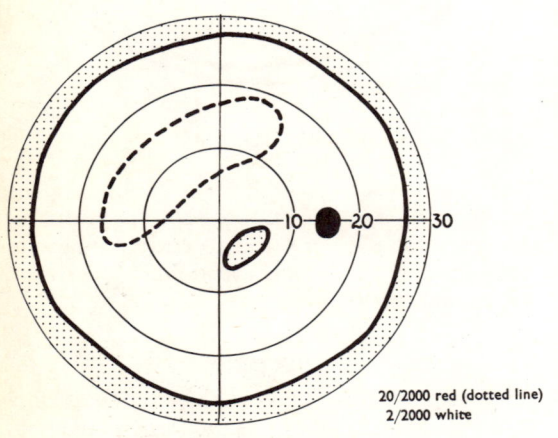

FIG. 36. Retrobulbar neuritis showing disproportion.

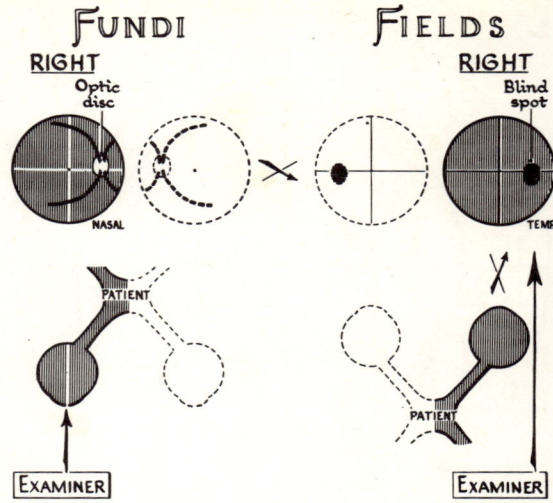

20/2000 red (dotted line)
2/2000 white

FIG. 37. Scheme to explain the custom of recording the visual field of the right eye on the right, and that of the left eye on the left.

SCOTOMATA

Scotoma means dark tumour. It indicates an area of relative blindness, particularly in the central field, which is surrounded by peripheral field in which vision is present. If the area of relative blindness extends to the periphery the term scotoma should not be used. Several types of scotomata are described.

A **positive scotoma** is one which appears to the patient to be black or coloured. For example, a large vitreous opacity will produce a black cloud in the vision. A vitreous haemorrhage may appear as a reddish cloud. The patient may complain of an orange patch in central serous retinopathy.

A **negative scotoma** indicates an area of defective vision of which the patient is not aware. The best example of this is the blind spot. We are not aware of any lack of vision in the area of the blind spot. It requires demonstration for it to be noticed. Negative scotomata are uncommon because most patients are aware of a 'hole' in the visual field.

A **relative scotoma** is an area in which the

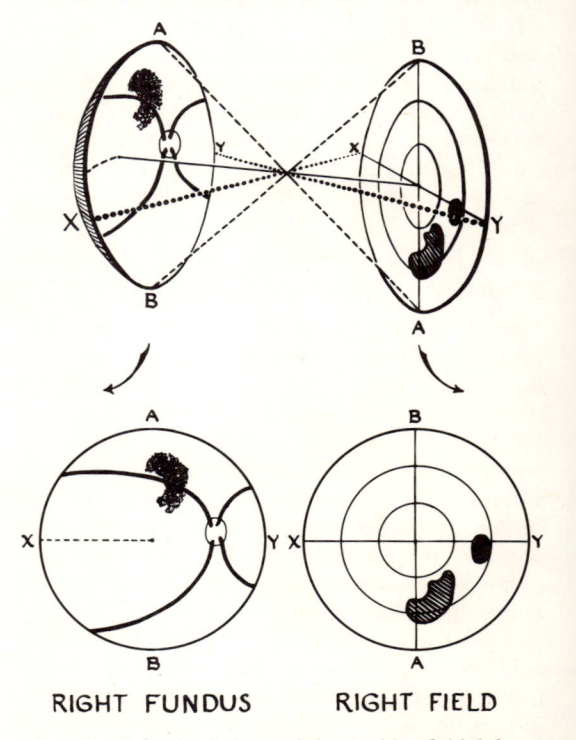

FIG. 38. A fundus lesion and the resulting field defect.

VISUAL FIELD CHART

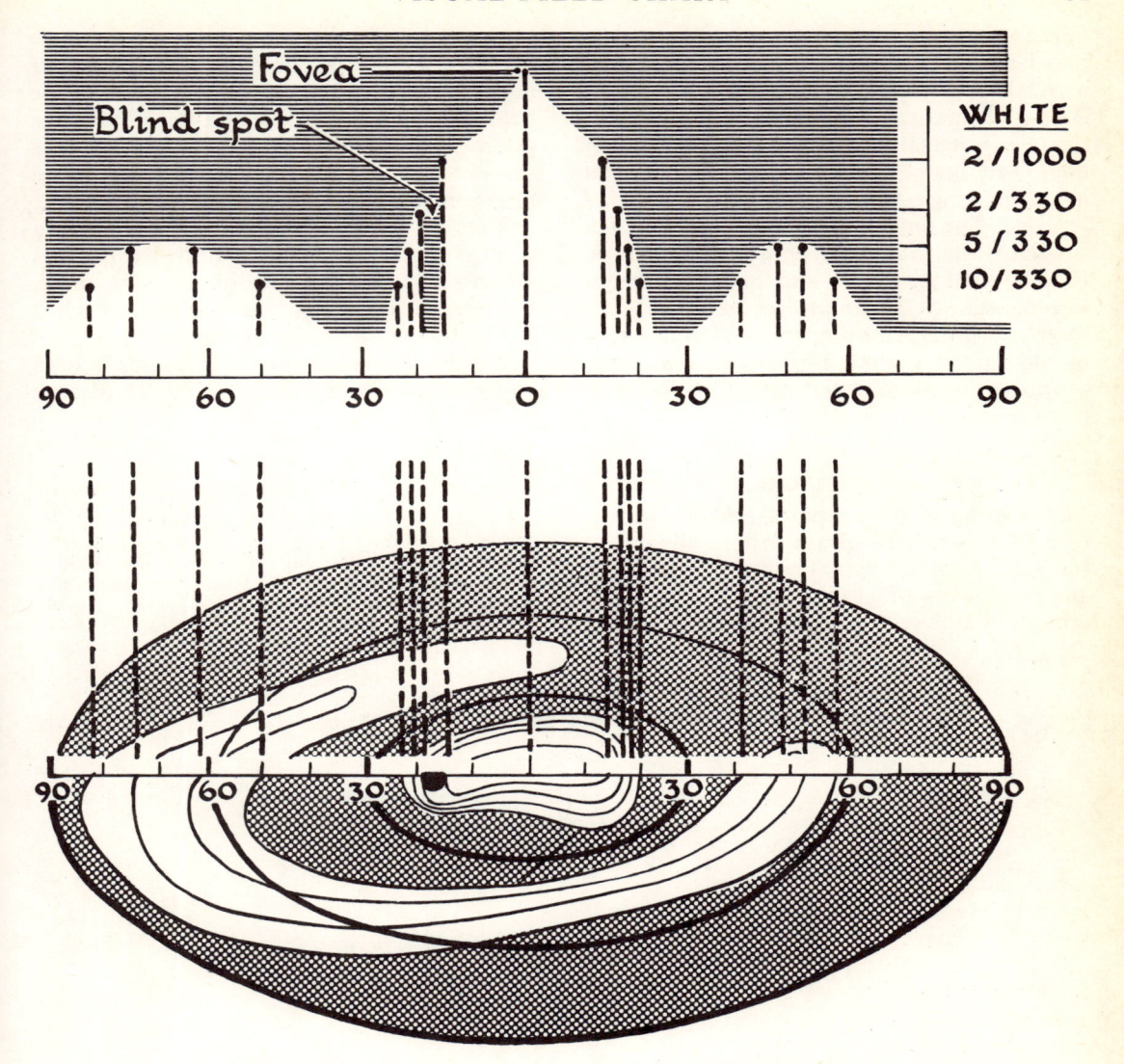

FIG. 39. A ring scotoma of retinitis pigmentosa, illustrating the steep and gradual slope of the margins.

retinal sensitivity is depressed so that colour is not properly recognized, e.g. a white target may appear grey, a red target may appear pink, or a green target may appear a dull white.

An absolute scotoma is one in which no perception of light is demonstrable.

Relating this to Traquair's hill of vision, a relative scotoma is a depression which has developed in the hill but not down to sea level, whilst in an absolute scotoma the depression has reached sea level.

SCOTOMATA AND VISUAL ACUITY

When the corrected visual acuity of an eye with no medial opacities is found to be reduced it means that the limbs of the test letter cannot be resolved by the retinal elements. In such a case a relative central scotoma can always be plotted providing the target and the illumination are reduced sufficiently. For example, if the vision is only 20/200 it is likely that a fairly large scotoma will be found with a 5/2000 white target. But if the vision is 20/60 a 5/2000 target may fail to elicit a scotoma and it may be necessary to use a 2/2000 target or even a 1/2000 white target to demonstrate a defect. Asking the patient to comment on differences of hue of a red target at fixation and in the four quadrants close to fixation [FIG. 140] is a great aid in directing attention to the defective area of the field. The area may then be analysed with smaller white targets and lower illumination. If the visual acuity is impaired an area of lowered sensitivity can always be found if the target and illumination are reduced sufficiently, providing the patient is intelligent and co-operative and the perimetrist sufficiently painstaking.

STEEP SLOPE AND GRADUAL SLOPE

The plotting of the shape of a field defect is usually adequate to give a definite diagnosis, but this is not enough. The defect should be analysed by plotting two or more isopters with targets of different sizes. Analysis by static, profile perimetry delineates precisely the slope of defects. Such an analysis gives a greater understanding of the nature and extent of the field loss and is invaluable as a record to assess progress. The use of stimuli of graded sizes shows whether the erosion or crater in the hill of vision has a steep or gradual slope.

The ring scotoma of retinitis pigmentosa is a good example [FIG. 39]. Centrally the isopters are close together, indicating a steep slope. Peripherally there is a gradual slope, which is shown by the isopters being farther apart.

The blind spot is the best example of a scotoma showing a crater with a steep slope [see FIG. 39].

REFERENCES

ARMALY, M. F. (1969) The size and location of the normal blind spot, *Arch. Ophthal.*, **91**, 192.

HARRINGTON, D. O., and HOYT, W. F. (1955) Ultraviolet radiation perimetry with monochromatic blue stimuli; method for early detection of conduction disturbance in retina and optic nerve, *Arch. Ophthal.*, **53**, 870.

5

APPARATUS FOR THE MEASUREMENT OF VISUAL FIELDS

The choice of the best method of testing and the most suitable equipment for plotting visual fields depends on the clinical evaluation of the type of visual field defect suspected and the purpose of the examination. The method and equipment must be so chosen as to allow the most accurate and reproducible examination in as short a period of time as possible. Gross homonymous hemianopias or quadrantopias may require merely the confrontation test. A simple standard perimeter is adequate if peripheral visual defects are anticipated or for visual field tests required for motor vehicle driving purposes. Such equipment is quite inadequate for detection of early changes in chronic simple glaucoma, residual fine defects of optic neuritis or early toxic amblyopia. The tangent screen or the hemispherical projection perimeters are required for this purpose. Perimetry with non-moving targets, called static perimetry, or profile perimetry is required for detailed analysis and for research into the development of field defects. The screening of entire populations in a specific survey or of ophthalmic patients as part of a routine eye examination requires the utilization of various screeners, but their limitations must be borne in mind.

THE CONFRONTATION FIELD TEST

The value of the confrontation test [FIG. 40] is not universally appreciated. Many visual field defects and the anatomical site of lesions may be diagnosed by the confrontation test alone. In patients who are bed-ridden or of low mentality, and in children, it is a most valuable examination. It is sometimes the only attainable form of field examination.

In confrontation testing the examiner attempts to compare the patient's visual field with his own. The blind spot can also be tested and compared with that of the examiner. The approximate extent of the normal visual field is learned after a few attempts at the confrontation test and a peripheral constriction can be recognized. An estimate of the blind spot confirms the patient's fixation and adds reliability to changes obtained in the peripheral parts of the visual field.

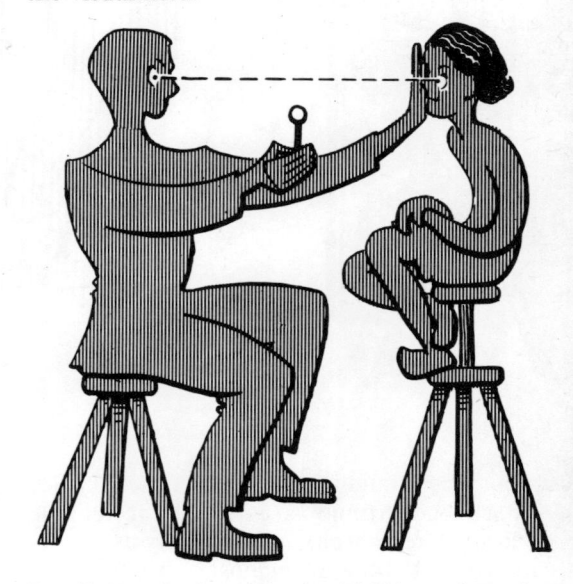

FIG. 40. Examination of the visual field by confrontation.

For this test it is often convenient to use a few hatpins with small coloured heads. A standard black holder with targets of varying sizes and colours is better. The background on which the target is moving is important. For example, if the room has white walls or the examiner is wearing a white coat, a white pinhead will show less clearly and the patient may

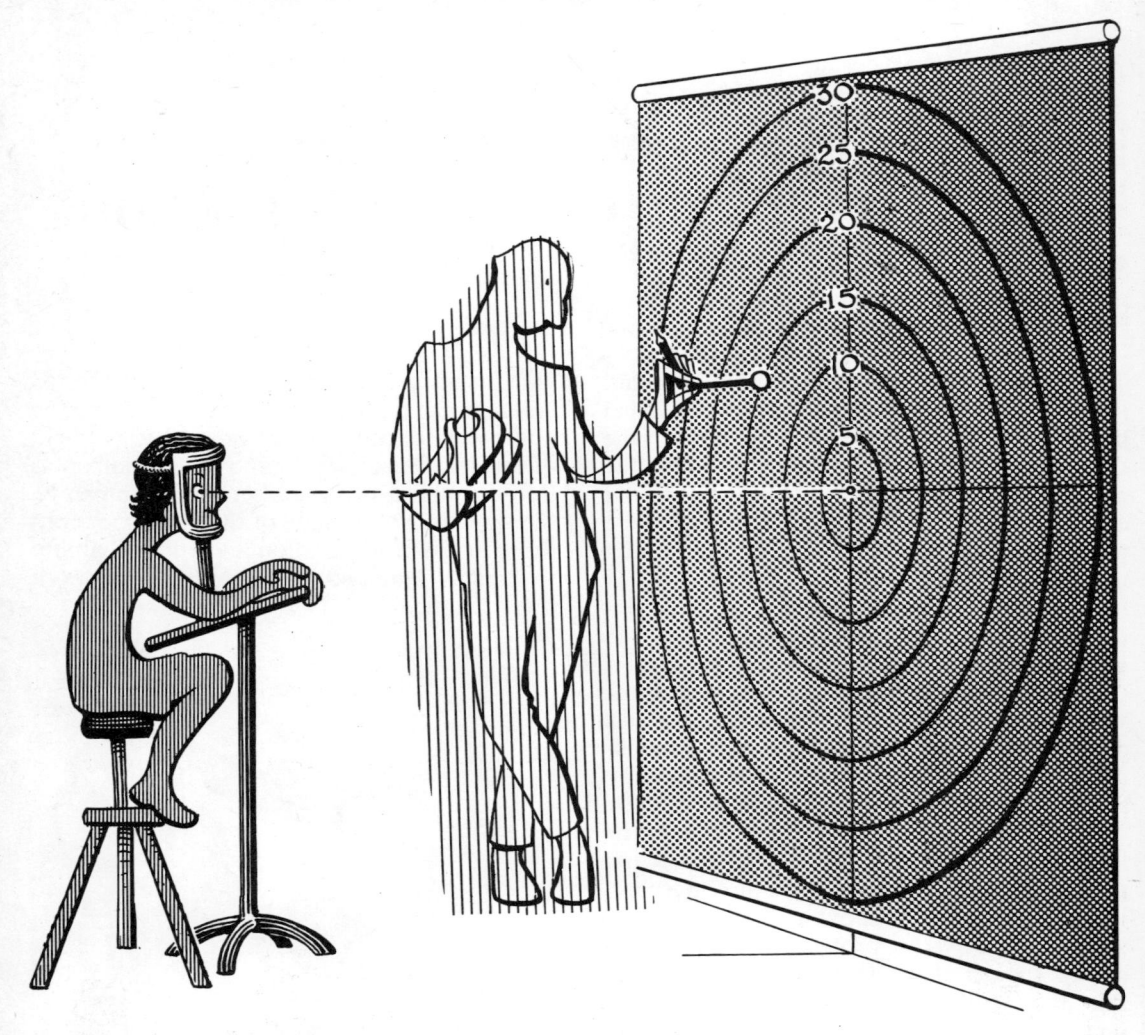

FIG. 41. Examination of the central field with the Bjerrum screen.

wrongly be thought to have a contracted field. A dark background is essential for reliable findings. A red hatpin is particularly useful because it will show up against a bright background which is found in so many examining rooms.

THE TANGENT SCREEN (BJERRUM SCREEN)

This is usually a black felt screen on which radial lines and 5 degree concentric circles are inconspicuously marked in the inner 30 degrees of the field [FIG. 41]. A 2 metre distance between patient and screen permits accurate examination of small defects. Many consulting rooms are not large enough to accommodate a screen of this size and a 1 metre screen is adequate for most diagnostic purposes.

The tangent screen is used to examine the field within 30 degrees from the fixation point. An increased distance of the patient from the screen increases the size of field defects and allows their evaluation in greater detail. Screens are therefore made for use at 1, or 2 metres.

The normal eye sees a 2 mm. white target at 30 degrees or even 35 degrees from fixation. Screens marked with isopters only to 25 degrees are therefore not satisfactory.

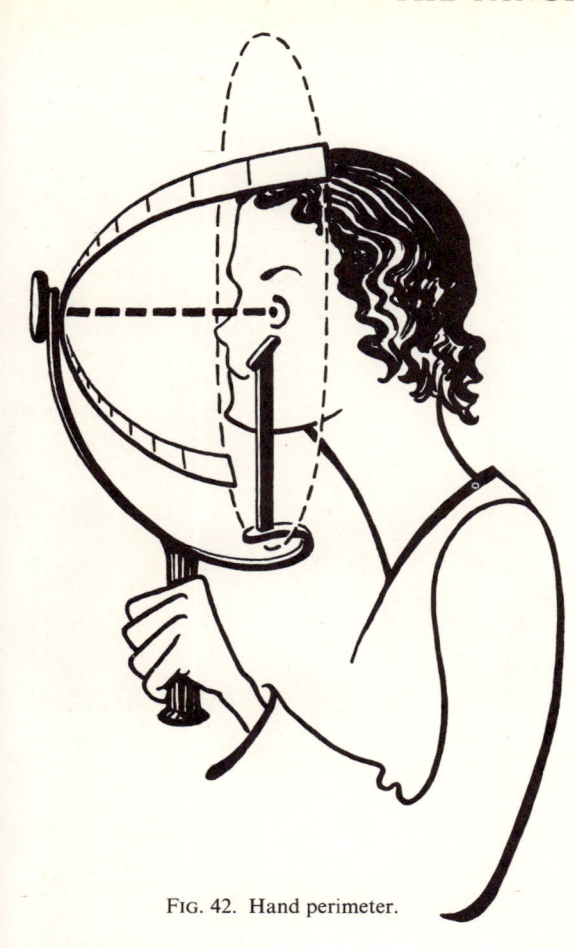

THE TANGENT SCREEN

The screen should be evenly illuminated and 7 foot candles of light are often called for. It is useful to be able to vary the background illumination and clinicians have to become accustomed to what is 'normal' with their own equipment. No reliance can be placed upon a comparison of fields obtained in different offices or hospitals under different conditions. Changes plotted by different observers should always be interpreted with caution.

THE PERIMETER

Numerous perimeters are available on the market, from the simple hand model [FIG. 42] which is valuable for visits to bed-ridden patients, to the self-recording perimeters in which a light is projected onto the inner surface of a half-sphere. In some of the more expensive types the target size, colour, and luminosity may be controlled by turning a knob.

The arc form of perimeter is in most common use [FIG. 43]. A metal strip curved into an arc with a radius of 330 mm. is mounted so that it rotates about its centre. The chin-rest is adjustable, so that the eye to be examined may be placed at the centre of the sphere of which the

FIG. 42. Hand perimeter.

Sets of targets for use with the tangent screen usually contain a series of white, red, green, and blue targets 1, 2, 3, 5, 7, 10, 15, and 20 mm. in diameter. These are made to fit into black wands which should have a mat surface so that they do not reflect light. With prolonged wear these wands often become shiny and should then be replaced or resurfaced. The targets tend to become dirty with use and should be renewed from time to time. It is desirable to be able to remove the stimulus from the patient's vision at will and it is therefore advantageous to use targets which are flat rather than spherical. The target may then be turned so that the unpainted edge is presented to the patient. This accomplishes the removal of the visual stimulus and permits confirmation of the limits of a defect which was plotted by moving the target from an area where it is not visible to one where it is visible.

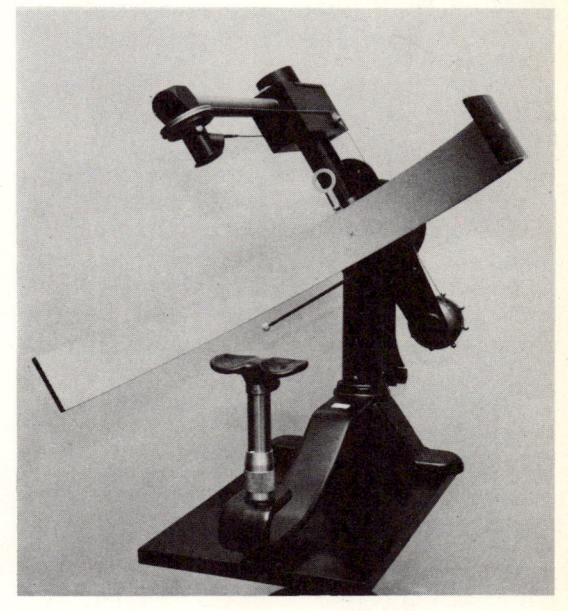

FIG. 43. Self-recording arc Vanderbilt perimeter (Curfax).

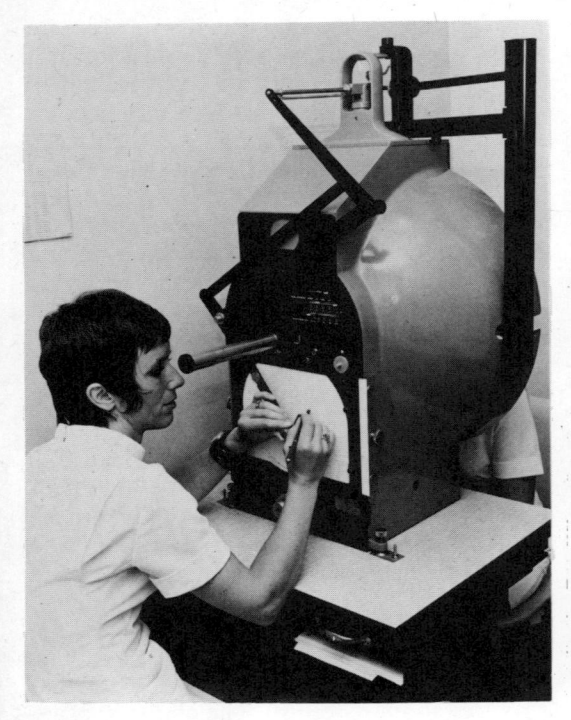

APPARATUS FOR THE MEASUREMENT OF VISUAL FIELDS

FIG. 44. The Goldmann hemispherical perimeter seen from the examiner's side.

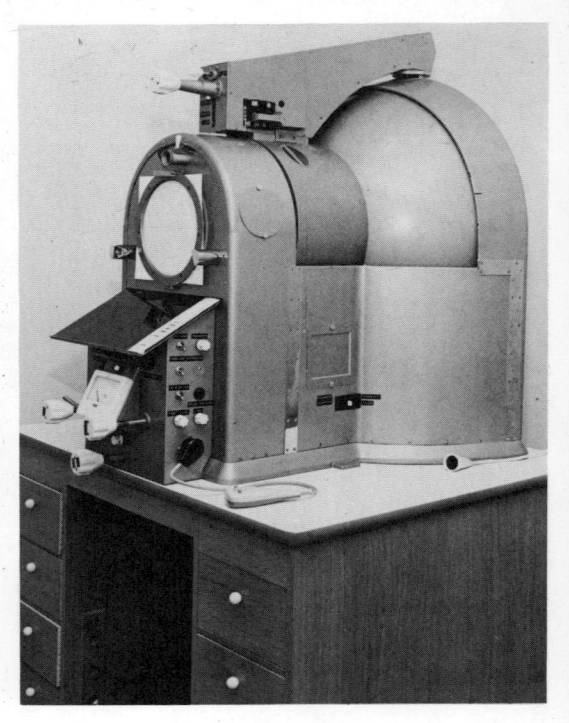

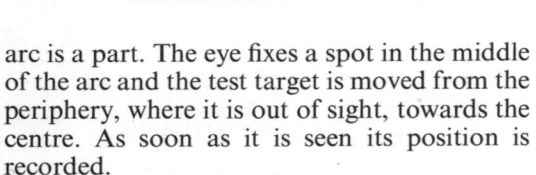

FIG. 45. The Tubingen perimeter seen from the examiner's side.

arc is a part. The eye fixes a spot in the middle of the arc and the test target is moved from the periphery, where it is out of sight, towards the centre. As soon as it is seen its position is recorded.

Test objects ranging from 1 mm. to 20 mm. in diameter and in white, red, green, and blue colours are usually provided. As soon as they become dirty they should be replaced.

The examination should be conducted in a moderately darkened room so that there is adequate contrast between the target and its surroundings.

The perimeter is seldom more useful than a confrontation test in establishing a diagnosis, but it is of great value in supplying records for the purpose of assessing progress. Almost all field defects are more easily discovered and analysed on the Bjerrum screen.

THE HEMISPHERIC PROJECTION PERIMETERS

During recent years a number of hemispherical perimeters with projected light stimuli have been designed. Of these the Goldmann perimeter (Haag-Streit) [FIG. 44] and the Tubingen (Oculus) perimeter [FIGS. 45 and 46] are the commonest in use. The background illumination, which is very important in all psychovisual testing, can be standardized and is therefore reproducible from one perimeter to another. The background illumination can also be varied from the usual photopic to mesopic and scotopic conditions. The stimulus can be altered in size and in intensity which allows a very much greater range of stimuli and permits the plotting both of central and peripheral visual fields without moving the patient. Fixation may be accurately monitored by the perimetrist through a telescope. The disadvantage is the short working distance of 330 mm. common to perimeters which condenses the central 30 degrees of the visual field into a small area. This makes the recording of small scotomata difficult. The Tubingen perimeter allows magnification of the inner 30 degrees onto a larger recording area. The short working distance makes fixation critical and correction of refractive errors becomes very important. An

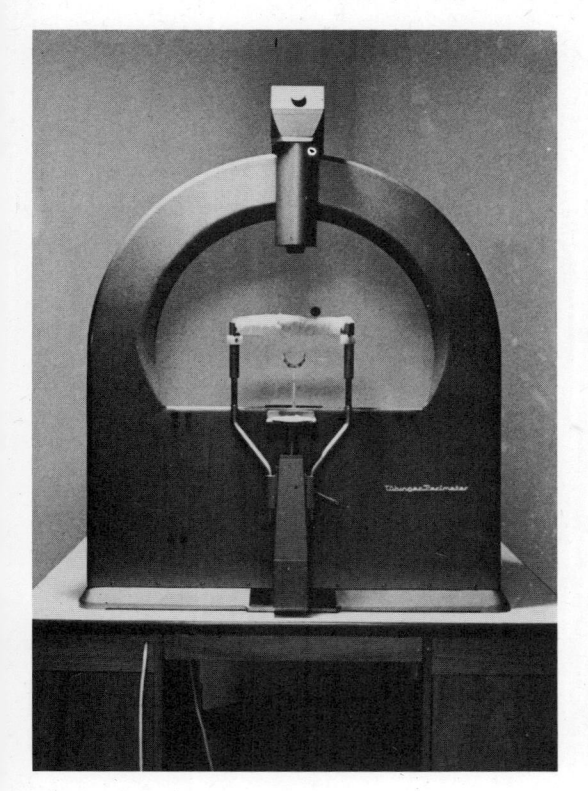

FIG. 46. The Tubingen perimeter seen from the patient's side.

improper understanding of these factors may produce artefacts which must be recognized and taken into consideration when interpreting visual fields.

The Goldmann perimeter [FIG. 44] is a tabletop instrument which is accurate for kinetic and static perimetry. It affords a remarkable speed of operation for kinetic perimetry and screening. The examiner sits behind the bowl and has complete control of the recording pantograph which controls the movement of the stimulus, the adjustment of its size (1/16–64 mm.^{2}), and its brightness, which can be reduced stepwise by 4 $\log^{10}$ units. The diffuse background illumination can also be calibrated. Colour filters can be added and a central scotoma device can be attached. The attachment to the pantograph for static perimetry allows examination of profiles along individual meridians but lacks the freedom of easy static perimetry in areas other than along meridians.

The Tubingen (Oculus) perimeter [FIGS. 45 and 46] was introduced by Harms and Aulhorn a decade ago. It is particularly useful for static profile perimetry but has the full capability of being used for kinetic perimetry. Fixation is accurately monitored and the fovea can be examined with ease and accuracy. The examiner has full control over the position of the target. Target sizes 5 minutes to 2 degrees of visual angle, changes in intensity of stimulus in 0·1 log unit steps, colour filters, intensity of background illumination, brightness and size of fixation device, duration of stimulus presentation, frequency of flicker, are all easily adjusted. The perimeter can also be used to measure dark adaptation of individual retinal areas, flicker fusion frequency, peripheral visual acuity, and response to simulated dazzle under night-driving conditions. The patient indicates his responses by means of a buzzer.

The chin rests of both perimeters can be adjusted and a supplemental lens holder is present to correct for the distance of the test object from the eye.

Both perimeters can be used for kinetic perimetry. The Tubingen perimeter has been designed for static perimetry whereas the Goldmann perimeter needs a special built-in system of filters for static perimetry and its movement is restricted to the testing of single meridians.

STEREOCAMPIMETER

This instrument for examination of the central field was introduced by Lloyd. It is designed for use on a table. The field is viewed through a stereoscope, which makes it appear to be at infinity and permits one eye to be occluded. The black field has a pattern of contrasting shades which aid fixation. The pattern seen with one eye differs slightly from that seen with the other, so that suppression may be detected.

This instrument is of special value in central scotomata. When central vision is lost, it is difficult to examine the field on the Bjerrum screen because steady fixation is impossible. With the stereocampimeter the eye under test is steadied by the fixation of the other eye, reinforced by peripheral fusion. An adjustable light source enables reduced illumination to be used, so that relative scotomata may be detected more readily. Specially designed targets are supplied with the instrument and the results recorded on special charts [FIG. 47].

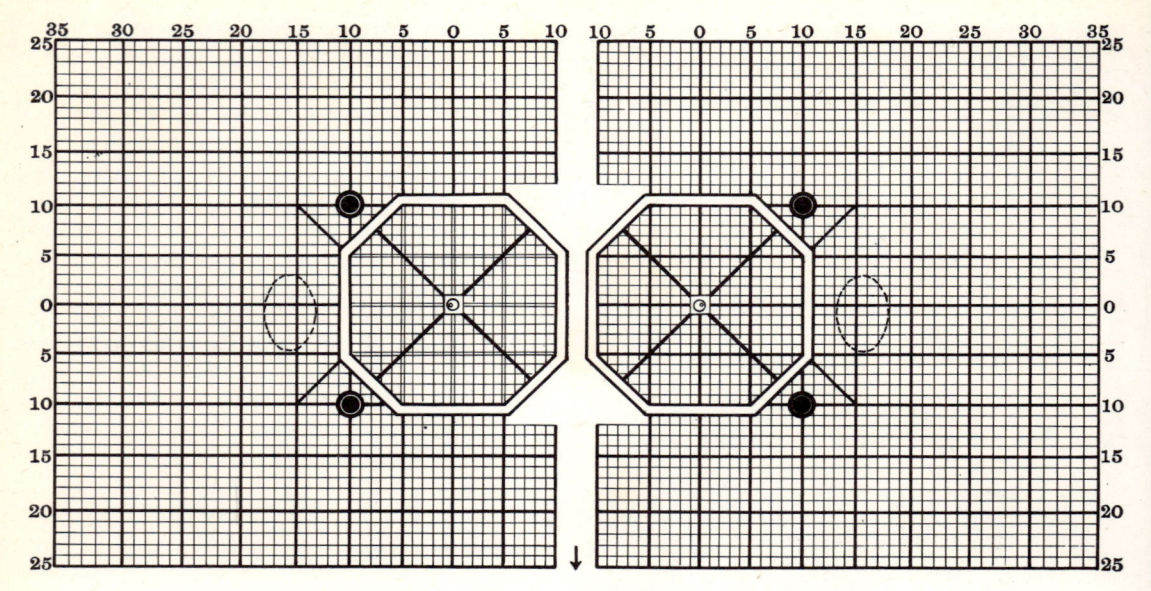

FIG. 47. Chart for use with Lloyd's stereocampimeter.

FLICKER FUSION PERIMETRY

If the frequency of flicker of a light-source is increased, a speed is reached at which the flicker disappears. This speed is known as the critical fusion frequency (C.F.F.), and it has been used by Miles in perimetry. He has designed an instrument called a Strobotac. It consists of a pointer with a light source at its end. The frequency of flicker of the light can be controlled. The critical frequency is measured by gradually reducing the frequency of flicker from a speed above the C.F.F. to that at which the flicker is just seen. This is the C.F.F. and it is recorded in various areas of the field. The normal C.F.F. is between 40 and 50 flashes per second. When a defect is present the C.F.F. falls to below 40 and may be as low as 10 or 20 flashes per second.

Miles claims that the retina may be capable of normal responses to standard methods of perimetry yet show a defect when examined this way. Moreover, although medial opacities and high refractive errors complicate ordinary perimetric procedures, they do not impair the reliability of this method. Some patients who find it difficult to co-operate fully when asked to say when a target becomes visible find it easy to say when the light begins to flicker.

Parsons *et al.* compared the results of flicker perimetry in 50 men with brain damage.

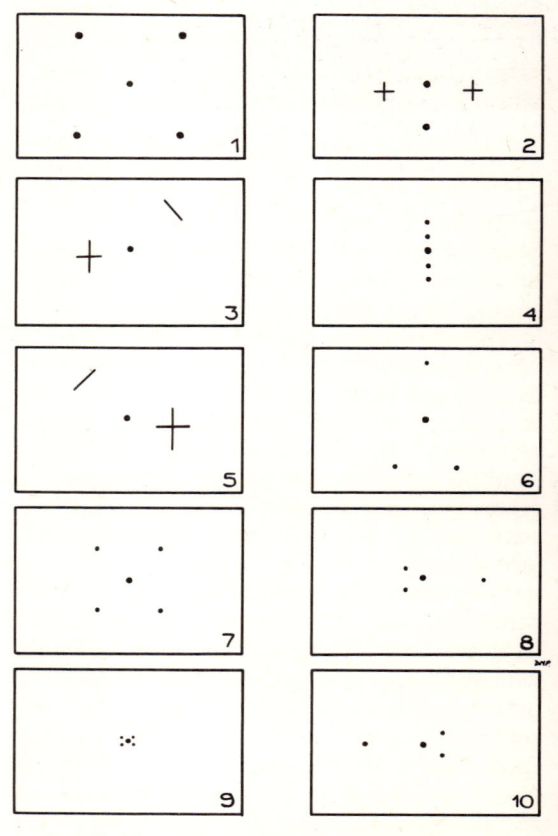

FIG. 48. The patterns of the Harrington-Flocks test.

THE MULTIPLE PATTERN TEST

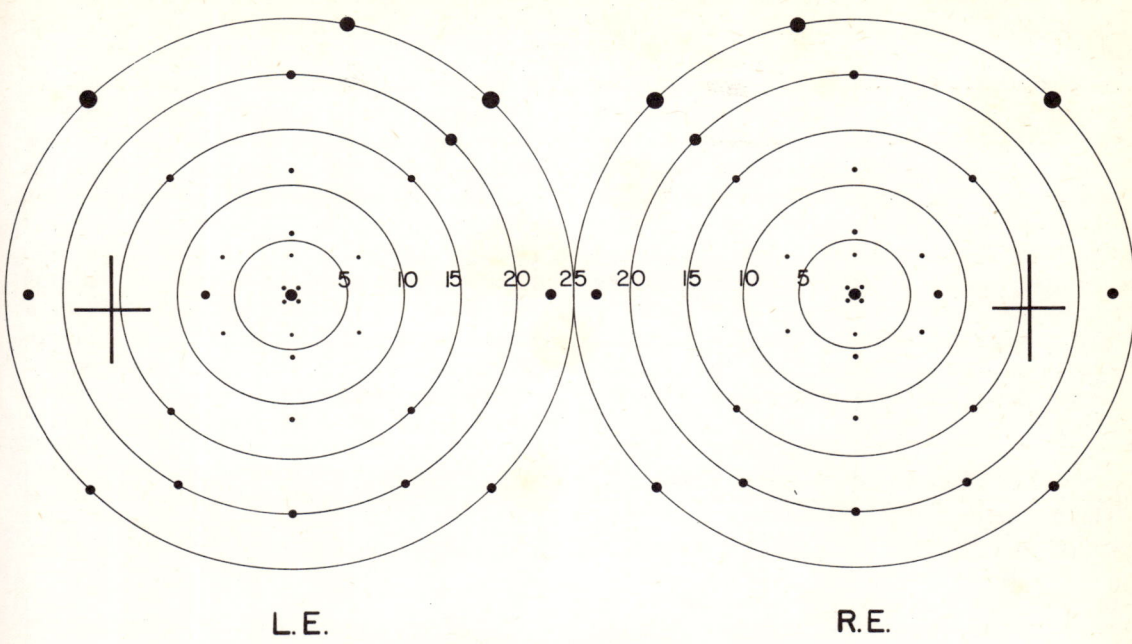

L.E.   R.E.

Fig. 49. Chart for use with the Harrington-Flocks test.

They found that flicker perimetry was more sensitive in detecting abnormalities in the visual field than routine perimetry.

THE MULTIPLE PATTERN TEST OF HARRINGTON AND FLOCKS

Most ophthalmologists examine the visual fields only when the history or clinical examination suggest a field defect. This must mean that early changes of significance are occasionally missed. It would not be possible to make a complete perimetric examination as part of every ophthalmic examination, because no busy ophthalmologist could afford the time. The Multiple Pattern Test has been designed by Harrington and Flocks to enable a relatively untrained person to exclude the commoner field defects.

The apparatus consists of a series of ten cards [Fig. 48]. These are presented in turn to each eye separately. On each card is printed with fluorescent sulphide ink a different pattern of two to four dots, lines, or crosses. They become visible only when illuminated with a flash of ultra-violet light. The flash is too brief to permit a change in fixation. The patterns are planned so that the central field of 25 degrees is examined. The lines and dots are placed in diagnostic areas of the field. When defects characteristic of special diseases are present, such as an arcuate scotoma in glaucoma, the patient fails to see the appropriate dot or line. Since more than one dot is presented at a time,

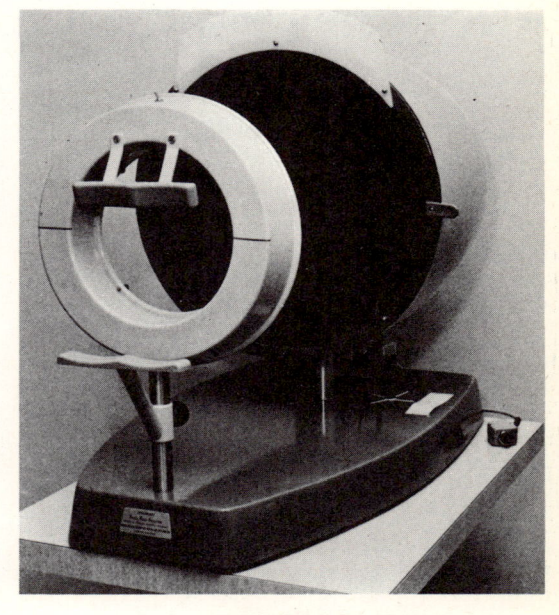

Fig. 50. The Friedmann analyser.

the extinction phenomenon may sometimes be discovered in areas in which no field defect can be demonstrated by standard methods. The patient is asked what he sees on each card in turn and the results are recorded on a composite chart [FIG. 49]. A nurse or a technician is able to carry out this test in three or four minutes with a patient of average intelligence.

It is, of course, a screening test, and is not infallible, but it is valuable. More early defects would be found if it became the custom in hospitals and consulting rooms for the nurse to use this simple test when taking the patient's visual acuity before examination by the physician.

THE FRIEDMANN ANALYSER

This instrument [FIG. 50] utilizes static perimetry for screening. The apparatus consists of a flash with a system of filters which allows control of the flash intensity. A shroud allows exposure of variable patterns located strategically in the central field. Defective areas can be recognized at a stage before they become absolute scotomata. The test can be rapidly performed by an assistant and is probably one of the better screening methods available at this time.

AMSLER'S CHARTS

Amsler's charts are valuable for the study of macular lesions. Intelligence and co-operation on the part of the patient are necessary. If defects are charted at intervals, the progress of a macular degeneration or the recovery of a central serous retinopathy may be recorded.

The charts consist of a series of cards of varying patterns. Each test card has a central fixation point at which the patient is asked to look. They are so designed that when held 30 cm. from the eye, the image of the square occupies a retinal area corresponding to that enclosed by the 10 degree circle on a tangent screen. The patient is asked to view each square in turn and draw what he sees on a recording chart [FIG. 51].

CHOICE OF INSTRUMENTS

The number of pieces of equipment available for perimetry is overwhelming. The choice must depend on the purpose of the examination and will clearly be different in a glaucoma clinic, research laboratory or private office. Expense, availability of space and the main use of the equipment must be considered.

For most offices a tangent screen, with reliable illumination, clean targets and a one meter distance will suffice and will, with the addition of a small perimeter, evaluate central and peripheral fields. The Goldmann perimeter adds the standardization of background illumination, versatility, monitoring of fixation and the ability to evaluate central and peripheral isopters at the same time. For neuro-ophthalmology the two metre tangent screen has some advantages.

For detailed analysis of glaucoma fields the

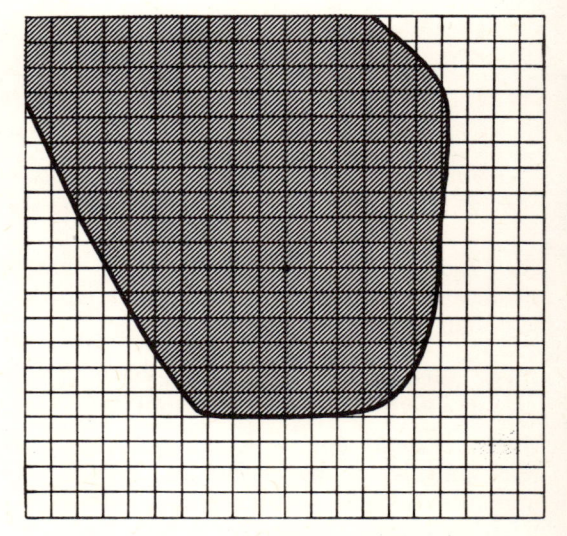

FIG. 51. Field defect due to a small macular haemorrhage, drawn by the patient on an Amsler recording chart.

Oculus perimeter is probably the most accurate equipment but a large tangent screen operated by someone who understands the nature of the glaucomatous defect is adequate.

Screening can be well done with the Friedmann analyser. It can be done even better with the Goldmann or Oculus perimeter though at much greater expense of time and effort. The Harrington-Flocks screener is adequate for gross disturbances.

There are many plotting devices and automatic attachments for the tangent screen but they do not add anything to careful perimetry with simple tools.

REFERENCES

FRIEDMANN, A. I. (1966) Serial analysis of field changes employing a new instrument, *Ophthalmologica (Basel)*, **152**, 1.

GOLDMANN, H. (1945) Grundlagen Exacter Perimetrie, *Ophthalmologica (Basel)*, **109**, 57.

HARMS, H. (1950) Entwicklungsmogeichkeiten der Perimetrie. V. Graefe, *Arch. Ophthal.*, **150**, 28.

HARRINGTON, D. O., and FLOCKS, M. (1954) Visual field examination by new tachystoscopic multiple-pattern method; preliminary report, *Amer. J. Ophthal.*, **37**, 719.

LLOYD, R. I. (1926) *Visual Field Studies*, New York.

MILES, P. (1950) Flicker fusion fields; technique and interpretations, *Amer. J. Ophthal.*, **33**, 1069.

6

VISUAL FIELD EXAMINATION

WHEN IS FIELD EXAMINATION INDICATED?

The ideal procedure would be to include a visual field test in every routine ophthalmic examination, but time is a precious commodity to every practitioner. A few conscientious ophthalmologists do so. Some use a perimeter and others use the Bjerrum screen or a simple confrontation test. The Harrington-Flocks screening test or the Friedman analyser have become popular, and are probably the best and least time-consuming screening tests. Many busy ophthalmologists believe, however, that the time spent on routine perimetry is relatively unrewarding. It may be impossible under many circumstances to evaluate every patient in this way.

The consensus seems to be that perimetry is mandatory only when indicated by the clinical history and ophthalmic examination.

HISTORY

The ophthalmologist is tempted to regard his patient as a piece of visual machinery. Perimetry is one field of investigation which leads away from this limited viewpoint towards the wider aspects of medicine.

The clinical history may be classified under three headings.

General Medical History

The patient should be questioned briefly concerning his general health and symptoms which might suggest such diseases as diabetes, hypertension, cardiovascular disease, haemodynamic crises, disseminated sclerosis, and syphilis.

Neurological History

An account of recent onset of headache which varies with changes in posture and is associated with vomiting may indicate raised intracranial pressure. Paraesthesiae, transient weakness of limbs, or other disturbances of function may be significant.

Ophthalmological History

Several conditions indicate that perimetry is essential.

A *head injury* may damage the visual pathway and cause field defects which indicate the site of the damage.

A complaint of *double vision* may lead to the discovery of a third, fourth, or sixth nerve palsy. Perimetry must always be carried out in these patients. The combination of chiasmal interference and one or more extra-ocular nerve palsies would indicate a middle cranial fossa lesion.

Complaints of *bumping into objects on one side*, a loss of vision or a blank space to one side, all suggest a homonymous hemianopia. Patients with a right homonymous hemianopia which encroaches on the central area have *difficulty in keeping to the appropriate line when reading*.

An intelligent patient with a paracentral scotoma may notice that he is unable to see a whole word at one time. Disturbance of the macular area of the retina by oedema or haemorrhage may lead to a complaint of distortion of central vision, a phenomenon best demonstrated by using Amsler's charts.

Very rarely visual hallucinations may occur. These hallucinations may be of flashing lights or colours, or of places, people, and faces. These may be caused by tumours or vascular lesions of the occipital, temporal, or parietal lobes which may involve the visual pathway.

Lesions in the region of the angular and

supramarginal gyri may cause patients to be unable to find their way home, or to recognize well-known locations. All such symptoms indicate the need for field examination.

OPHTHALMOLOGICAL EXAMINATION

Several clinical findings may require perimetry for elucidation.

Pallor of the optic disc, unless unilateral, is seldom adequate evidence for a diagnosis of optic atrophy without the demonstration of a field defect. If the optic discs appear to be pale in any patient a perimetric examination is essential.

Cupping of the optic disc, or a rise in ocular tension on routine tonometry, indicates that the central fields must be examined to exclude glaucoma.

The slightest suggestion of papilloedema demands a perimetric examination followed by X-ray of skull and possibly referral to a neurologist.

In **retinal and choroidal diseases,** the finding of a characteristic field change is not only confirmatory evidence, but a valuable record for the future assessment of the rate of progress of the disease. Occasionally, new blood-vessel formation, or an attenuated artery, may be seen in the fundus, suggesting that it is the site of an old vascular accident. The nature of the lesion may sometimes be diagnosed with certainty only by demonstrating a characteristic scotoma, e.g. a scotoma with a straight horizontal edge in branch arterial occlusion.

Unilateral proptosis may be caused by an orbital tumour, an intracranial tumour invading the orbit, or by endocrine exophthalmos. Perimetry may give some assistance in diagnosis in these cases. This is particularly true of a meningioma of the sphenoidal ridge which is involving the orbit.

X-RAY EXAMINATION

Sometimes an X-ray of the skull will show anomalies which indicate the need for a field examination. Examples of these are listed below.

Signs of Raised Intracranial Pressure

1. Separation of sutures in children.
2. Erosion of the dorsum sellae, particularly in adults.

Localizing Signs

1. Displacement of a calcified pineal gland to one side.
2. Local erosion or hyperostosis of bone. Of particular interest to the ophthalmologist are erosion of the clinoid processes and hyperostosis of the sphenoid ridge.
3. Enlargement of optic foramina. This should be sought in cases where a glioma of the optic nerve is thought to be dilating the optic canal.
4. Tumour calcification. This is common in craniopharyngiomata and occurs in about 10 per cent of intracranial gliomata.
5. The 'egg-shell' outline in the wall of a cystic craniopharyngioma or an aneurysm of the circle of Willis.

THE FIELD EXAMINATION

The fields are usually investigated only after the history has been taken and the eyes thoroughly examined. If these suggest the presence of a field defect, they will also indicate the type of defect that should be sought, e.g. a cupped disc will suggest glaucomatous field defects. It is therefore most important to know what type of field defect to look for and how to demonstrate it. For example, consider a patient in the early stages of glaucoma. If glaucoma is suspected and he is examined with a 3 mm. white target on a 330 cm. perimeter, and the blind spot is then plotted on the Bjerrum screen, normal readings will be found. Thus time is wasted and early field defects are missed. Such a person should be examined for paracentral scotomata, for arcuate scotomata and for a nasal step, using a Bjerrum screen with a 2 mm. white target or other equipment which will accurately test the central field [see Chapter 9].

The shape of a field defect is its most important feature. In the majority of cases this is best demonstrated with a 2 mm. white target on a

2 metre Bjerrum screen or its equivalent on a hemispherical perimeter. Although the diagnosis of most conditions can be made from an accurate chart of the shape of a defect with one isopter, this is not a complete perimetric examination. The defect should be analysed. This means that two or three isopters should be plotted, using stimuli of varying sizes to indicate the 'slope' of the edge of the defect.

There are four all-important rules for efficient visual field examination.
1. The examiner should know from his preliminary examination of the patient's eye what type of field defect to seek.
2. The patient must be made to understand fully what is expected of him. The blind spot should be plotted first to show him what is expected, and to assess the patient's reliability.
3. The observer should watch the patient's eye to make sure that it is not moving to look for the target.
4. In all doubtful responses the examiner should assess reproducibility and patient fatigue by moving the target from non-visible areas to visible areas and then reversing the direction

CONFRONTATION TEST

It many cases it is wise to perform the confrontation test first. This will often indicate the site of the lesion, e.g. in cases of retrobulbar neuritis or advanced bitemporal hemianopia.

The examiner sits or stands facing the patient, a little less than one arm's length away [FIG. 40]. The observer closes one eye and the patient's opposite eye is covered. The patient is asked to look steadily at the open eye of the examiner and in this way any wavering of fixation of the eye under test may be seen.

Throughout this test the pinhead is held about one foot from the patient's eye. The white pinhead is moved inward from a point outside the patient's field of view. The patient is asked to say 'Yes' as soon as he catches the faintest glimpse of it. This is repeated at intervals around the circumference of the patient's field of vision and any defect of the periphery can be noted. A homonymous hemianopic defect would quickly be discovered by this method.

A red pin is often best for exploring the central area between 5 and 30 degrees of an imaginary line between the patient's eye and the examiner's eye. It is moved methodically through the four quadrants of the central area and the patient is asked whether the hue is different in any position. If in one situation the red appears pale or hazy, then a relative or absolute scotoma is present. The central scotoma which occurs in retrobulbar neuritis is most rapidly discovered in this way.

Asking the patient to count fingers in the four quadrants with the fingers held about 30 degrees from fixation is often a useful modification of the confrontation test. Field defects caused by glaucoma, retinal detachment and cerebral vascular lesions are readily demonstrated in this way. Technicians easily learn this simple technique and may save the time of the ophthalmologist by drawing his attention to the defect.

If optic atrophy is present and the vision so reduced that a pinhead cannot be seen at all, the hand or a sheet of white paper should be used. Even with such poor vision, the patient may be able to see the sheet of paper in the temporal field, although he cannot see it in the nasal field. An ophthalmoscope light may be used in the same way. As the light is moved from the nasal field to the temporal field, the patient may say that the light has been turned off. A sheet of white paper or the ophthalmoscope light used in this way may also establish the diagnosis when the perimetric examination is hampered by corneal or lenticular opacities.

In many cases the diagnosis can be made by the confrontation test. If a defect is found it should be analysed and recorded by using the Bjerrum screen or the perimeter. This analysis will give greater information about the state of the disease and supply a record for assessing progress. If no defect is discovered with the confrontation test, further examinations with the screen and perimeter may reveal one.

BJERRUM SCREEN TEST

A 2 mm. white target used with the 2 metre Bjerrum screen is a most useful threshold target.

In order to increase the contrast of the white target against the black screen some perimetrists don a black gown and black gloves for a screen test. It is inadvisable to wear a white coat but a dark suit is quite adequate.

Chalk, or pins with black heads, may be used to mark out the isopters on the screen during the test. At the end of the examination these isopters are transferred to a chart. It is, however, both quick and simple for the examiner to hold the chart in one hand and the target rod and a pencil in the other hand [FIG. 41]. It is as easy to make a mark on the chart with the pencil as it is to stick a pin in the screen or mark it with chalk. When the chart itself is marked the recording is complete at the end of the test and a secretary may ink it in later for a more permanent record.

The patient sits at the appropriate distance (i.e. 1 or 2 metres) from the screen with one eye covered by an occluder, or a pad and strapping. He is asked to look steadily at the central white spot with the uncovered eye, and to say 'Yes' as soon as he catches the faintest glimpse of the target out of the corner of his eye. The examiner stands by the side of the screen, half facing the patient in order to ensure that the patient's fixing eye does not wander. It is wise to plot the blind spot at the beginning of the examination. This gives an indication of the reliability of the patient as a witness and demonstrates to him what he is expected to do.

Starting well outside 30 degrees from fixation, the examiner moves the white target slowly towards the centre until the patient indicates that he can see it. This position is recorded on the chart and the test is repeated at 15 degree intervals around 'the clock'. The 2 mm. white target should normally be seen at or about 30 degrees from fixation.

The test object should not be moved with a vibratory motion. This causes an increase in the effective visual angle, so that the target is seen sooner than it should be.

Scotomata are not always easy to detect. With an intelligent patient it is best to move the target slowly towards the centre of the screen along each of the tested meridians in turn. If it disappears at any point a scotoma is present. This method will fail with patients who persist in watching the target.

A scotoma may sometimes be discovered by placing the 2 mm. white target in different situations in the central field and asking the patient if he can still see it even when he looks at the fixation spot. This procedure may prove more effective than asking him to say when the target disappears.

If one suspects that the patient is saying he can see the target when he should not, his reliability can often be checked by turning the target so that its edge faces the patient. If he still maintains he can see it, his future answers should be suspected and double-checked.

For a long time it has been customary to use a rod with a target at its end. This has the disadvantage that the patient can often see the rod by the reflection of light on its surface. This gives him a guide to the position of the target and lessens the reliability of the test. This difficulty may be overcome by using a flashlight or torch especially designed so that the size, luminosity and colour of the light projected on the screen may be varied. A black screen is unsuitable for this purpose and a special grey one is used. Greater versatility may be obtained by arranging for the illumination of the screen to be variable. In this way minimal defects may be discovered by using targets of medium size, e.g. 5/2000 white, but with reduced illumination. However, unless one uses this technique fairly often in order to learn the normal responses, the significance of a minimal defect found in this way is difficult to assess.

Another useful method developed by Harrington is a target illuminated by ultra-violet light which can be flashed on and off. When patients tend to follow a moving target this technique will often supply more reliable answers. A black screen is used with a luminescent target on a black rod. The target may be illuminated by an ultra-violet light held in the examiner's other hand, or better still by a battery in the handle of the holder of the target.

When using a coloured target the point to be recorded on the chart is the point at which the patient recognizes the true colour of the target. It is essential to explain to the patient that as the target moves towards the centre of the screen, he will not at first be able to determine its colour. As it moves farther inwards he will suddenly recognize its hue. At this point he should say 'Yes'.

Sometimes a scotoma may be revealed by placing a 10 mm. red target in different situations at equal distances, e.g. 10 degrees, from the fixation point, and asking the patient to state whether there is any change in hue. If he says it is pink or brown in any area, a relative scotoma is present and requires analysis. This test may be carried out almost as well on confrontation.

VISUAL FIELD EXAMINATION

The most satisfactory perimetric examination is a tangent screen test done by the ophthalmologist himself. Seldom will use of the perimeter reveal a defect not found on the tangent screen.

THE PERIMETER

The standard arc perimeter is used mainly to provide a record of the peripheral field. It is of little value for diagnosis except in cases of retinitis pigmentosa or rare cases with defects situated outside the 30 degree isopter. Almost all defects are discovered most readily by using the confrontation test and the Bjerrum screen.

The patient is comfortably seated before the instrument, with the chin on the rest, so that the eye to be tested is at the centre of the sphere of which the arc of the perimeter is a part [FIG. 43]. The other eye is covered.

It is usual to start with the 3 mm. white target and to move it slowly inwards from the extreme periphery, where it is out of sight, to the centre. Larger targets may be used as required. Each meridian is examined in turn at intervals of 30 degrees. As in the case of the screen test the point at which the target is first seen is recorded. The target is then moved on towards the centre, and if it disappears at any point the area should be analysed.

ANALYSIS

When a field defect has been discovered it must be analysed. If no time is available or the patient is tired he should return at a convenient time. The defect should be plotted with at least three isopters. In most cases it is best to move the target from the area where it is not seen to the field where it is visible.

For example, in a case of chiasmal compression due to a chromophobe adenoma of the pituitary gland, the essential changes in the field would be revealed by a 3 mm. white target on the perimeter, together with a 2 mm. white and 15 mm. red target on the 2 metre Bjerrum screen. More isopters may be plotted, but these three or three similar ones are essential.

CHARTS

Simple charts are available for recording the results of the examination with the Bjerrum screen [FIG. 52]. On these the circles should be marked out to 30 degrees because early changes are sometimes found just outside the

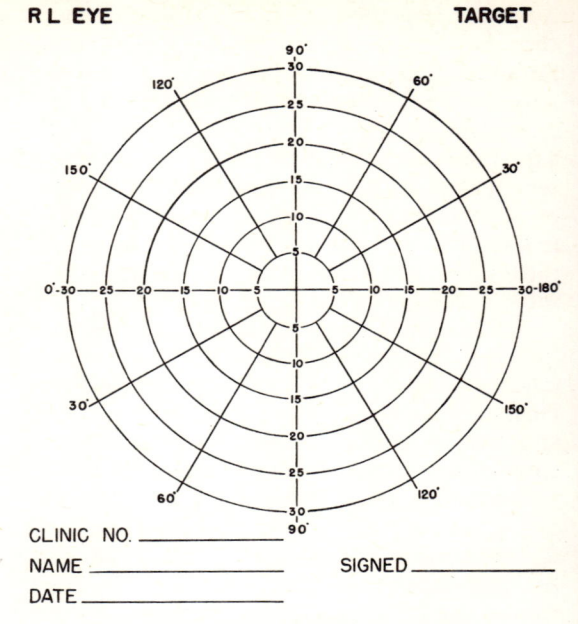

FIG. 52. A standard Bjerrum screen chart.

25 degree circle. Most perimeters are self-recording and each has its own special chart. Many perimetrists prefer to have the visual fields of both eyes recorded on one sheet [FIG. 53]. This has merit when both eyes have associated field defects as in bilateral hemianopia, but has none when one eye is normal. The majority of ophthalmologists record the results of the central and peripheral field examinations on separate charts and file them together. Others, particularly neurosurgeons, dislike having to refer to two different charts. They prefer to have all the isopters recorded on one. But if the Bjerrum screen findings are added to the perimeter chart a considerable reduction results and significant features may be less defined. Since the Bjerrum screen findings are usually of greater significance than the perimeter findings, this practice is not satisfactory.

In an attempt to solve this problem Walker introduced a chart in which the central isopters are farther apart than the peripheral isopters [FIG. 54]. The distance between 0 and 10 degrees is twice that from 80 degrees to 90 degrees, and between them the intervals are graduated. Even with the Walker charts, however, the central field is relatively too small to be satisfactory and both the screen and peri-

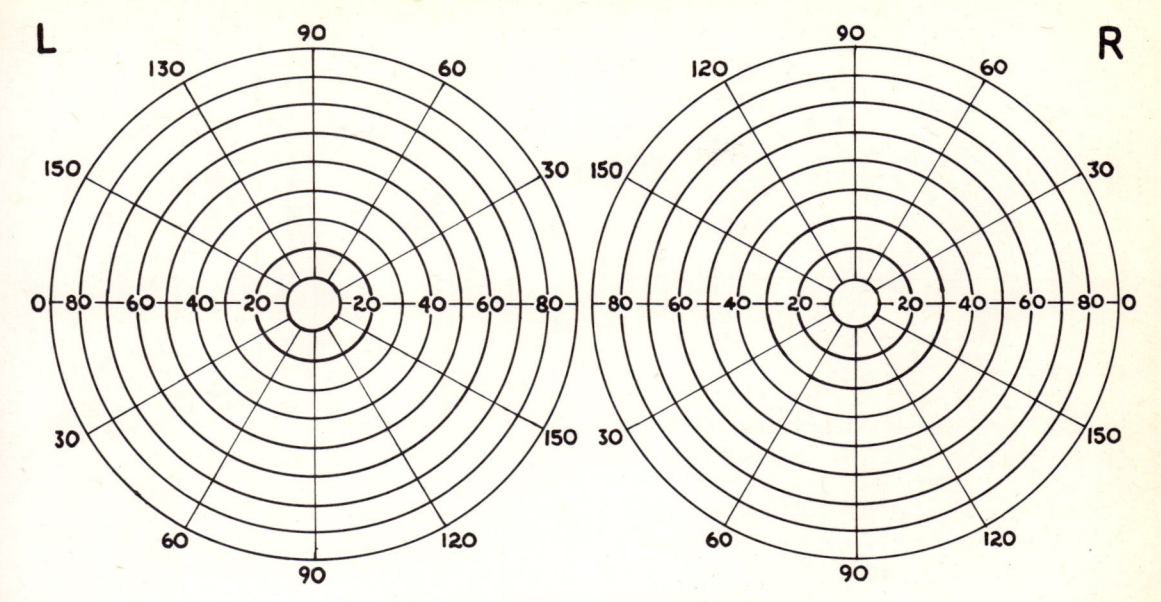

FIG. 53. A standard perimeter chart.

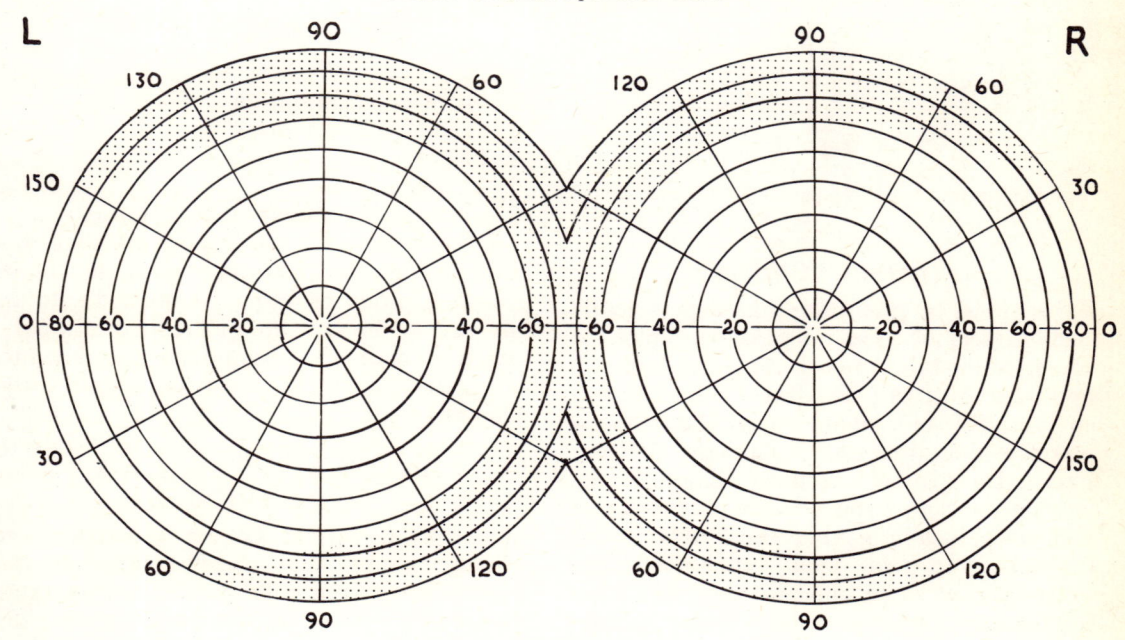

FIG. 54. Walker's chart.

meter findings must be transcribed by hand.
    Crick has suggested a further modification. His chart is based upon a parabolic projection [FIG. 55]. The central isopters are more widely spaced than those in Walker's chart and there is a gradual narrowing of the spaces between them towards the periphery. He has also designed an attachment which fits some of the standard perimeters and permits mechanical recording.

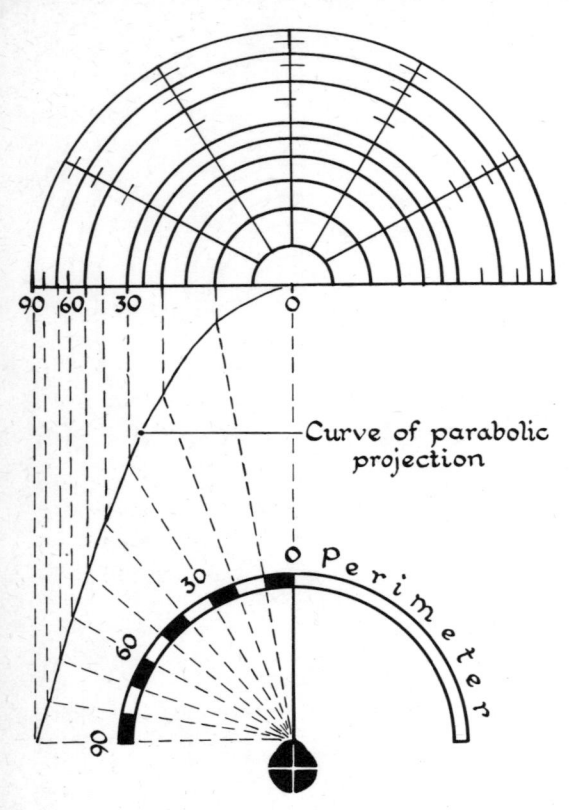

FIG. 55. The principle of the parabolic projection chart (Crick).

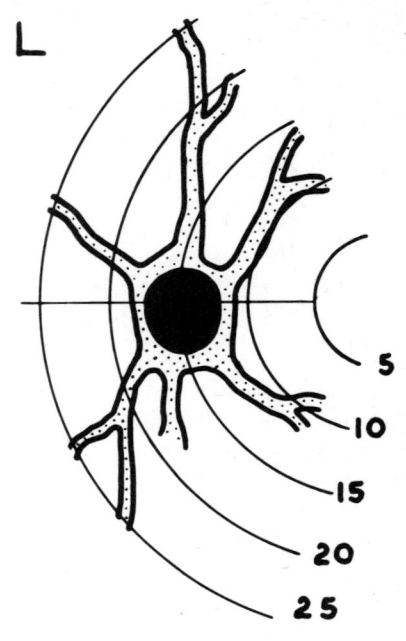

FIG. 56. A normal angioscotoma.

ANGIOSCOTOMETRY

It has long been known that if sufficiently small targets are used it is possible to plot the course of the blood vessels radiating from the optic disc [FIG. 56]. This can be done with a co-operative and intelligent patient using a 1 mm. white target and the 2 metre Bjerrum screen. The 5 metre screen is even more satisfactory. As can be imagined, however, it is a very time-consuming procedure. Evans studied this subject in great detail, but little further work has been done since. He used the Lloyd stereocampimeter with targets made by heating the end of fine silver wires to produce little balls. He emphasized that angioscotometry is not the plotting of the shadows cast by the retinal blood vessels. He claimed that in normal people the angioscotomata widen as a result of a number of diverse conditions:
1. Digital pressure on the eyes. Pressure on one eye causes widening of the angioscotomata of both eyes.
2. Suspending expiration.
3. Jugular vein compression.
4. Fright.
5. Menstruation.
6. Cervical sympathetic stimulation.

Evans advanced the hypothesis that this phenomenon resulted from depression of function in a group of retinal elements due to an increase in the pressure of the fluid in a perivascular space. This technique was claimed to be of great value in the study of cases of early glaucoma.

INATTENTION OR LACK OF AWARENESS

This was called by Bender the extinction phenomenon. It may be regarded as an exaggeration of a normal response. A severe pain in one area of the body will cause a lesser pain elsewhere to be disregarded. Similarly a faint light in one area of the visual field may not be noticed if there is a brighter light shining in a different area. This lack of awareness results from a difference in intensity of the stimuli.

A defect in the sensory mechanism may result in a phenomenon resembling this normal response. If the sensory mechanism is defective, the simultaneous movement of two lights in different areas of the visual field may result in only one being seen. Yet if each is moved separately, each is seen. This occurs particularly in lesions of the retrogeniculate pathway. A hemianopia not demonstrable with a single stimulus in routine perimetry may be revealed by the use of two stimuli. A simple way of demonstrating this phenomenon is to stand facing the patient, with arms outstretched. The patient keeps both eyes open and looks directly at the examiner. He is asked to say which finger moves. Each quadrant of the visual field is explored by first twitching a finger of one hand and then a finger of each hand simultaneously. If the movement of each finger separately is seen but only one is noticed when both fingers are moved at the same time, the phenomenon of extinction exists. This test is really a refinement of the confrontation test.

Various improvements may be introduced. A 5 mm. white test object mounted in a black holder may be held in each hand. The perimeter arc may be used in association with two white test objects. An assistant will be needed to hold the second target if a screen is used, particularly a 2 metre screen. This test for the extinction phenomenon is usually performed on the binocular field, but the visual field of each eye may also be examined separately. Two targets are used, so that two different areas may be stimulated at the same time. In this way doubtful paracentral scotomata may sometimes be defined more exactly.

When examining a patient for inattention in the binocular field or making use of the phenomenon to elicit a doubtful defect in the monocular field, one must bear in mind that this is a relative test. The patient may occasionally notice the test object in an area which usually exhibits the extinction phenomenon. But if he fails to see the movement of the target three out of four times, it may be said that inattention is present.

SOME CAUSES OF APPARENT FIELD DEFECTS
MEDIAL OPACITIES

Diffuse opacities of the cornea or lens cause generalized contraction of the isopters and aggravate any defects which may be present. If the corneal opacity is well-defined and limited to the temporal area of the cornea it will tend to cause a defect in the temporal field. On the other hand, a discrete posterior cortical opacity of the lens on the temporal side will tend to produce a defect in the nasal field. When medial opacities reduce the visual acuity, it is wise to use larger targets or to increase the illumination on the targets. Dilating the pupil in these cases usually decreases the size of the defect.

If the vision is very poor, a fairly reliable estimate of the state of the visual field may be obtained with two flashlights, using one for fixation and one as the target. The use of flicker fusion perimetry and static perimetry are of especial value when medial opacities are present.

In cases of reduced visual acuity a pinhole disc is often useful in rapidly distinguishing medial opacities from macular lesions. In medial opacities a pinhole often improves vision but in macular lesions vision is usually decreased.

APHAKIA

The visual field of an eye with uncorrected aphakia is contracted because the visual acuity is poor. Although it is possible to examine the peripheral field with large targets, e.g. 5/330 white or 7/330 white, with considerable reliability, several degrees of constriction must be expected. Since vision is so blurred in uncorrected aphakia a special fixation device such as a circle or a cross often aids fixation. During examination of the central field the patient must wear his spectacle correction. Targets of 1 or 2/2000 white may be used, but again the isopters will be constricted by at least 5 degrees. The inherent spherical aberration of an aphakic correction prevents the examination of the visual field outside 25 degrees. Bifocals tend to produce a false inferior defect but this can be avoided by asking the patient to tilt the head down so that the eye looks through the upper part of the lens.

Contact lenses provide the best solution to this problem. The patient may wear his own contact lenses or may be fitted with a trial lens. But even with a contact lens there is a 20 to 30 degree constriction of the peripheral isopters compared with the normal phakic eye. Due to changes in the optical system the blind spot in an aphakic eye corrected with a contact lens is the same as in a phakic eye without correction,

THE DULL PATIENT

It is usual to move the target from a 'blind' to a 'seeing' area. When a patient is mentally retarded, the reaction time is slow and the visual field will appear contracted. If this is suspected, the 2/2000 white isopter should be plotted by moving the target centrifugally from a seeing to a blind area and asking the patient to say when the target disappears. This isopter should not be more than 5 degrees larger than the first. If there is a big gap between the two isopters it is due to a slow reaction time. This occurs in dull and mentally defective patients, but it should be remembered that it is also found in patients with toxaemia, arteriosclerosis, cerebral tumour, brain abscess, or raised intracranial pressure from any cause. A slow reaction time may thus give an alert perimetrist a clue which may lead to the diagnosis of a serious disease.

MALINGERING

This is found particularly in patients seeking compensation and in young men hoping to avoid military service. A concentrically contracted field is usually found. Targets of all sizes are seen abruptly at the 'edge' of the area of vision. The slope of the defect is therefore steep. A diagnostic feature is that the area of the field on the 2 metre screen within which the target is seen tends to remain constant whether the patient is $\frac{1}{2}$, 1, or 2 metres away, no matter what size of target is used [FIG. 57]. Thus the isopters at different distances are inconsistent.

HYSTERIA

Like malingering, this condition usually gives rise to contracted fields with steep margins. Plotting the field at different distances from the screen will likewise reveal inconsistencies. The size of the visual field should vary directly with the distance and the target size but in hysteria it usually remains constant as in malingering [FIG. 57]. In pathological conditions the edge of the field is often irregular but in hysteria it is usually smooth.

Spiral fields are also common in hysteria [FIGS. 58 and 59]. These result when the target is moved centripetally from a 'blind' to a 'seeing' area. If the target is moved centrifugally from a 'seeing' to a 'blind' area the spiral may be reversed.

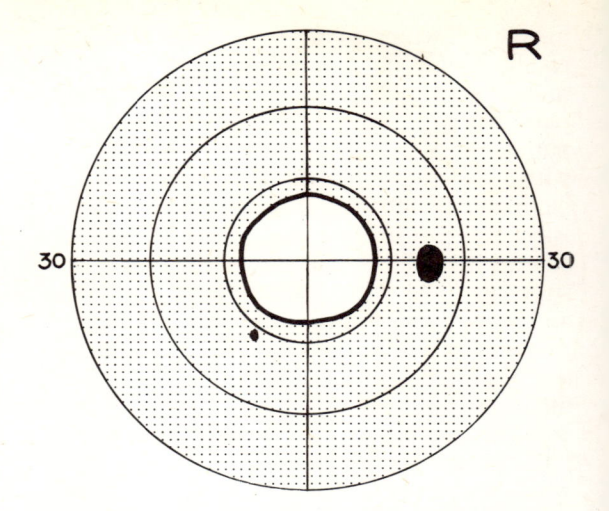

FIG. 57. Visual field chart of a malingerer. All targets were seen just within the 10 degree circle whether the distance was $\frac{1}{2}$, 1 or 2 metres.

These patients are often very susceptible to suggestion. If, when moving the target centripetally, the examiner suggests by leading questions that it cannot yet be seen, the patient may agree. A spiral field then results. If the target is being moved centrifugally and the examiner suggests that it has not yet disappeared the patient may again agree, so that the spiral is reversed. Occasionally a hysterical or malingering component may be added to a genuine defect. This may make field recording difficult, but the functional element can usually be separated from the organic by charting the fields with different targets on both the perimeter and the screen at 1 and 2 metres. Inconsistencies due to the functional component will become apparent when these charts are compared.

Many of these patients are below average intelligence and tend to be somewhat hostile and unco-operative. For example, during examination of their ocular movements they will not put forth sufficient effort to move the eyes fully to the right or to the left and both accommodation and convergence will be found to be deficient.

Whilst contraction of the field is the usual change in hysteria, bilateral scotomata have

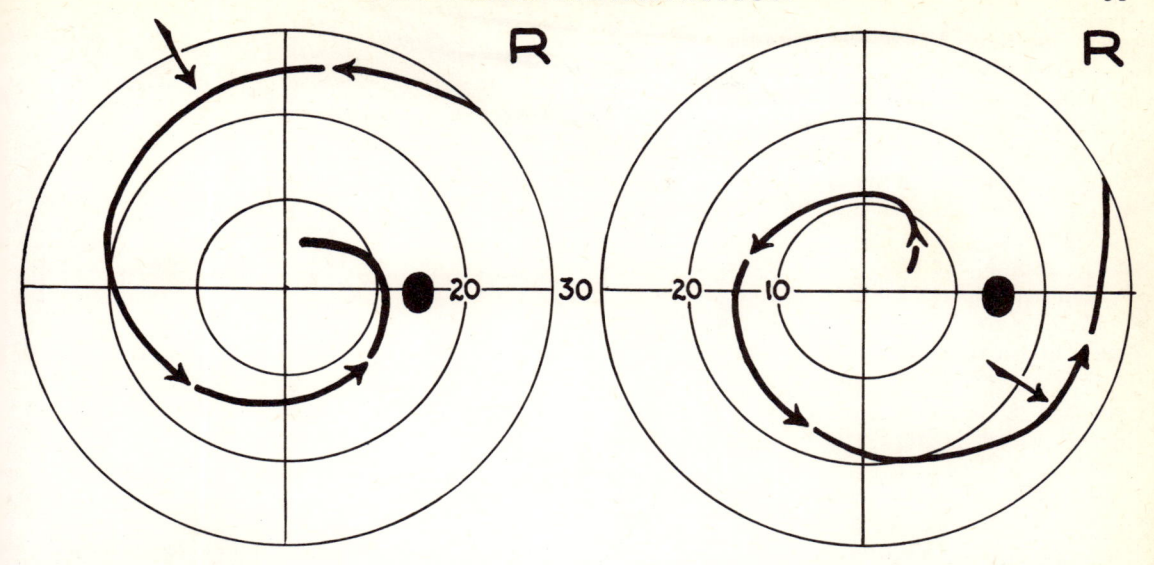

THE FIELD EXAMINATION

FIG. 58. A spiral field in hysteria, plotted centripetally.

FIG. 59. 'Reversing a spiral' plotted centrifugally.

been reported. These may give rise to great difficulty in diagnosis because scotomata almost always have a pathological basis. The diagnosis of hysteria may be made if optic atrophy does not develop, fixation is not eccentric, the patient appears to function well despite apparent poor sight, he shows no anxiety despite the defective vision and, finally, no deterioration occurs with time.

It is customary to consider malingering and hysteria as two separate entities. But many cases are seen in which the patient's motives are so confused and his insight so clouded that a psychiatrist's help is required to assist in the diagnosis.

PTOSIS

Ptosis may cause flattening of the upper part of the field. A ptosed lid should be raised during the field examination [FIG. 60].

HEAD TILTING

If the patient's head is tilted towards the left shoulder the right blind spot is elevated. When the head is tilted to the right shoulder the right blind spot is lowered. Thus if the head is tilted to the left during the plotting of the upper margin of the right blind spot and to the right during the plotting of the lower margin, the blind spot will have a false appearance of enlargement [FIG. 61].

THE ENLARGED BLIND SPOT

Enlargement of the blind spot may be found in a number of conditions including papilloedema, drusen of the nerve head, opaque nerve fibres, coloboma of the disc, inferior conus, inverted disc or a nasally directed scleral canal, juxtapapillary choroiditis, temporal crescent of myopia and atrophy of the peripapillary choroid. These anomalies can be

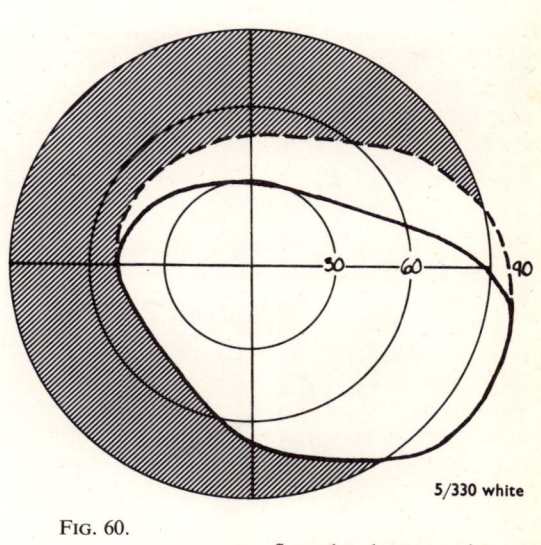

FIG. 60.

5/330 white

——— flattening due to ptosis.
- - - - - field on raising upper lid.

seen ophthalmoscopically. The enlargement of the blind spot may be irregular but it usually corresponds to the area of the disturbance. Papilloedema produces enlargement of the blind spot in all directions. When small threshold targets are used the blind spot is found to enlarge with age but enlargement is not necessarily found with large targets. Some of the anomalies enumerated may be associated with a nerve fibre bundle scotoma.

With an intelligent patient the course of the main blood vessels may be plotted for a short way from the blind spot with a 1 or 2 mm. white target at 2 metres, but these are unlikely to be confused with a true enlargement of the blind spot.

The blind spot may be elongated superiorly and inferiorly in the presence of a glaucomatous defect but this is seldom the early specific change of the disease. Baring of the blind spot, especially superiorly but also inferiorly, occurs with the use of threshold stimuli. It must be remembered that stimuli which are above the threshold for a normal young eye may be threshold or below the threshold of an ageing eye or an eye with opacities of the nuclei. Threshold changes must therefore be interpreted with great care.

USE OF REDUCED ILLUMINATION

Scotomata due to lesions of the retina and to conduction defects are more obvious when plotted with white targets in reduced illumination. It is sometimes possible to demonstrate a doubtful scotoma with certainty by diminishing the light on the screen. A means of graduating the illumination of the Bjerrum screen is therefore of great value.

Good lighting is required for the recognition of colour. Reduced illumination should not be used when plotting colour isopters, because this results in marked contraction. Field defects are so greatly aggravated when coloured

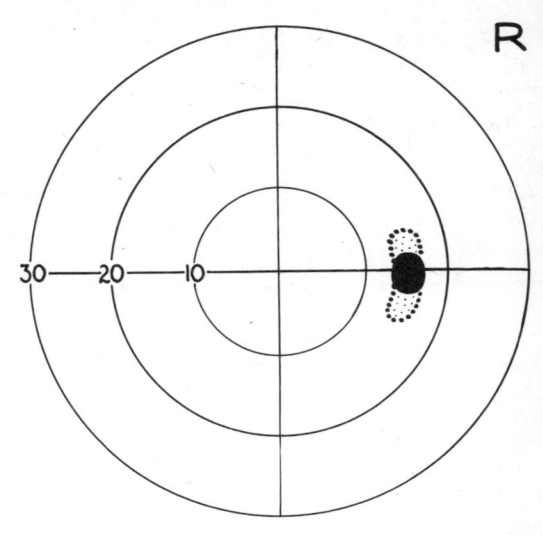

FIG. 61. False enlargement of the blind spot due to head tilting.

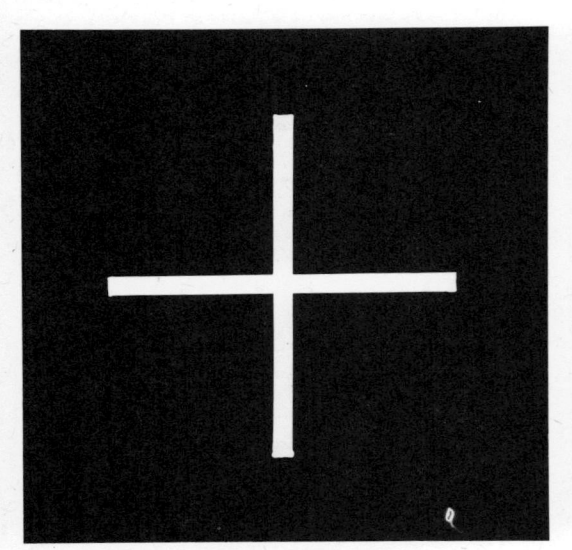

FIG. 62a. Fixation target—a cross.

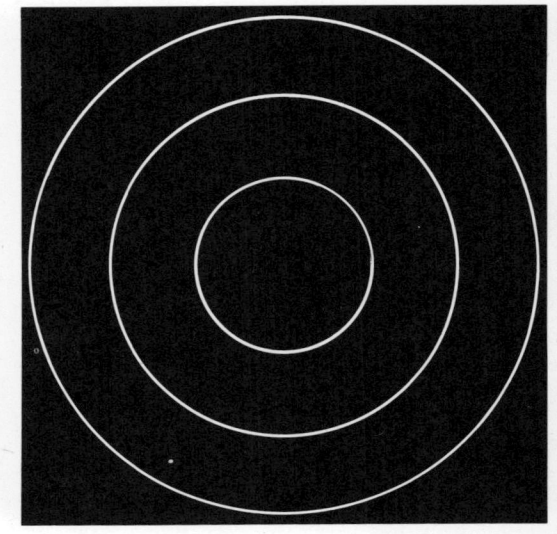

FIG. 62b. Fixation target—concentric circles.

targets are used with reduced illumination that they are unreliable.

PLOTTING A CENTRAL SCOTOMA

It is often very difficult to plot a central scotoma accurately because the patient is unable to gaze steadily at the fixation target. If it is suspected that the patient's eye is wandering and the defect which has been plotted is incorrect, plotting the blind spot quickly confirms or disproves one's suspicions. Various methods may be adopted in these cases.

1. The confrontation test will often give adequate information, providing small targets are used.
2. It is sometimes useful to make use of eye-hand co-ordination by placing the tip of the patient's right index finger on the fixation target and asking him to look at his finger-nail. This can be done only with the perimeter or the smaller scotometer models.
3. The phenomenon of completion may be used by providing a large fixation target composed of a cross or concentric rings [FIGS. 62a and b]. If the eye can see the outer pattern of the target it may 'complete' the pattern, and fix the centre steadily.
4. Red-green goggles may be used. In the case of a patient having a central scotoma in the right eye, the left eye fixes a green fixation target light through a green glass. The central field of the right eye is then plotted with a red test light. This method is valueless if a marked degree of heterophoria is present.
5. The phenomenon of polarization of light may be used in a similar manner. Goggles with polarized lenses are worn. The fixation light and the target light are polarized at right angles to each other. Thus the fixation light is seen with one eye and the test object is seen with the other. Like the red-green goggle method it is valueless if heterophoria is present.
6. Stereoscopic devices are the most valuable means of plotting central scotomata. Lloyd's stereocampimeter has been described and is probably a good instrument for this purpose. Static perimetry can also be helpful in these situations.

REFERENCES

BENDER, M. B. (1952) *Disorders in Perception*, Springfield, Ill.

CRICK, R. P. (1957) A system of visual field testing and recording using a parabolic projection, *Trans. ophthal. Soc. U.K.*, **57**, 593.

EVANS, J. N. (1948) Angioscotometry, in *Modern Trends in Ophthalmology*, p. 141, 2nd series, ed. Sorsby, A., London.

WALKER, C. B. (1917) Quantitative perimetry, *Arch. Ophthal.*, **46**, 537.

7

STATIC PERIMETRY

An important function of perimetry is the evaluation of the progress of certain disease states. The improvement in the visual field or its deterioration may be factors on which adequacy of therapy or even necessity for surgical interference in certain diseases may be decided. This is particularly true in glaucoma, the toxic amblyopias and in some neurological disturbances. In order to make such important decisions meaningfully accurate and reproducible perimetry is mandatory.

Kinetic perimetry was introduced for this purpose and is carried out by plotting many isopters with different stimuli. This allows an estimate of the slope of the contour of the visual island and helps in the assessment of the steepness of a visual field defect. The closer the isopters the steeper the slope of the contour of the island, whereas the farther they are apart the more gradual the slope [FIGS. 34 and 63]. This is analogous to the contour lines joining those points of the same height above sea level used in contour maps. A similar map of the visual field can be obtained by measuring the differential threshold of very many points of the visual field with stationary stimuli and then joining all those points in the visual field which have the same threshold [FIG. 64]. Such a procedure gives the isopters and indicates topographically the contour features of the visual field.

The measurement of thresholds with stationary targets is called static, threshold or profile perimetry. It is usually recorded not as isopters but along meridians in which the vertical cross-section of the island of vision is recorded. The actual slopes are therefore graphically presented in this method of field testing. It is not necessary to keep to the meridians as any area of visual field can be analysed by static perimetry. The depth and width of the disturbance in an abnormal area can be established in terms of the increase in threshold values and the slope of the edges of the defect can be accurately determined and graphically portrayed.

An inspection of the profile of the island of vision along the horizontal meridian [FIG. 65] reveals the peak to be at the fovea. The nasal slope is steeper than the temporal slope and there is a more gradual slope of the field between 5 and 20 degrees from fixation. A second plateau occurs between 30 and 70 degrees on the temporal side, less marked in the nasal part of the visual field. This flattening of the contour is well marked in the vicinity of the blind spot [FIG. 66]. Opacities in the media [FIG. 67], refractive anomalies [FIG. 68] and marked miosis [FIG. 69] all produce a decrease in light sensitivity of the whole island resulting in a flattening of the contour which is more marked in the central than in the peripheral field. It can also be seen that small changes in the over-all differential threshold of the eye produce large changes in the isopter where the slope of the visual island is gradual. This is shown in FIGURE 69 where a small change in threshold produced by miosis caused marked contraction of the isopters which could easily be misinterpreted. Flattening of the visual field contour also occurs as a result of adaptation of the eye to a diminishing background illumination. In the mesopic state where the background illumination is reduced to 0·001 apostilb the contour becomes increasingly flat as the more peripheral rod areas gain in sensitivity and reach the threshold values of the cones [FIG. 70].

In areas in which the slope of the contour of the visual field is less steep, kinetic perimetry involving the use of moving stimuli which are only just above the threshold for that part of the visual field, produces a great inconsistency in responses because the patient has difficulty in distinguishing the stimulus from the background [FIG. 71]. Small scotomata can easily be missed in such areas with moving targets.

STATIC PERIMETRY

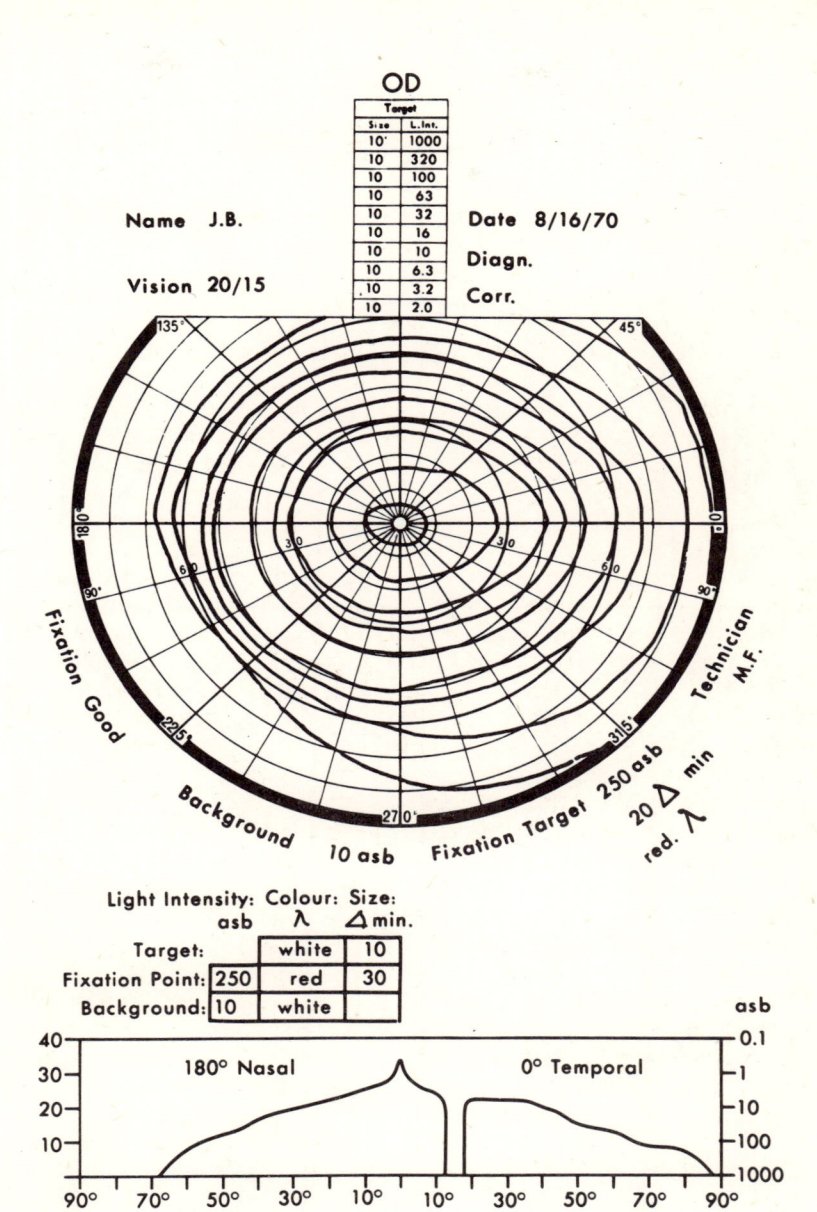

OD

Target	
Size	L. Int.
10'	1000
10	320
10	100
10	63
10	32
10	16
10	10
10	6.3
.10	3.2
10	2.0

Name J.B.
Vision 20/15
Date 8/16/70
Diagn.
Corr.
Technician M.F.
Fixation Good
Background 10 asb
Fixation Target 250 asb
20 △ min red. λ

	Light Intensity: asb	Colour: λ	Size: △ min.
Target:		white	10
Fixation Point:	250	red	30
Background:	10	white	

180° Nasal — 0° Temporal

FIG. 63. Perimetry on a normal subject carried out with multiple stimuli. The profile perimetry along the horizontal meridian shows the various slopes of the 'visual island'. It can be seen that where the slopes are most gradual the isopters are most separated.

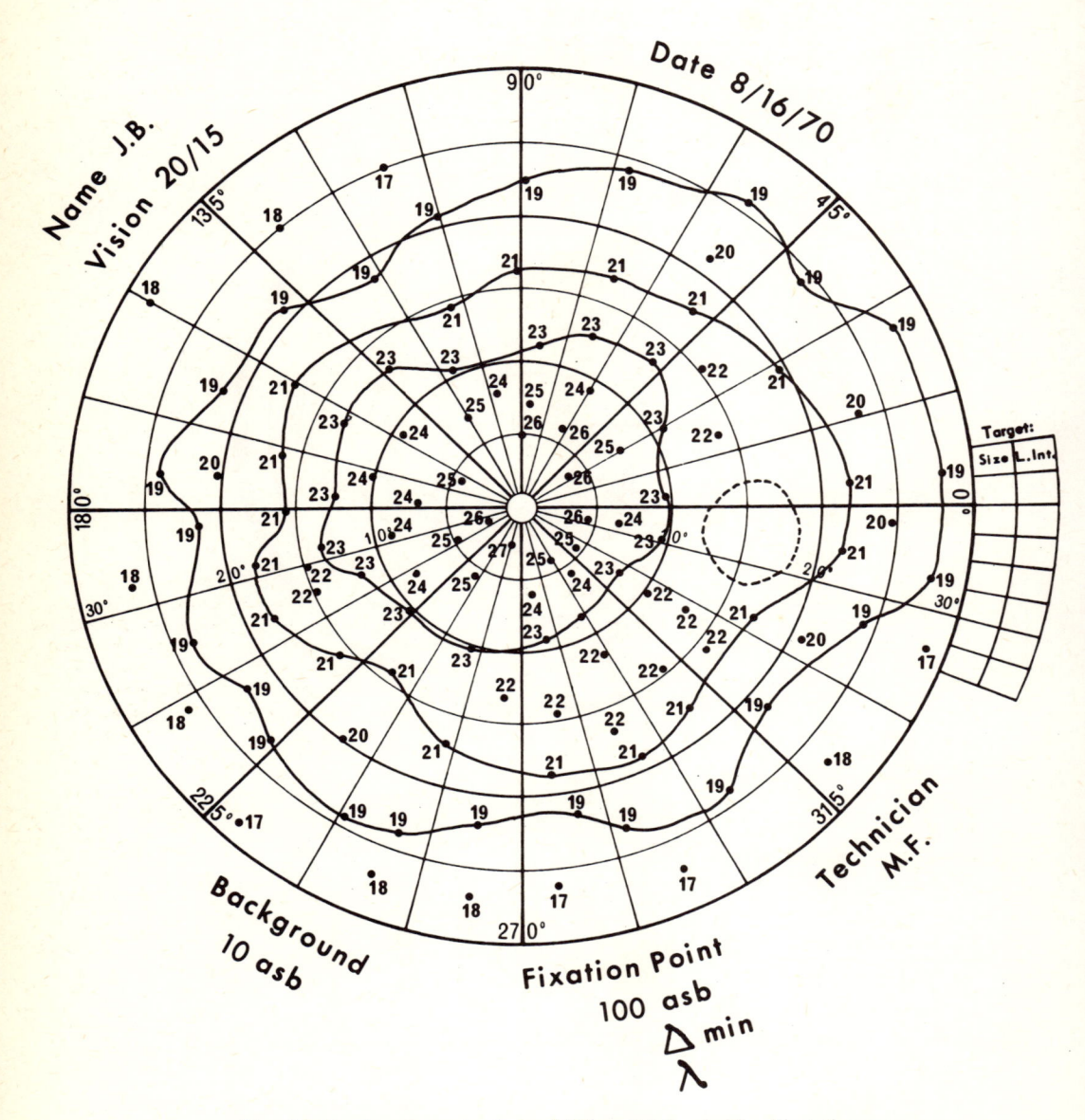

FIG. 64. Random determinations of differential thresholds with stationary targets. Those points having the same thresholds have been joined by lines, thus delineating the isopters.

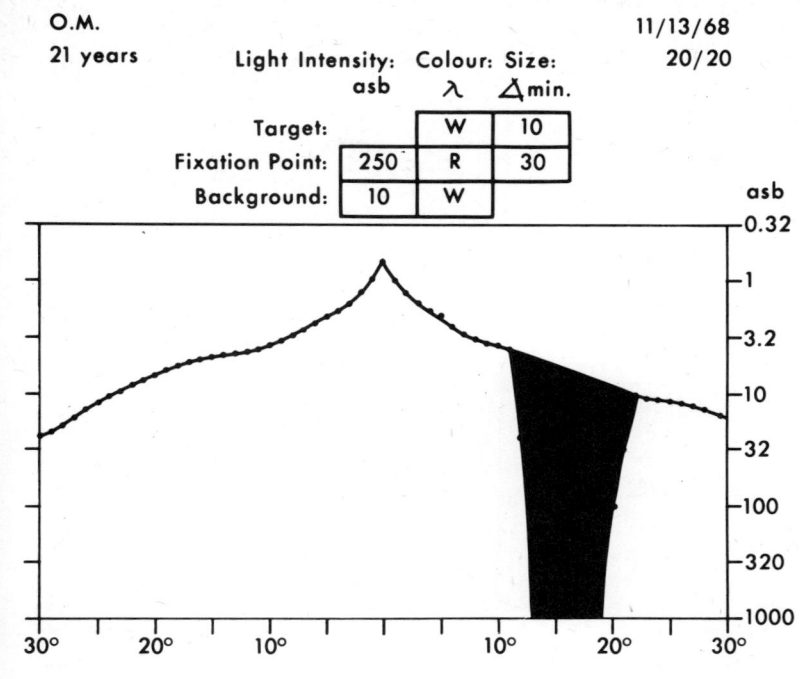

STATIC PERIMETRY

O.M.
21 years

11/13/68
20/20

	Light Intensity: asb	Colour: λ	Size: △ min.
Target:		W	10
Fixation Point:	250	R	30
Background:	10	W	

Pupil: 4 mm.   Fixation: Good   Technician M.F.

FIG. 65. Central profile of the visual island charted along the horizontal meridian. The actual locations along the meridian in which the differential thresholds were tested by non-moving stimuli are indicated with dots. The central portion near the fovea has steep slopes which become more gradual 5–20 degrees from fixation, particularly along the edges of the blind spot.

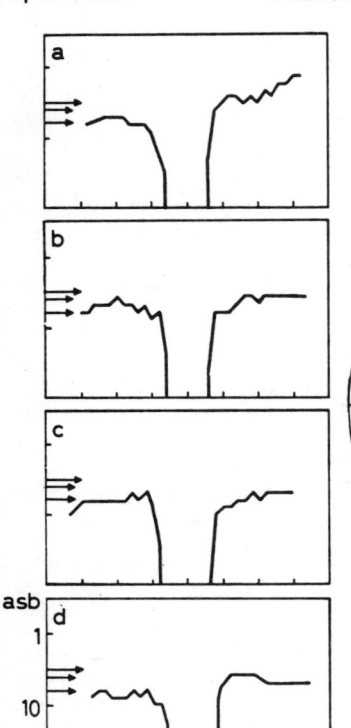

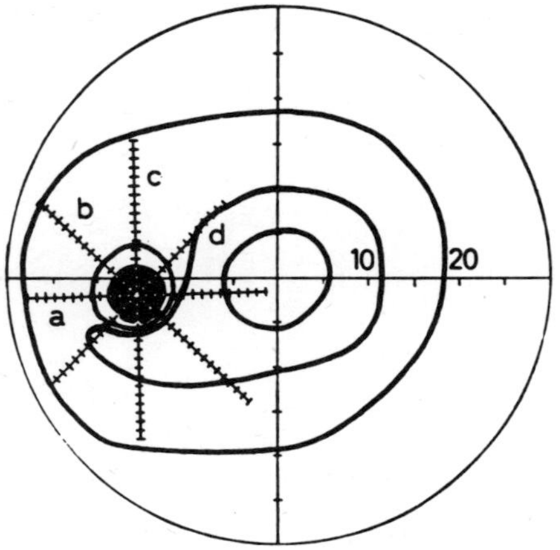

FIG. 66. Static analysis of the contour of the visual field in the areas surrounding the blind spot showing that the blind spot is surrounded by areas of minimal slope. Testing with moving threshold targets becomes difficult and imprecise. (Reproduced by kind permission of E. Aulthorn and H. Harms.)

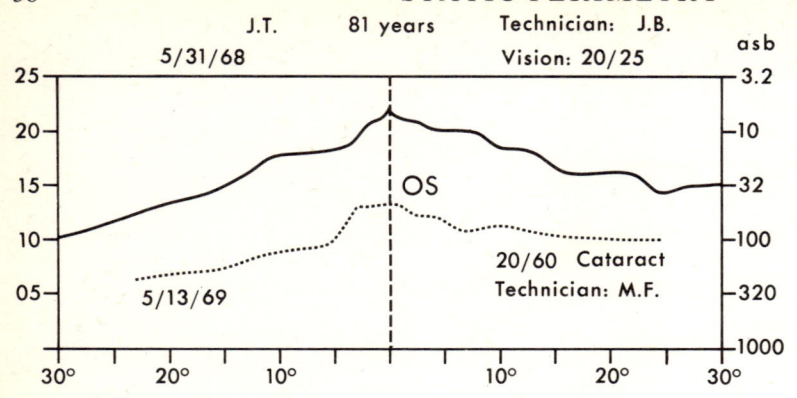

FIG. 67.
Static profile of vertical meridian through fixation in a patient with uniocular cataractous change in the left eye reducing visual acuity from 20/25 to 20/60. The cataract produced a lowered differential threshold with special flattening of the central portion of the profile.

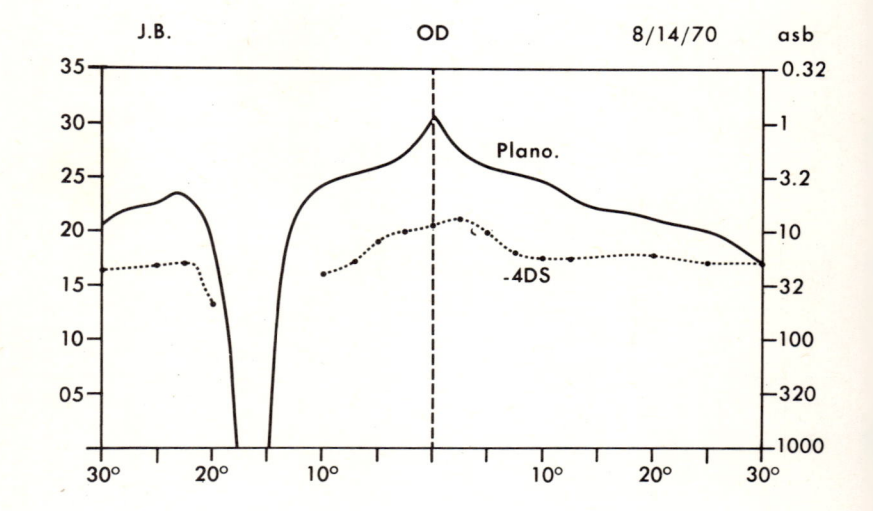

FIG. 68.
Static profiles of horizontal meridian in a young adult showing the effect of a refractive change. The central portions of the visual field are particularly affected.

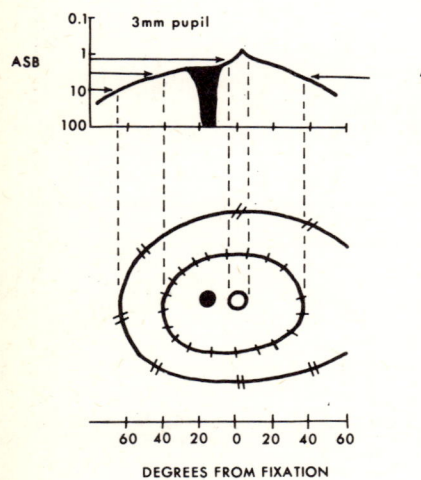

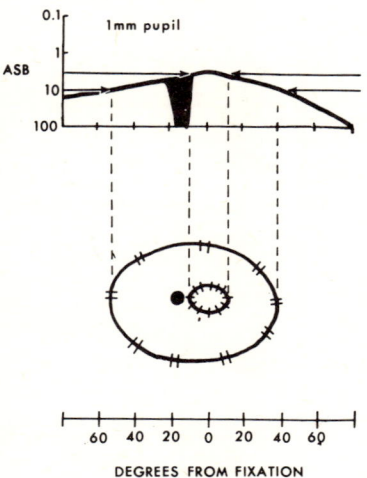

FIG. 69.
Kinetic perimetry carried out with three targets and the corresponding static profile of the horizontal meridian show that when the pupil changed from 3 to 1 mm. in diameter there was only a slight rise in differential threshold (evidenced by a lowering of the profile) yet the isopters showed a very marked change because of the very gradual slope of the areas tested.

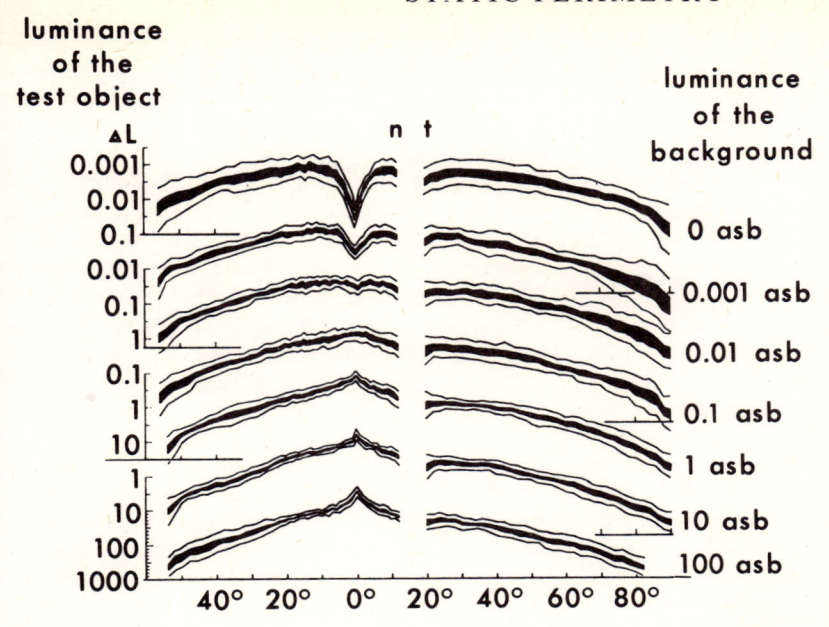

FIG. 70. Profiles of horizontal meridian in ten normal subjects carried out with eight different background illuminations. The lower profiles show the characteristic photopic profiles, the top profile shows the scotopic profile in which the peripheral rod-containing portions of the retina have a lower threshold than the fovea. The mesopic state with background illuminations between 0·1 and 0·01 ASB is characterized by a flattening, indicating equal light sensitivity between fovea and surrounding retina. (Reproduced by kind permission of E. Aulthorn and H. Harms.)

FIG. 71.
The upper profile shows the inconsistency of responses in the flat portion of the contour when tested with moving threshold targets (kinetic perimetry). The patient's responses are indicated by the Xs. A small relative scotoma on the nasal side was missed with the stimuli used. The lower profile shows the contour clearly and demonstrates the relative scotoma when tested with threshold static perimetry.

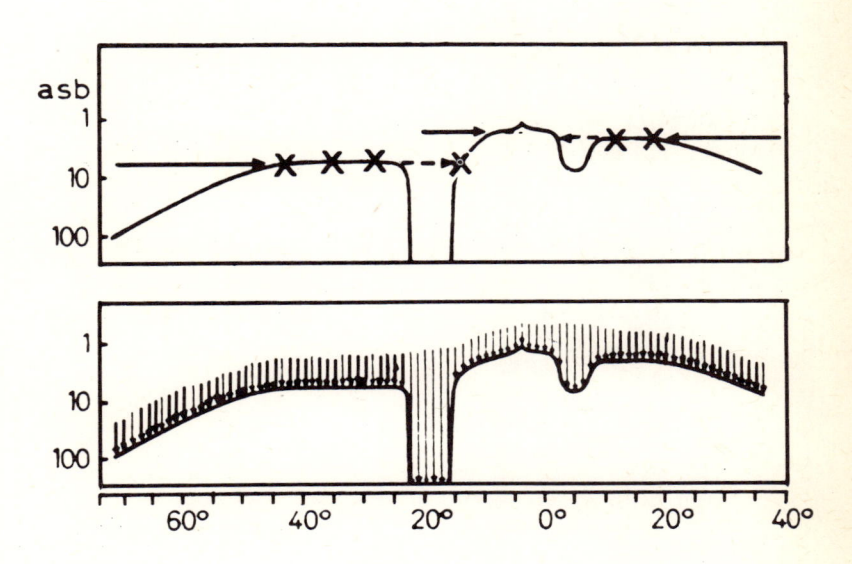

The use of stationary targets obviates some of the difficulties and allows more consistent responses in these areas. The mapping of small scotomata, which are easily overlooked with moving targets, becomes possible. This is particularly important in the areas around the blind spot and when opacities [FIG. 67] produce the flattening of contour in the central visual field which is so often the site of expected visual field changes.

Static perimetry can be carried out on any perimeter fitted with a system of filters which allows small step-like changes in the illumination of the stimulus. After the blind spot has been mapped with kinetic targets to ascertain reliability of fixation a meridian is selected for testing. It has been shown that a small projected stimulus subtending 5–10 minutes of arc, with a photopic background of 10–15 apostilb produces optimal results. The threshold at 1–2 degree intervals along the meridian is established by using one-second flashes of sub-threshold intensity increasing them in steps of 0·1 log unit until the patient indicates that he has seen the stimulus. A few areas must be tested repeatedly in order to ascertain the scatter of responses for the individual tested. Once the profile of the meridian has been plotted one can examine any other parts of the visual field with stimuli which have been established by the profile to be above the threshold for the area to be examined.

Static perimetry is time consuming but yields reliable and reproducible information. Patient acceptance is good and patients are often less tired than after an equivalent lengthy kinetic examination because they know which area is being tested instead of having to concentrate on the entire visual field. Fixation is as important as in kinetic perimetry and, as the test is a subjective one, patient co-operation is as important as in other psychovisual tests.

Static perimetry is of greatest use in glaucoma [see Chapter 9] but is also of value particularly as a research tool in studying many other conditions such as centroserous retinopathy, toxic amblyopia, and small paracentral scotomata caused by lesions of the postgeniculate pathway.

REFERENCE

AULHORN, E., and HARMS, H. (1967) Early visual field defects in glaucoma, in *Glaucoma Tutzing Symposium*, ed. Leydhecker, Basel.

8
TYPES OF FIELD DEFECTS

Field defects should be considered in four main groups, depending upon the anatomical site of the lesion in the visual pathway. The defects in each group show special characteristic features. These four basic patterns should be constantly borne in mind when examining a patient. They are:

1. Retinal lesions.
2. Retrobulbar lesions.
3. Chiasmal lesions.
4. Retrochiasmal lesions.

RETINAL LESIONS
Retinal lesions cause field defects which have the following characteristics:
1. They may correspond to the course of the retinal nerve fibres or to the area of supply of the retinal blood vessels.
2. They may cross the physiological vertical midline through the fovea.

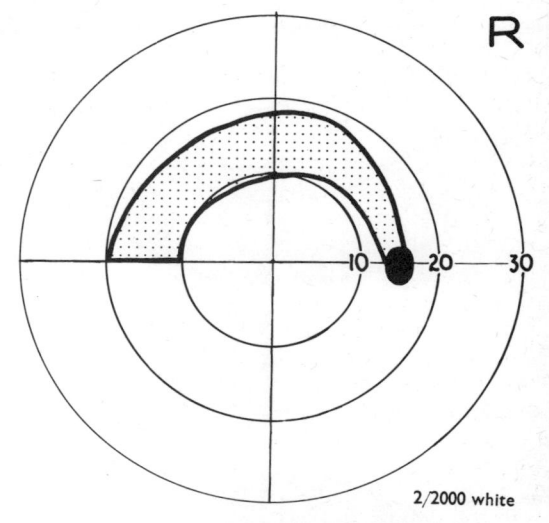

FIG. 73. The arcuate defect which is characteristic of glaucoma.

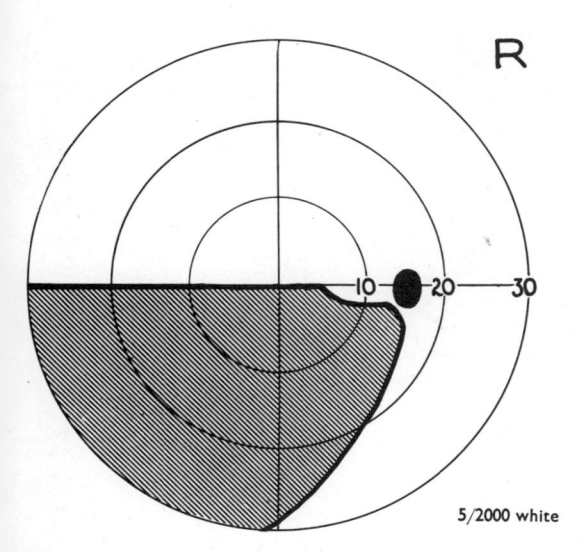

FIG. 72. Field defect in occlusion of the right superior temporal artery.

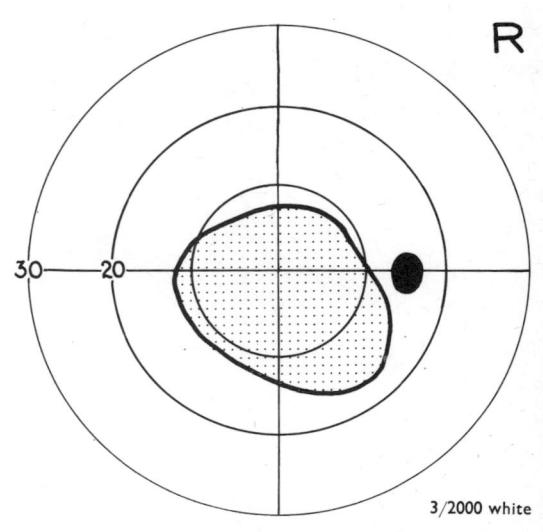

FIG. 74. A central scotoma due to retrobulbar neuritis.

61

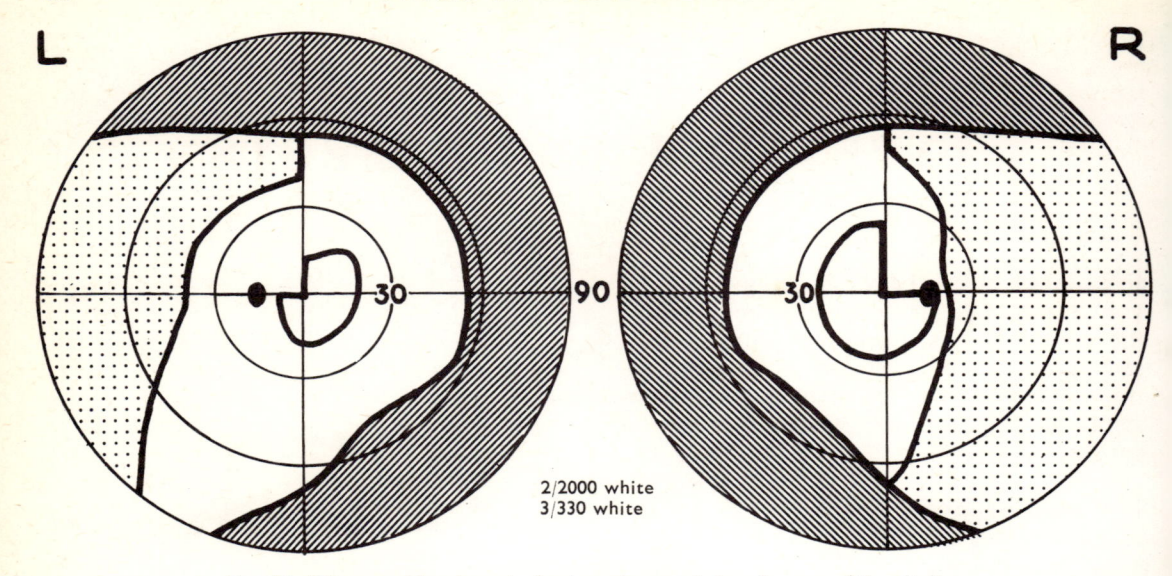

FIG. 75. Bitemporal hemianopia due to a chromophobe adenoma of the pituitary.

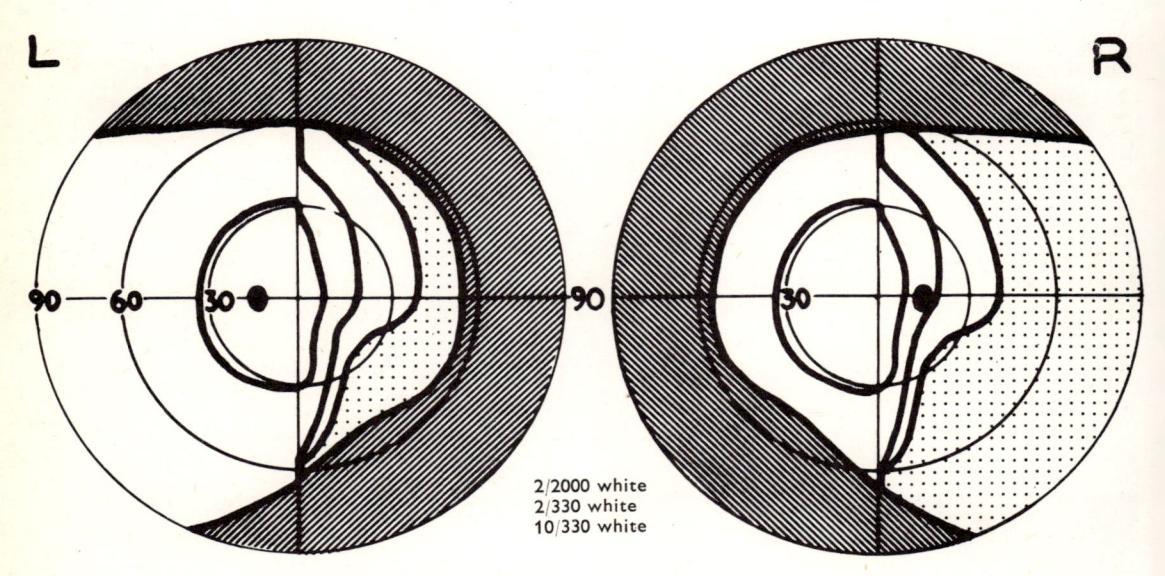

2/2000 white
3/330 white

FIG. 76. Right congruous homonymous hemianopia caused by a glioma of the left occipital region.

2/2000 white
2/330 white
10/330 white

RETINAL LESIONS 63

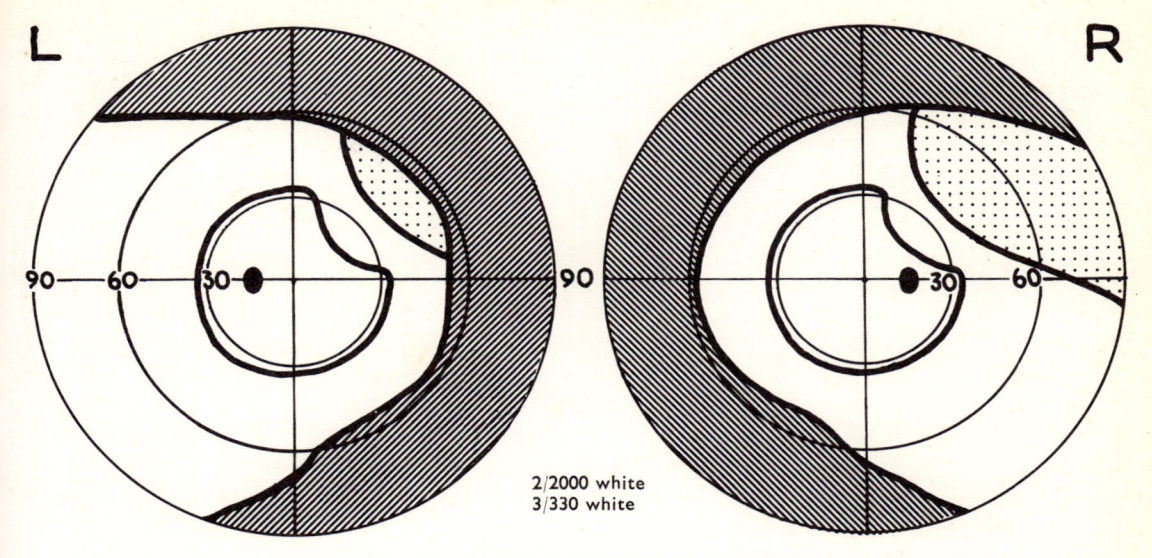

2/2000 white
3/330 white

FIG. 77. Right upper congruous homonymous quadrantopia due to a tumour involving the lower radiation fibres in the left temporal lobe.

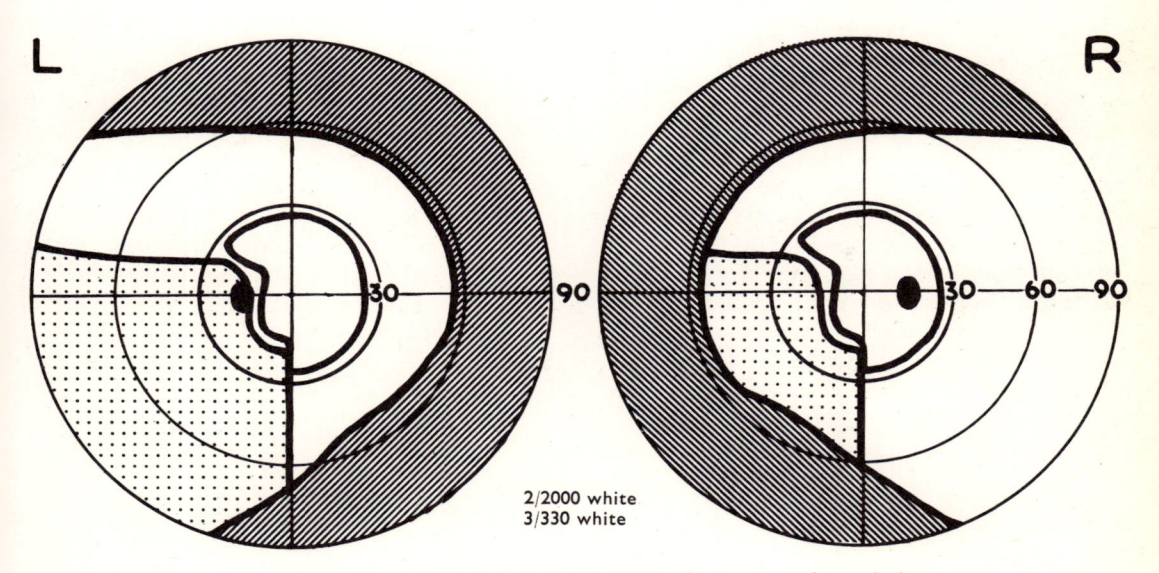

2/2000 white
3/330 white

FIG. 78. Left lower homonymous quadrantopia due to a vascular occlusion.

3. They correspond to inflammatory or degenerative lesions seen with the ophthalmoscope.

These features may be illustrated by occlusion of the superior temporal artery when the field loss corresponds to the area supplied by the artery and crosses the physiological midline [FIG. 72]. Arcuate defects which commonly occur in glaucoma conform to the course of the retinal nerve fibres and also cross the midline [FIG. 73]. It should be borne in mind that arcuate scotomata may occur in many other conditions [see p. 66].

RETROBULBAR LESIONS

Retrobulbar lesions, whether due to inflammation or compression, usually give rise to central scotomata [FIG. 74]. It is important to note that the scotoma in these cases typically occupies both sides of the physiological midline. If a field defect is limited to one eye, the site of the lesion must obviously be anterior to the chiasma. The only exception to this rule is the rare lesion in which the uniocular portion of the binocular field is affected [p. 155].

CHIASMAL LESIONS

Chiasmal lesions give rise to bitemporal defects or heteronymous hemianopia, but they are seldom symmetrical. The field loss is usually more advanced in one eye than the other. If the pressure upon the chiasma is in the midline from below, then the defect begins in the upper temporal quadrant, progresses to the lower temporal quadrant, and thence to the inferior nasal quadrant. If the pressure is from above, the field is lost in the following order: the lower temporal quadrant, the upper temporal quadrant, and finally the lower nasal quadrant. In each case the upper nasal quadrant is the last to be lost. The chiasma is more commonly compressed from below than from above. The most frequent cause is a chromophobe adenoma of the pituitary [FIG. 75].

LESIONS BEHIND THE CHIASMA

Damage to the optic tract, the optic radiation, or to the visual cortex, will produce homonymous hemianopia. Lesions occur less frequently in the optic tract than in the optic radiation or cortex. When the lesion is behind the lateral geniculate body the field defects usually show two characteristic features, namely: (1) congruity; (2) macular sparing.
1. Congruity means that the edge of the defect is identical in shape in both eyes [FIG. 76]. Incongruity, in which the defects are not identical, suggests a tract lesion.
2. Macular sparing is the term given to a field defect in which the central area is intact for about 5 degrees around the fixation point.

In temporal lobe tumours, the inferior bundle of optic radiation fibres which end below the calcarine fissure is often damaged. This causes a superior homonymous quadrantopia of the opposite field [FIG. 77].

Vascular lesions of the optic radiations often occur. The superior bundle of nerve fibres in the optic radiation is particularly prone to be damaged. This causes inferior homonymous quadrantopia with macular sparing [FIG. 78].

PART III

FIELD DEFECTS AND THEIR INTERPRETATION

9
GLAUCOMA

One of the main areas of applied perimetry lies in the detection of the field defects of chronic simple glaucoma and the accurate charting of their progression. In angle closure glaucoma, disturbances in vision and the visual field do, of course, occur but are overshadowed by the more dramatic events in the eye. Examination of the visual field therefore forms an unimportant part of the evaluation of the acute attack but may be of significance in the follow-up to assess damage to the posterior segment of the eye resulting from the very high intraocular pressure.

CHRONIC SIMPLE GLAUCOMA

The characteristic visual field defects in chronic simple glaucoma occur as a result of damage to individual bundles of nerve fibres at the optic nerve head. Chronic simple glaucoma is the most frequent cause, but not the only cause, of nerve fibre bundle defects. The other causes of nerve fibre bundle defects have been listed by Harrington.

Lesions at the Optic Disc
1. Juxtapapillary choroiditis
2. Myopia with peripapillary atrophy
3. Colobomata and pits of the optic nerve
4. Drusen on the optic nerve
5. Papilloedema with increased intracranial pressure
6. Optic atrophy secondary to papilloedema
7. Papillitis
8. Retinal arterial plaque on the disc
9. Papilloedema in malignant hypertension
10. Occlusion of central retinal artery

Lesions in the Anterior Part of the Optic Nerve
1. Ischaemic infarct and segmental atrophy in the optic nerve due to arterial occlusion
2. Carotid and ophthalmic artery occlusion
3. Cerebral arteritis
4. Retrobulbar neuritis
5. Electric shock
6. Exophthalmos

Lesions in the Posterior Part of the Optic Nerve and Chiasma
1. Meningioma at the optic foramen
2. Meningioma of dorsum sellae
3. Pituitary adenoma
4. Opticochiasmatic arachnoiditis

Perimetric techniques for work in glaucoma must be so designed as to:
1. Delineate the earliest characteristic nerve fibre bundle defects which would indicate glaucomatous damage.
2. Plot the size and density of the scotomata so that any change can be recorded accurately and reproducibly.

Experiments with acute and chronic artificially elevated intraocular pressures have shown that generalized changes in retinal sensitivity occur and may lead to a contraction of the isopter, baring of the blind spot and even depression localized to the Bjerrum region. Similar changes occur as a result of ageing, miosis, particularly in the presence of lens opacities, and uncorrected refractive errors.

THE SIGNIFICANCE OF BARING OF THE BLIND SPOT

Baring of the blind spot [FIG. 79] denotes a difference in retinal sensitivity above and below the optic disc. In most normal individuals

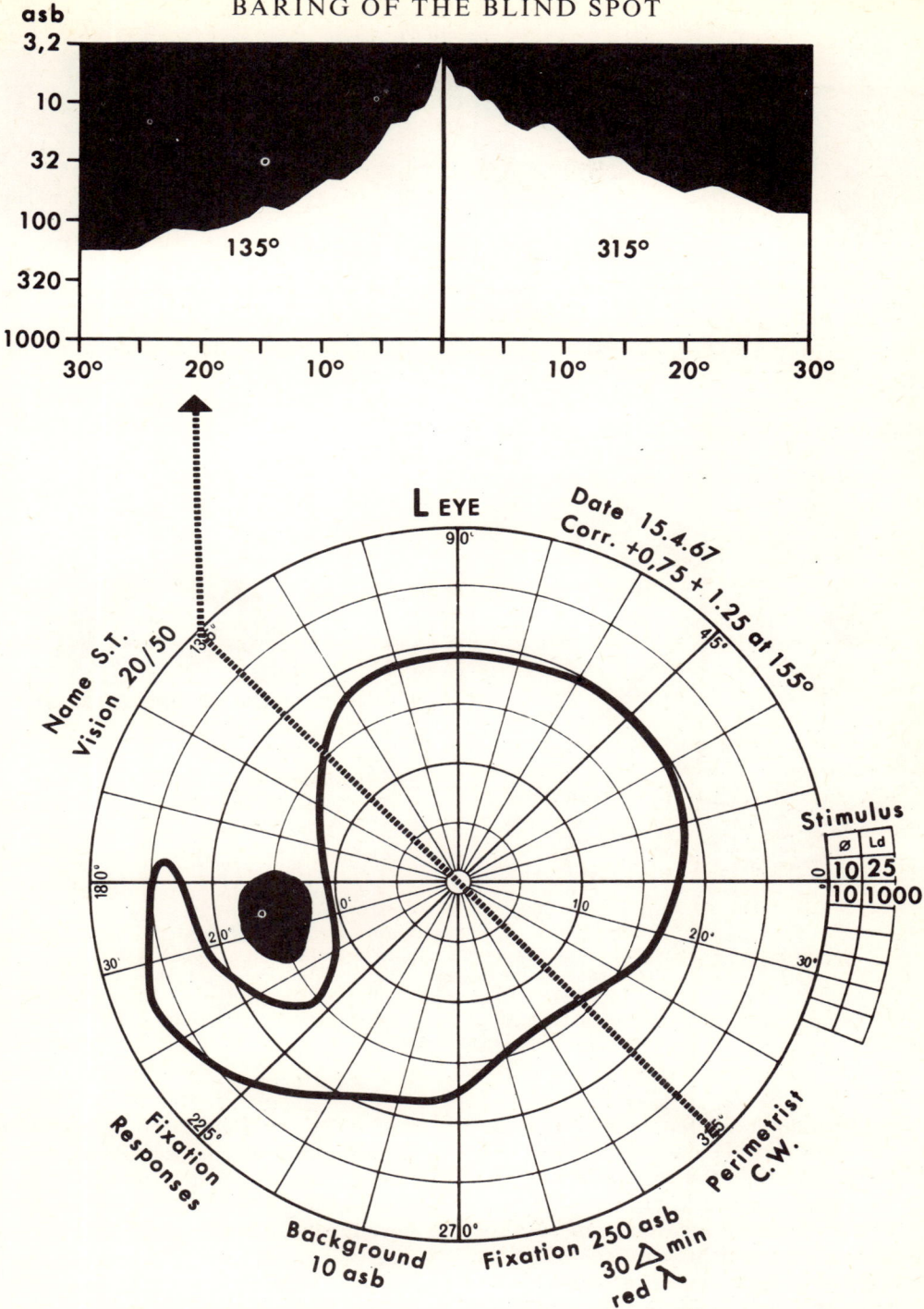

FIG. 79. Upper baring of the blind spot in a patient with a slight lens opacity but no evidence of glaucoma. The profile perimetry 135–315 degrees shows a slightly lowered sensitivity to light in the upper temporal part of the visual field but no evidence of a nerve fibre bundle defect.

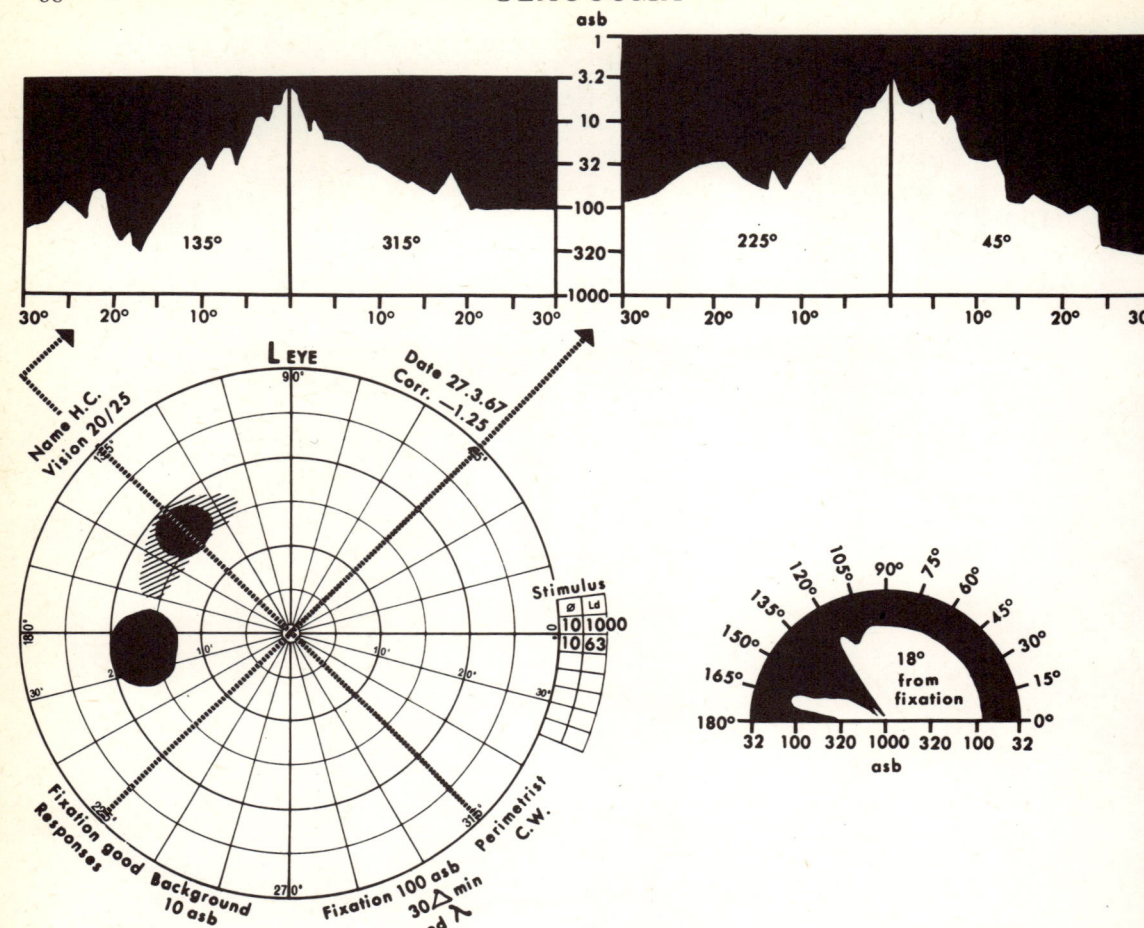

FIG. 80. A dense relative paracentral scotoma in the Bjerrum region above the blind spot. The scotoma is surrounded by a less dense scotomatous area and is separated from the blind spot. This is demonstrated more clearly by circular static perimetry. In this the threshold levels were measured in the upper half of the visual field on an arc 18 degrees from fixation, graphically shown in the lower right diagram.

there is a very slight difference, the portion below the optic disc being very slightly less sensitive to light than the corresponding area above. By using a stimulus of threshold value for the more sensitive area one can bare the blind spot in the less light sensitive area of the visual field. The selection of threshold targets can therefore produce baring in almost all normal individuals. An arcuate scotoma also produces baring of the blind spot and is, of course, a very significant finding. The finding of baring of the blind spot to small stimuli, while it may be significant, is usually not an indication or a precursor of an arcuate defect. It must be remembered that in the presence of miosis, ageing of the lens, etc. targets which are above the threshold in the normal eye may become threshold level at a later stage for the same eye. Many of the glaucoma patients and suspects belong to the age group where lens changes are common and the addition of the iatrogenic small pupil may lead to baring of the blind spot even to larger stimuli. It is essential to view baring of the blind spot with

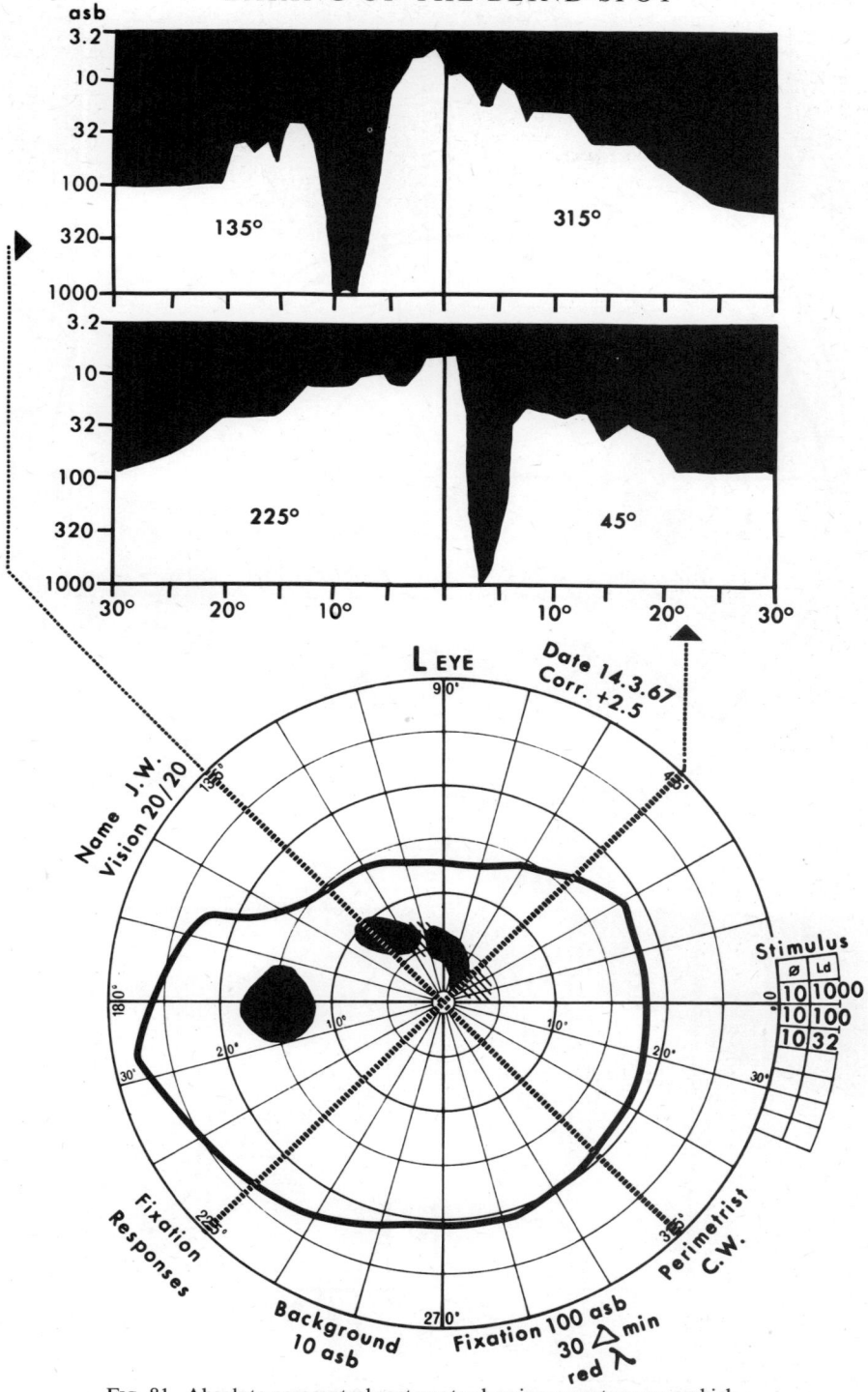

FIG. 81. Absolute paracentral scotomata showing arcuate course which arches over fixation but encroaches on the area 3 degrees from fixation on the nasal side. The absolute nuclei are surrounded by a zone of relative disturbance but the scotoma does not join the blind spot.

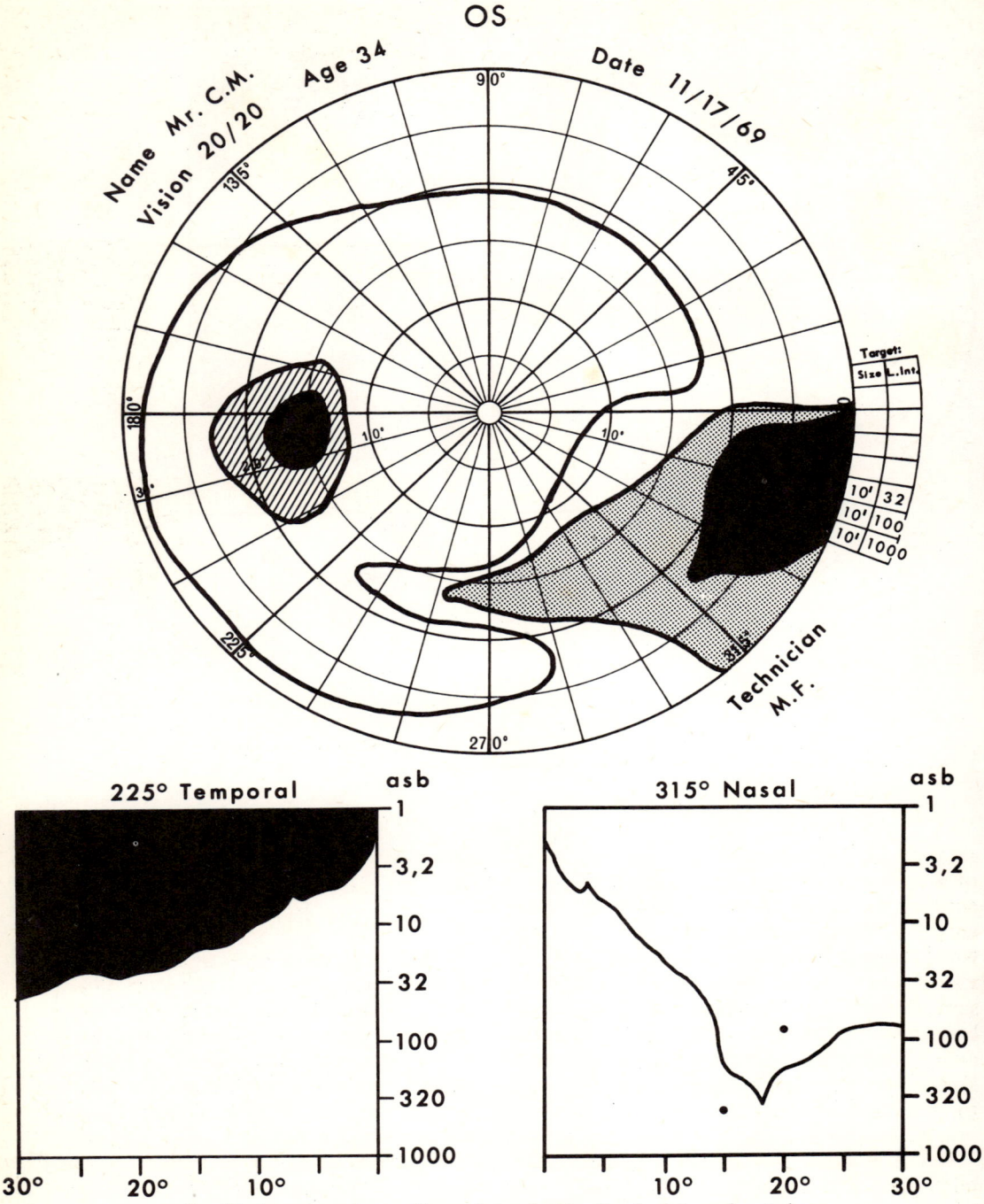

Fig. 82. Arcuate scotoma with nasal step showing the absolute nucleus to be 20 to 30 degrees from fixation. The arcuate nature can be seen from the shape of the scotoma. The 315 degree profile shows a deep relative defect extending from 14 to 22 degrees. The 225 degree profile shows no scotoma which indicates that the scotoma does not join the blind spot.

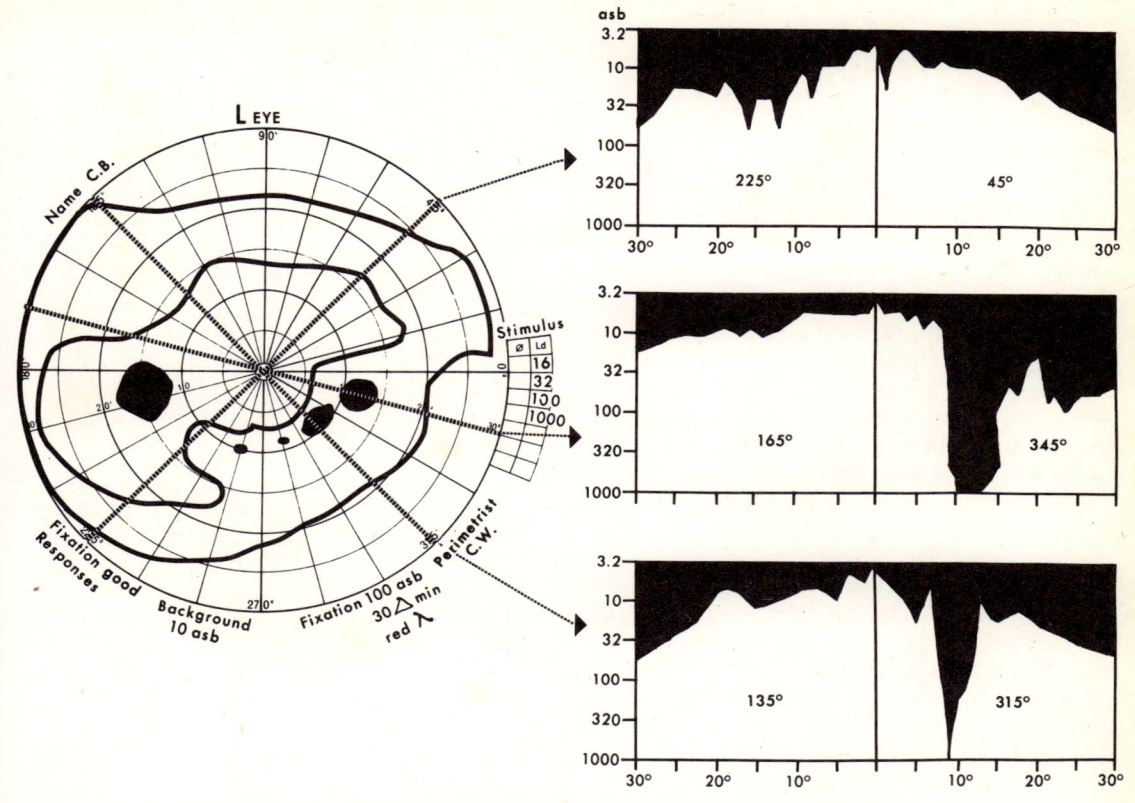

FIG. 83. Multiple absolute scotomata in the inferior Bjerrum area. In the 225 degree profile (upper left) a relative disturbance is shown, indicating that the scotoma does not appear to join the blind spot. A nasal step is evident.

extreme caution before considering it as a sign of progression of the disease and to take into account the age and visual acuity of the individual. A baring of the blind spot to a 3/1000 white target in a 30-year-old patient with 20/15 vision is likely to be due to pathology, but the same finding in a 65 year old with 20/40 vision has quite a different significance. Careful analysis of baring of blind spots by quantitative kinetic perimetry or static perimetry is required to demonstrate the presence of nerve fibre involvement [FIG. 79].

Relative sector-like scotomata joining the blind spot and running up and nasally but usually not to the nasal horizontal meridian may be due to refraction defects. These occur particularly in myopic individuals in whom the lower part of the fundus has an unusually pale appearance [see p. 164]. The placing of additional concave lenses before the eye abolishes the scotoma.

NERVE FIBRE BUNDLE DEFECTS

All sector-shaped defects of the visual field are nerve fibre bundle defects but in chronic simple glaucoma it is the superior and inferior pole of the optic nerve head, and particularly the superotemporal and inferotemporal parts, which seem to be most vulnerable to damage. The nerve fibre bundle defects involve the arcuate fibres which arch above and below the fovea to end along the horizontal raphe which is situated temporally to the fovea. In the visual field, therefore, it is represented by the horizontal meridian extending nasally from fixation to the periphery of the field. The size, shape and location of the nerve fibre bundle scotoma will depend on the extent and site of the dam-

age to nerve fibre bundles at the optic nerve head. Nerve fibre bundle defects may produce three types of perimetric findings:
1. Circumscribed paracentral defects in the distribution of the arcuate fibres.
2. Nasal steps.
3. Classical arcuate scotomata.

CIRCUMSCRIBED PARACENTRAL DEFECTS

Circumscribed paracentral defects can occur either in the temporal or in the nasal part of the Bjerrum area. They tend to be elongated circumferentially along the course of the nerve fibres. On the temporal side of the central field they occur in the classical Bjerrum region between 10 and 20 degrees from fixation in areas which constitute an upward or downward arcuate projection from the appropriate pole of the blind spot [FIG. 80]. Their location on the nasal side is very different. The scotomata can come to within 2 degrees of fixation [FIG. 81] or alternatively lie up to 30 and even 40 degrees away from fixation [FIG. 82]. The defects are often absolute when first discovered, or show deep, relative nuclei surrounded by areas of less dense involvement. The dense nuclei are often multiple along the course of a nerve fibre bundle [FIG. 83]. The width of the scotoma can vary from 2 to 10 degrees on the nasal side but it is always much narrower on the temporal side. The nasal horizontal meridian often limits a nasal scotoma [FIGS. 82, 84 and 85]. A relative disturbance can often be traced to a varying extent towards the blind spot indicating its arcuate nature [FIG. 82].

NASAL STEPS

All complete arcuate scotomata go round to the nasal horizontal meridian producing a nasal step [FIGS. 84 and 85]. By means of static perimetry absolute or deep relative scotomata can be plotted along the course of the nerve fibre bundles which terminate at the horizontal nasal meridian corresponding to the nasal step [FIG. 86]. The shape of the nasal step and its width depend on many factors. In the periphery of the visual field it is often wedge shaped [FIG. 87]. In the mid-periphery it tends to be closer to a right angle [FIG. 88]. Nearer to fixation the nasal step assumes the characteristics of an obtuse angle consistent with the shape of the nerve fibre bundles reaching the horizontal nasal meridian at that point [FIGS. 87 and 88]. A nasal step, when present, may be evident in some isopters but not in others, depending on the nerve fibre bundles damaged [FIG. 88]. The width of the nasal step, in degrees, is also variable and no arbitrary rule which assigns significance to a particular size of nasal step is strictly accurate. Nasal steps of some isopters are very frequently found in association with arcuate or paracentral scotomata. Only rarely (1·6 per cent) is a nasal step found as the only field defect of glaucoma, i.e.

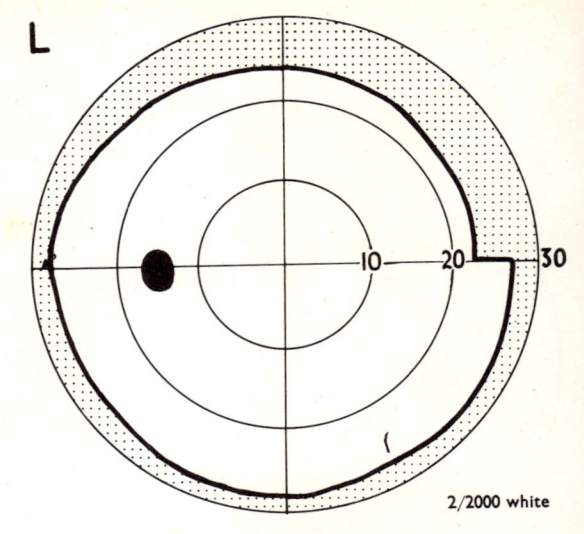

FIG. 84. Nasal step in glaucoma.

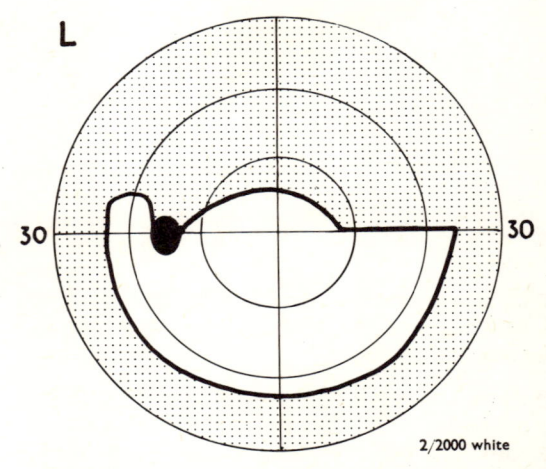

FIG. 85. A combination of extensive arcuate defect and a nasal step.

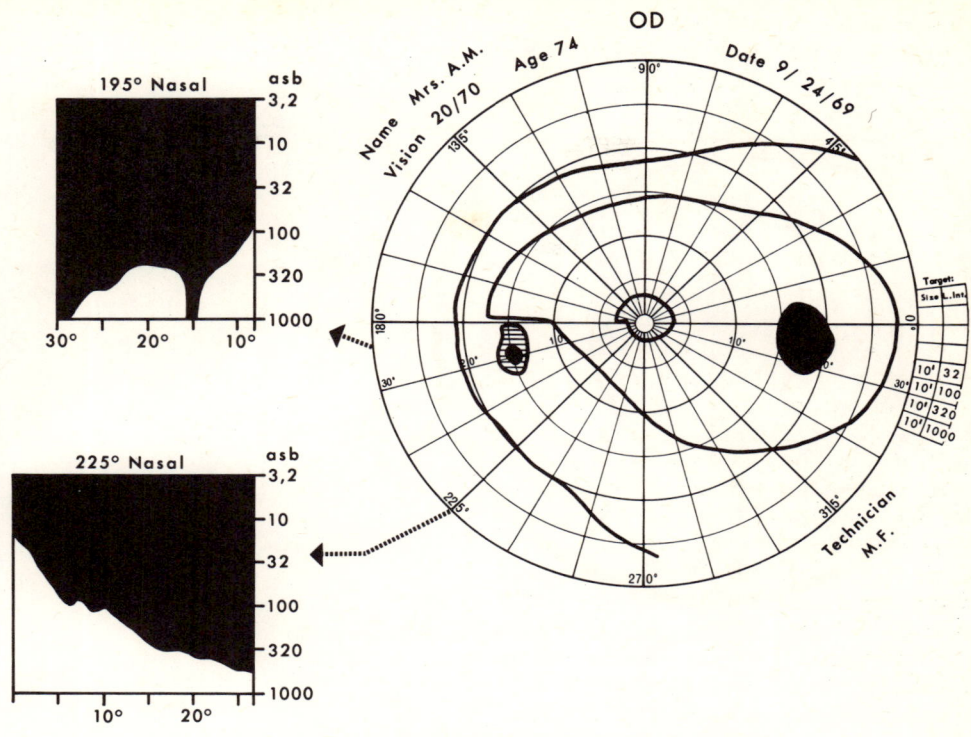

FIG. 86. Absolute paracentral scotoma producing a nasal step which is not present in the more peripheral isopters but is reflected in a more central isopter.

without paracentral or arcuate scotomata. It is a very useful corroborative sign when other defects are doubtful.

ARCUATE SCOTOMA

An arcuate scotoma may be relative or absolute. In the temporal portion of the field it is narrower because all nerve fibre bundles converge onto the blind spot. It spreads out towards the nasal side and may come to within a degree or two of fixation on the nasal horizontal meridian and be very wide along this meridian [FIGS. 89 and 90]. It is often accompanied by separate absolute nuclei, situated along the nasal horizontal meridian peripheral to the arcuate scotoma. These cause nasal steps in the peripheral isopters [FIG. 90]. The arcuate scotoma with its sharp nasal horizontal border often goes all the way to the blind spot [FIG. 90]. It may be separated from the blind spot by an area of normal function [FIGS. 82 and 91], or alternatively it joins the blind spot

through an area of relative impairment. The fact that these scotomata do not necessarily join the blind spot, and if they do, are rarely densest near the blind spot, suggests that they do not usually arise from the blind spot. Arcuate scotomata above and below usually show a nasal horizontal step between them and when complete take the form of a ring scotoma [FIG. 92]. Rarely arcuate scotomata cease abruptly at the vertical meridian but any cut-off along the vertical meridian should be treated with suspicion and a chiasmal lesion should be suspected [FIG. 93].

PROCEDURE FOR DETECTION OF EARLY DEFECTS

With the knowledge of the early characteristic field changes of chronic simple glaucoma one can design a testing procedure for the detection of the early visual field defects of this condition. Armaly has suggested the following test routine [FIG. 94]:

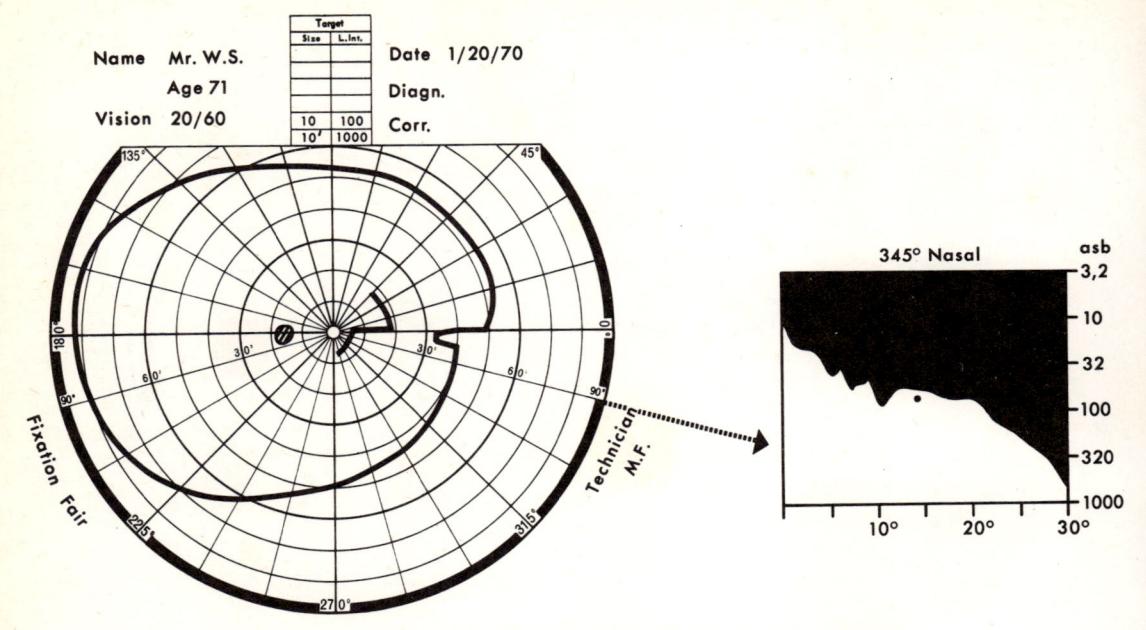

FIG. 87. Relative scotoma shown in the 345 degree profile 10 degrees from fixation, reflecting a nasal step in the corresponding area. There is separate involvement of nerve fibres 30 degrees from fixation, evidenced by a wedge-shaped scotoma producing a nasal step.

1. An accurate plotting of the blind spot.
2. Examination for a nasal step.
3. A thorough search of the circumferential areas 5, 10 and 15 degrees from fixation with small targets for the presence of paracentral defects.

Such testing on the tangent screen or on the Goldmann perimeter will find the great majority of early glaucomatous visual field defects which then have to be subjected to a careful analysis of extent and depth. This forms a baseline from which the progression, arrest or unusual improvement of field defects may be judged.

PATHOGENESIS OF FIELD DEFECTS

The nerve fibre bundle defects found in glaucoma occur as a result of interference with the blood supply at the optic nerve head. It would appear that the blood supply to the nerve head comes predominantly from the posterior ciliary arteries, through the circle of Zinn and through the peripapillary choroid. Fluorescein angiography has shown that the choroidal supply is more segmented than was assumed. The perfusion of the nerve head will depend on the balance between the intraocular pressure and the intravascular pressure in the small vessels of the choroid and on the state of the arterioles supplying this area. Artificial rises in intraocular pressure have more effect on the choroidal and particularly the peripapillary choroidal circulation than on the retinal vessels. A chronic interference with the perfusion of the papilla probably leads to the disc changes seen in chronic simple glaucoma with enlargement of the optic cup at the expense of the neuroretinal rim and the atrophy which accompanies the field loss. More acute interference with the circulation leads to ischaemic optic neuropathy with small haemorrhages on the optic disc with loss of nerve fibre bundles but without the increase in the size of the optic cup [FIG. 95, PLATE 1A, and FIG. 96]. Such interference may be due to emboli, arteritis, shock, arteriosclerosis, severe anaemia from blood loss and probably other events. It is likely that such minor acute episodes are superimposed on the chronic perfusion changes of the nerve. In some patients one can trace multiple causes all leading

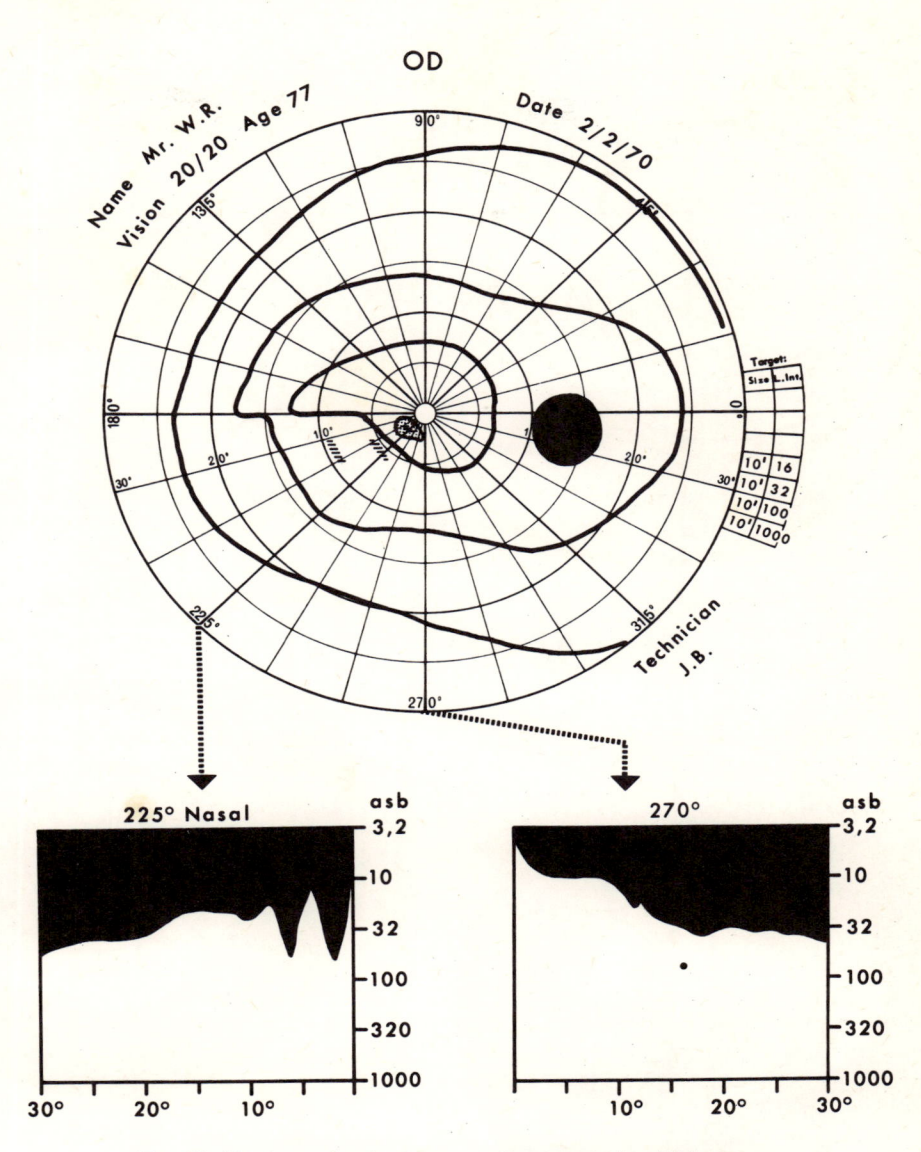

FIG. 88. Nasal step showing paracentral scotomata 4 and 8 degrees from fixation. The scotomata do not extend to the vertical meridian 270 degrees. The peripheral isopter is not involved.

GLAUCOMA

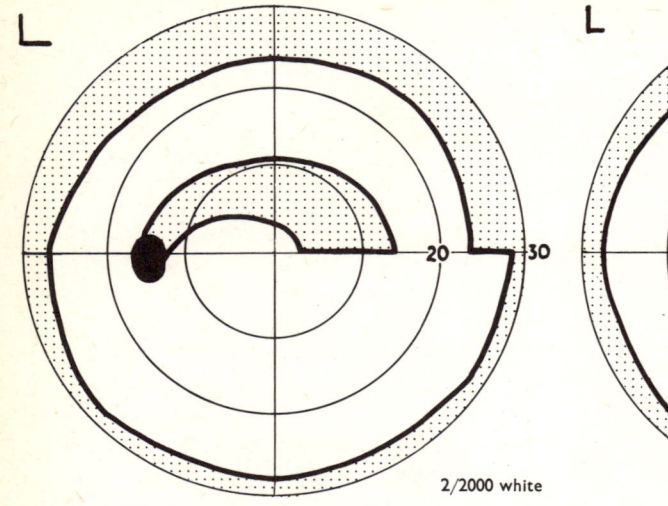

FIG. 89. Arcuate scotoma.

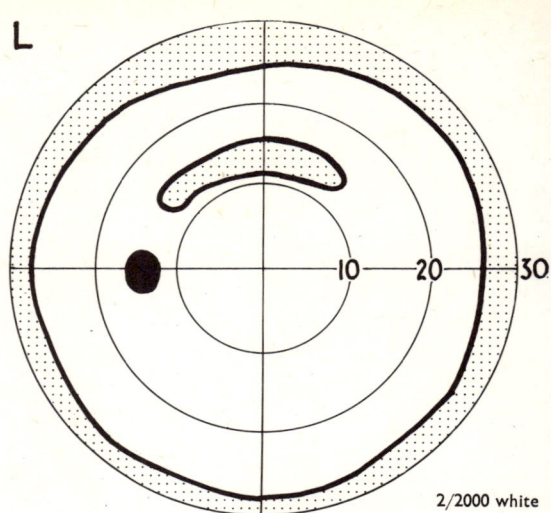

FIG. 91. Relative paracentral scotoma not joining the blind spot but showing arcuate course.

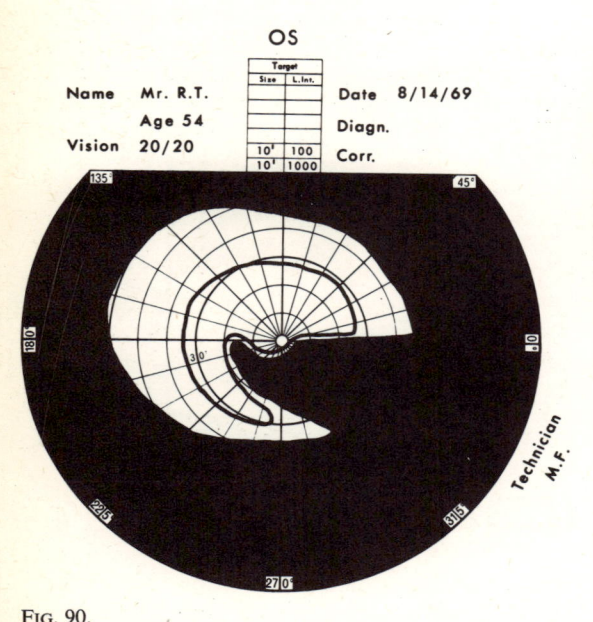

FIG. 90.
The right eye shows a nerve fibre bundle arcuate scotoma joining the blind spot. The scotoma is narrow on the temporal side but widens nasally coming to 2 degrees from fixation. There is additional evidence of involvement of more peripheral arcuate bundles shown by the wedge-shaped scotoma with nasal step in the peripheral field. The left eye shows an absolute arcuate defect 'breaking through' to the periphery.

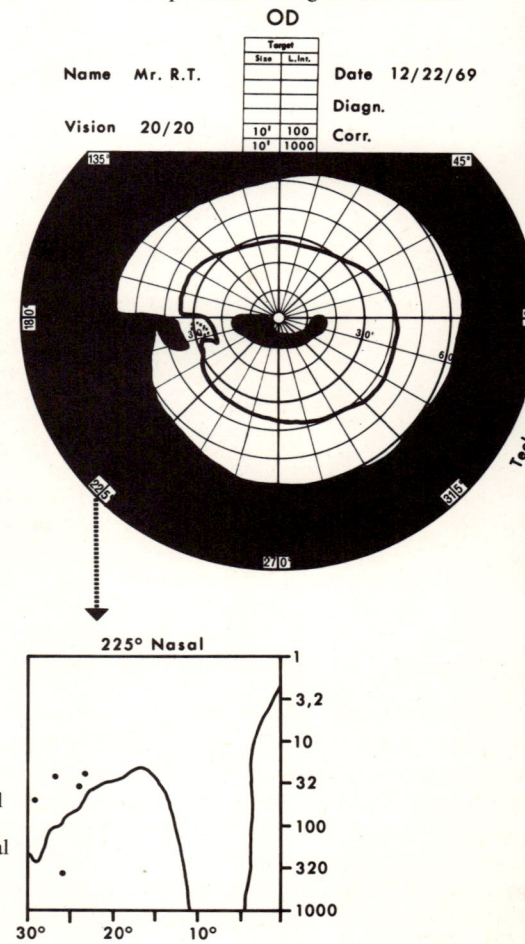

PROCEDURE FOR DETECTION OF EARLY DEFECTS

FIG. 92. A developing ring scotoma.

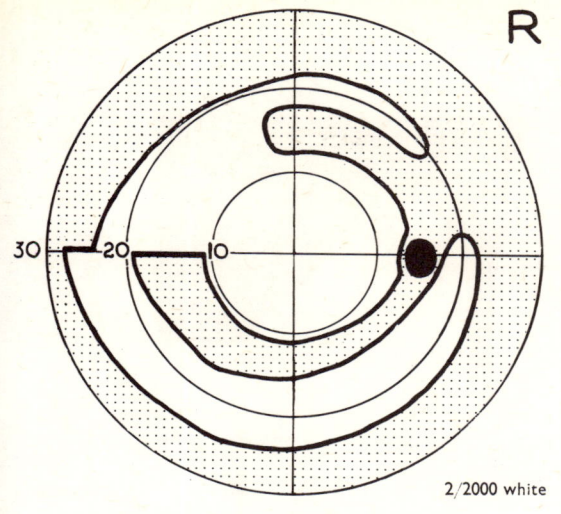

FIG. 94. Armaly's method of screening for glaucoma.

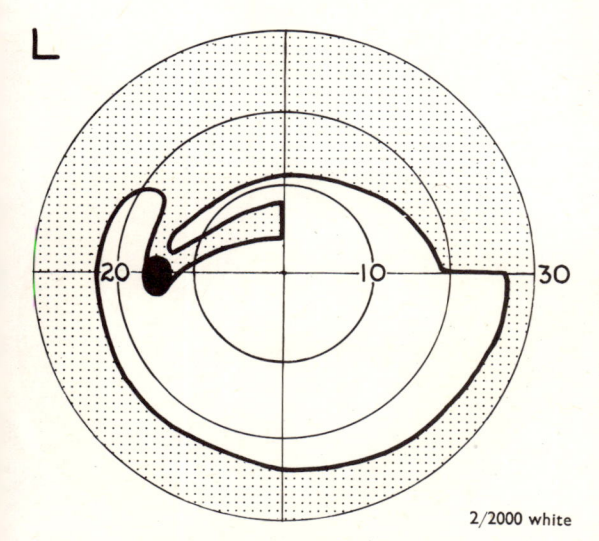

FIG. 93. A scotoma ending at the physiological midline presumably due to damage to the nasal retinal fibres which arise from ganglion cells between the optic disc and the fovea.

to progression of the defects of the visual field.

PROGRESS OF VISUAL FIELD CHANGES

There are probably two ways in which a visual field defect progresses in chronic simple glaucoma. The first is a sudden step-like occurrence of fresh visual field defects of the nerve fibre bundle type. These are most likely to occur in proximity to previous defects because the affected part of the optic nerve head is poorly perfused and vulnerable to further changes. Progression of this kind could therefore produce fresh absolute or deep relative nuclei in the course of the same nerve fibre bundle, which would gradually convert the isolated paracentral scotomata into the classical arcuate scotoma [FIGS. 97, 98, 99, 100 and 101]. Secondly, if damage occurs to adjacent bundles a gradual increase in width of the original visual field defects in a peripheral direction can lead to the 'breaking through' of the scotoma to the periphery [FIG. 90].

Scotomata can occur independently of the original signs of damage in other parts of the field [FIG. 101]. Such fresh visual deficits may occur in the other half of the visual field, gradually leading to an upper and lower involvement of the arcuate fibres with a characteristic ring-shaped scotoma. This scotoma almost always retains a nasal step, because of the asymmetry of the independent bundles involved [FIGS. 92, 102, 103 and 104]. The ring gradually spreads to the more peripheral areas and towards the centre. Fixation is often spared for a long time and, even when the upper or the lower scotoma encroaches on its nasal side to within a degree or two of fixation, foveal function may remain perfectly normal with good visual acuity. Even when a central island of vision is the only remnant, a nasal step can often be plotted [FIG. 105]. However, in some fields the central island, though not symmetrical, does not show the characteristic nasal step. The central island of

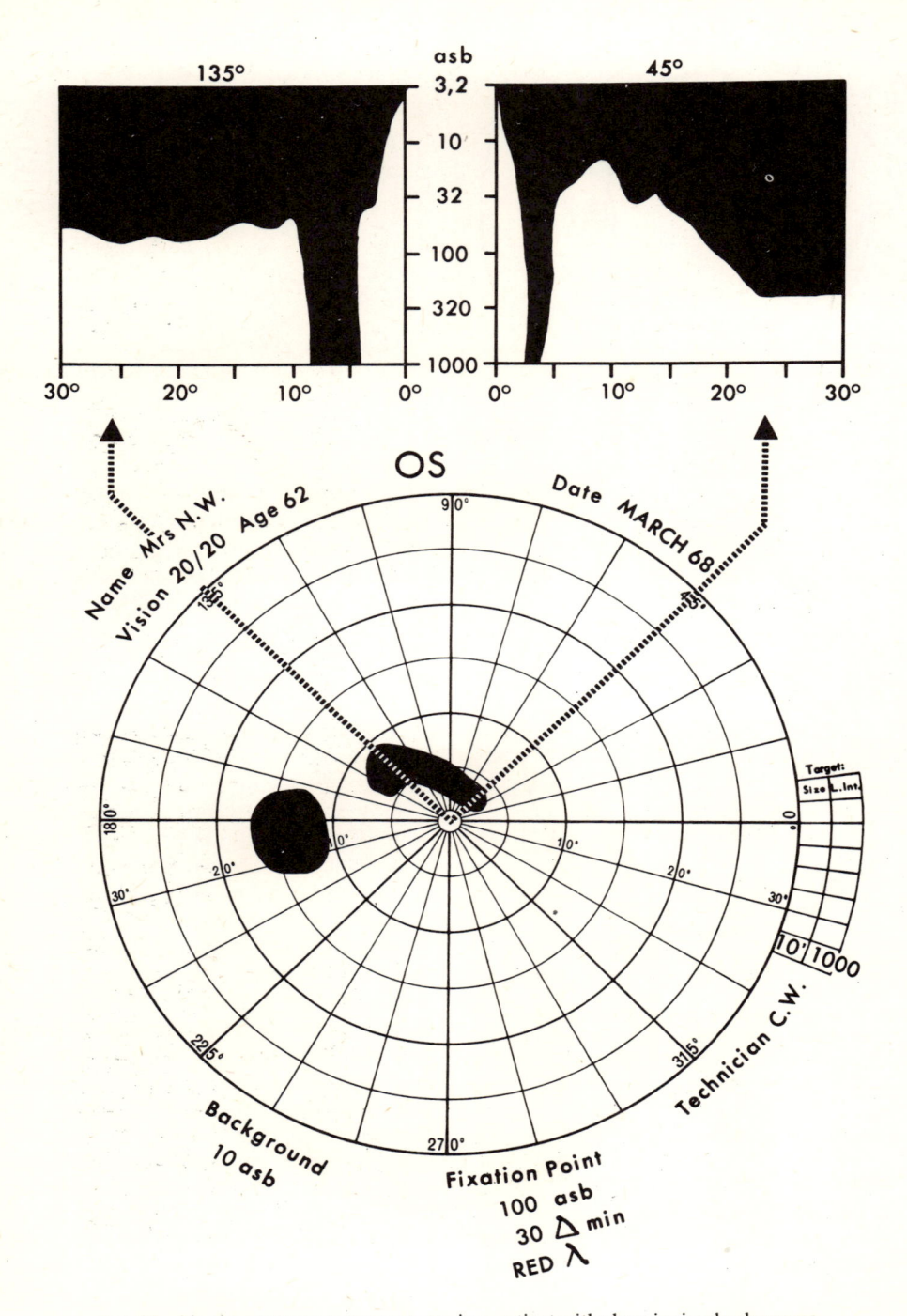

FIG. 95. Absolute upper arcuate scotoma in a patient with chronic simple glaucoma.

PLATE I

A

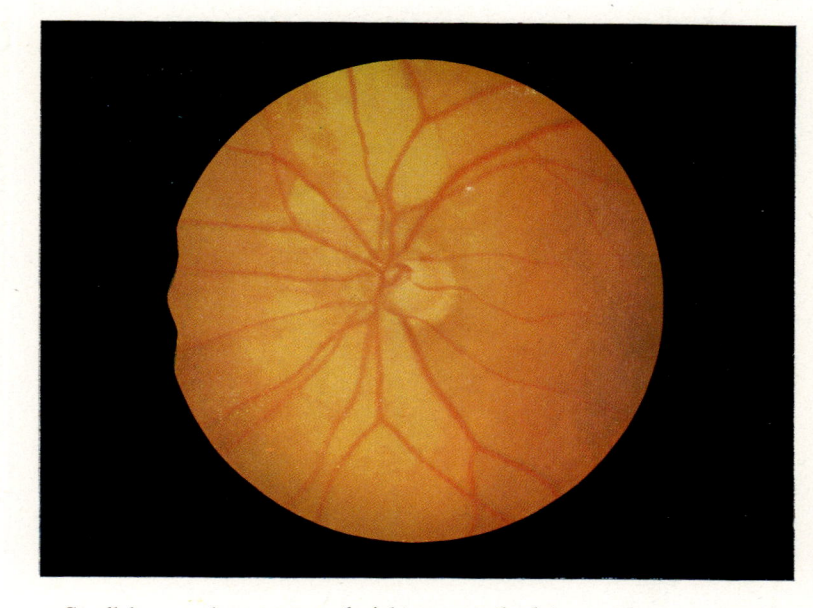

Small haemorrhage appeared eighteen months later on the upper outer portion of neuroretinal rim in patient whose earlier field is shown in Fig. 95

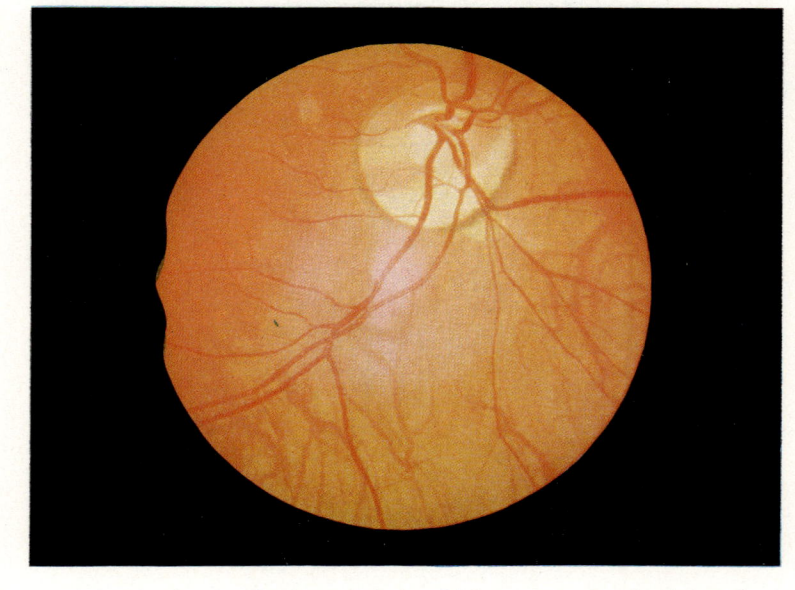

B

Myopic fundus showing increased choroidal pattern and pallor below the disc. This is the appearance which is characteristically seen in patients who show visual field defects due to partial ectasia in myopia

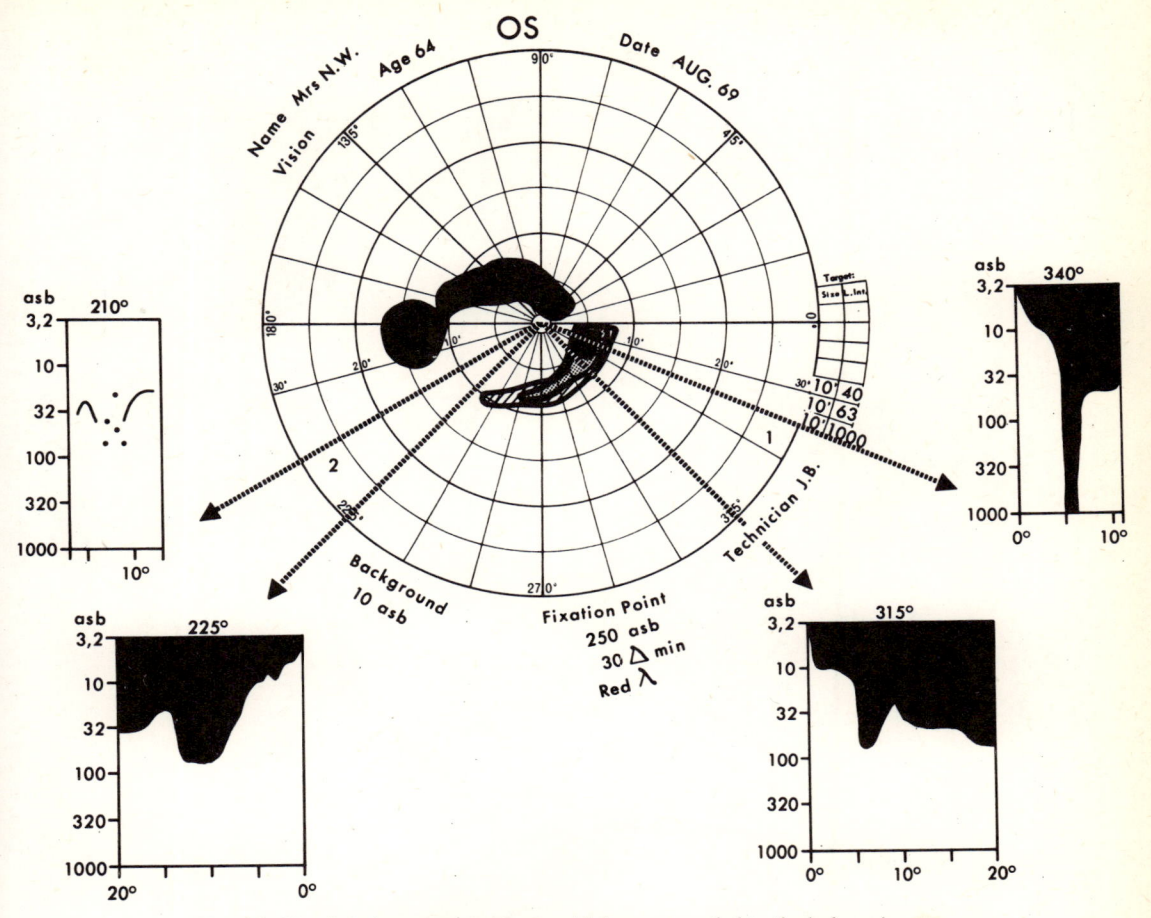

FIG. 96. New inferior arcuate scotoma which corresponded to the ischaemic area shown by the haemorrhage in PLATE 1A.

vision is often accompanied by some sight in the temporal visual field which may disappear before central vision is finally abolished. Occasionally the central area is lost first and the temporal area persists [FIG. 104].

The normal way of progression is a change in density of existing scotomata and the conversion of surrounding relative scotomata into areas of absolute defect. It is not clear whether this manner of change occurs as a result of a gradual deterioration of function or step-like episodes of involvement of fresh nerve fibre bundles as previously outlined.

Static perimetry lends itself to the recording of changes in visual defects of chronic simple glaucoma and finds its main application in glaucoma work. The time involved in plotting static perimetry is well worthwhile in this disease because of the consistency and reliability of the responses which one obtains. The information gives greater confidence in the findings of deterioration on which further medical or surgical therapy has to be planned.

Isolated paracentral scotomata in the Bjerrum area can occasionally disappear with successful medical or surgical reduction in intraocular pressure [FIG. 106]. This change is slow and rather infrequent. It indicates that certain types of damage are reversible, possibly because of a reversible impairment of

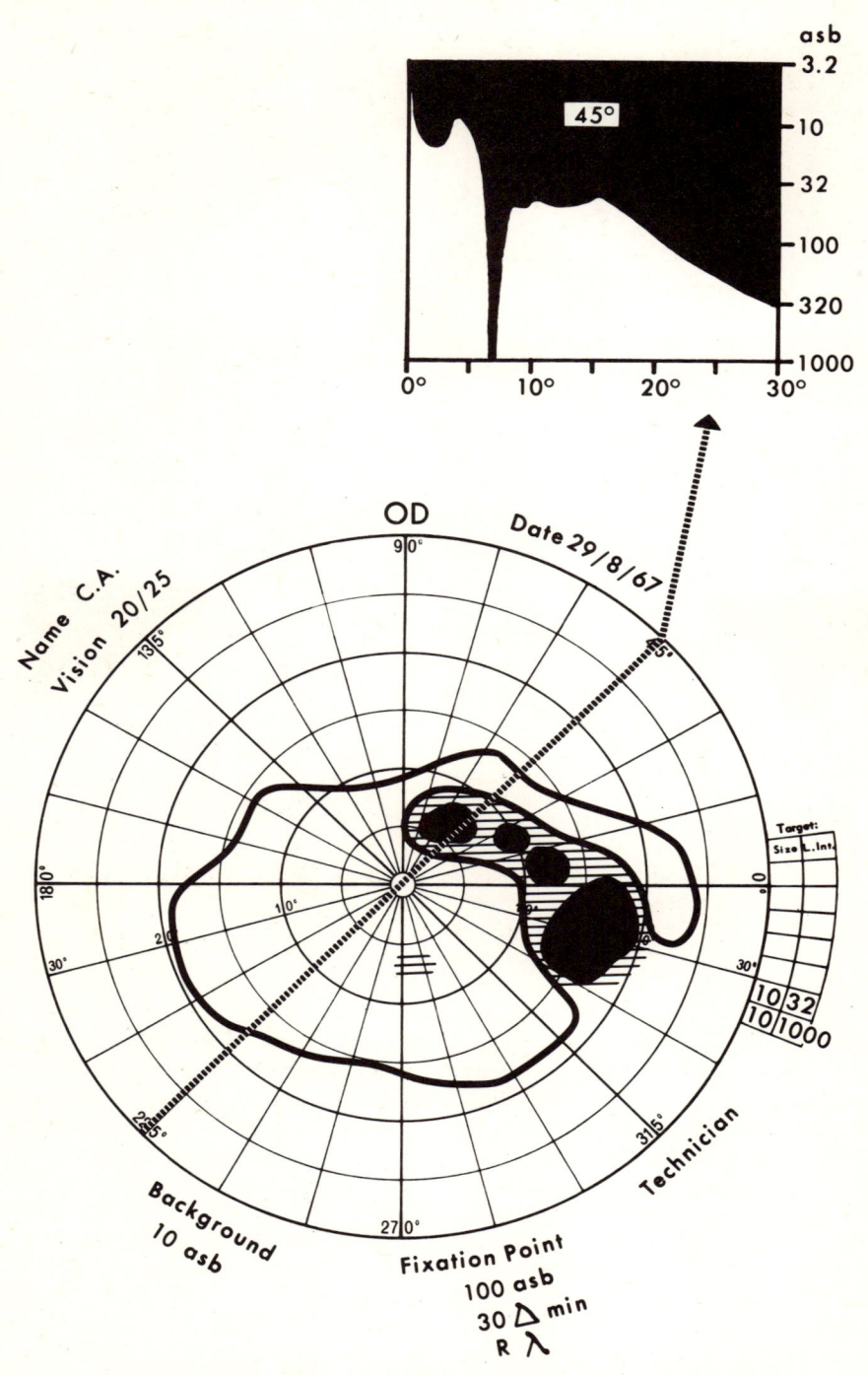

Fig. 97. Multiple absolute nuclei in an arcuate scotoma. Profile 45 degrees shows the absolute nucleus to be very narrow.

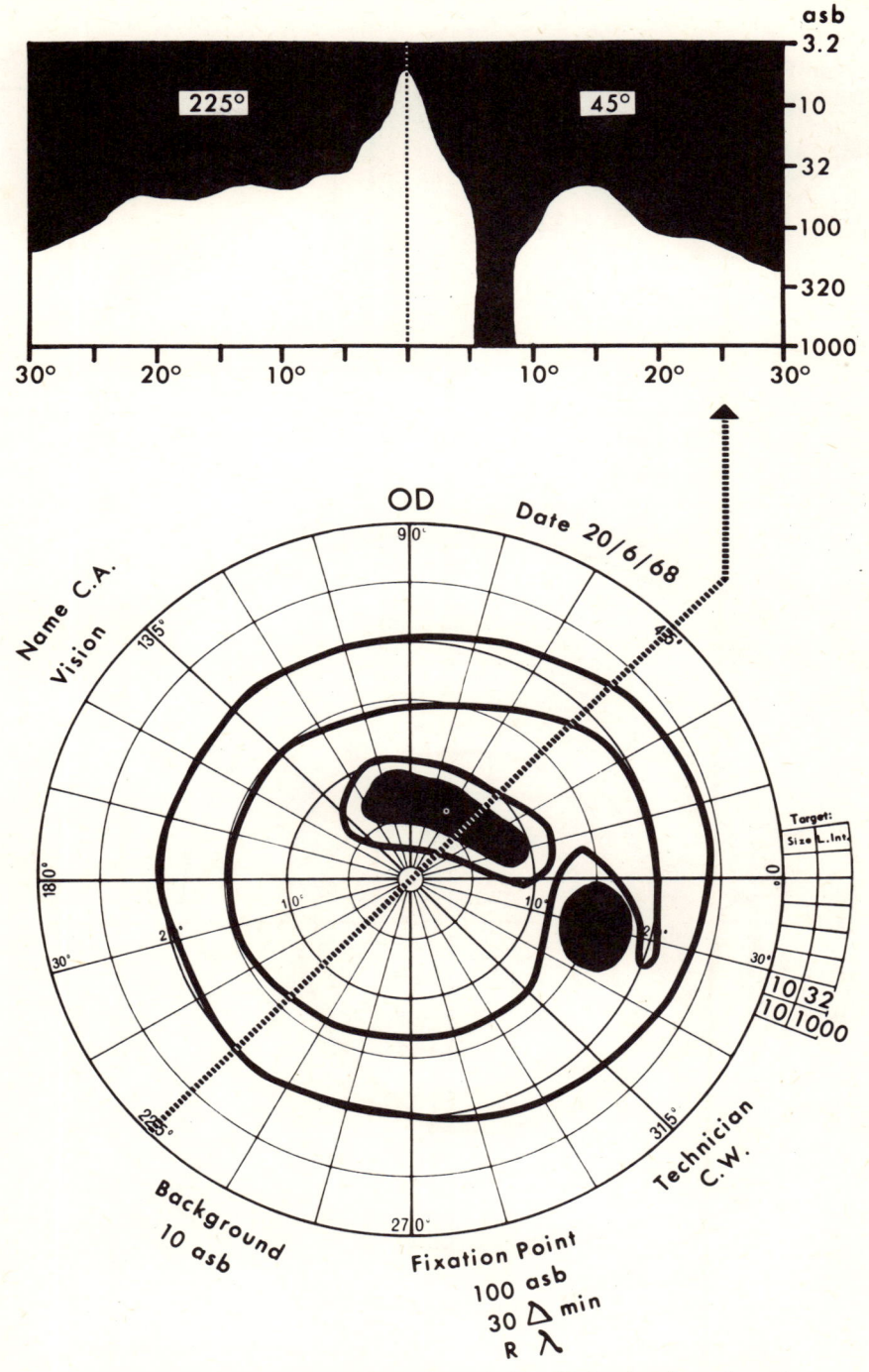

FIG. 98. Progression of field defect shown in FIG. 97 showing the coalescence of absolute nuclei into a larger and wider absolute scotoma. See profile 45 degrees.

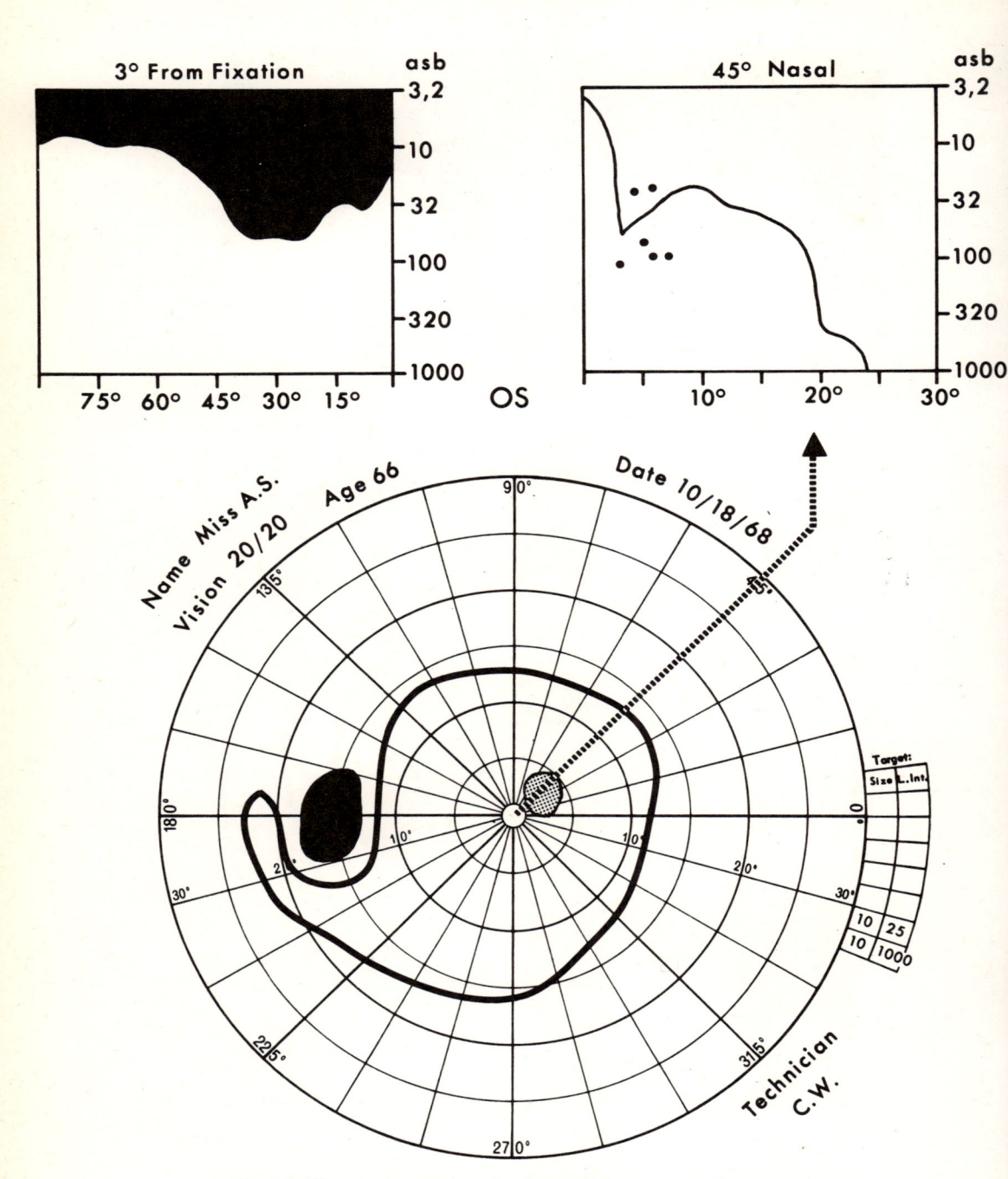

FIG. 99. Glaucomatous patient showing a relative paracentral scotoma 4 degrees from fixation on the nasal side. The upper left diagram records the findings of circular static perimetry on an arc 3 degrees from fixation in the upper nasal quadrant of the visual field.

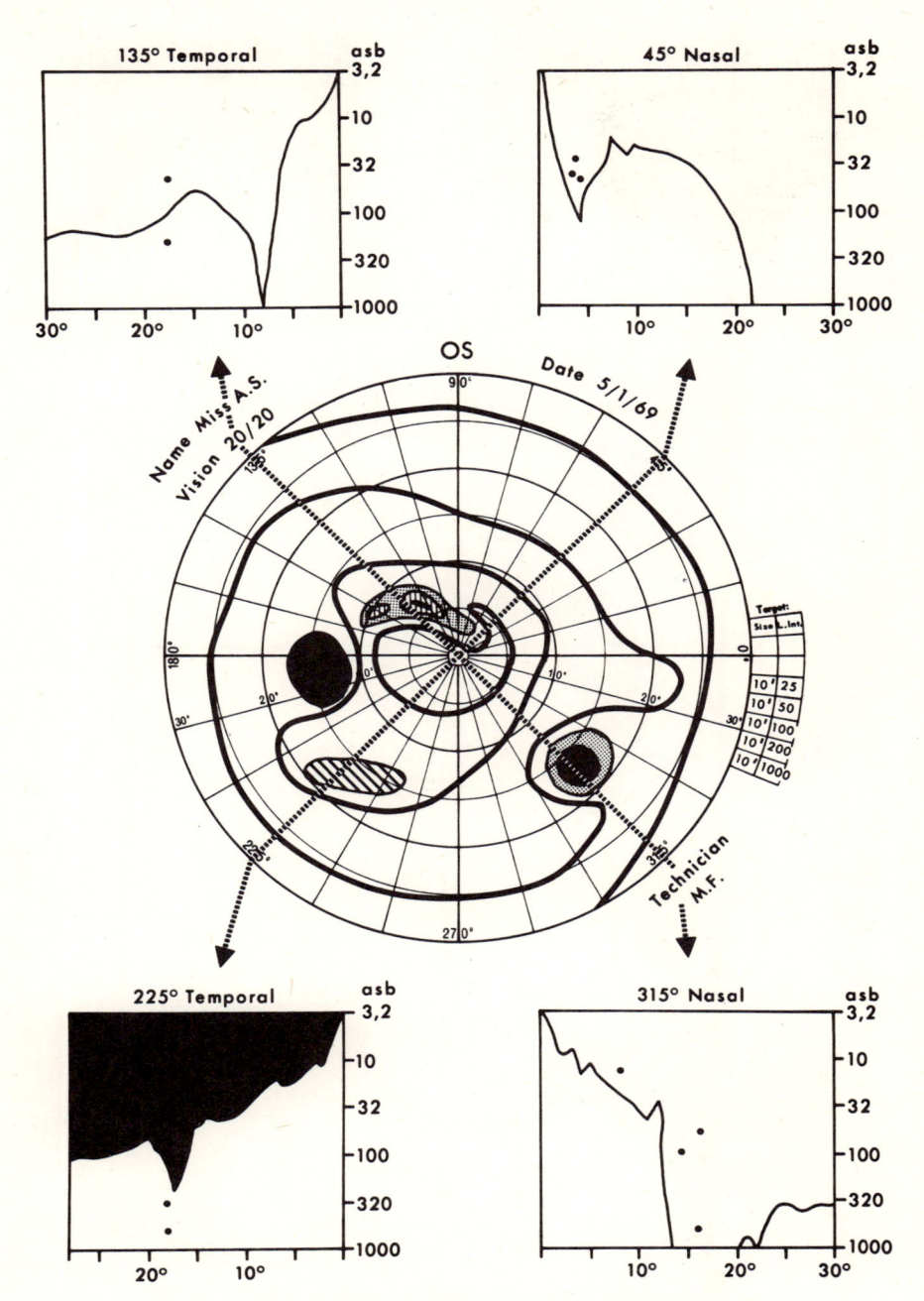

FIG. 100. Progress of visual field defect shown in FIG. 99. The relative scotoma now shows arcuate features with an absolute nucleus. There is a new inferior paracentral scotoma nasally and a relative disturbance on the temporal side (profile 225 degrees).

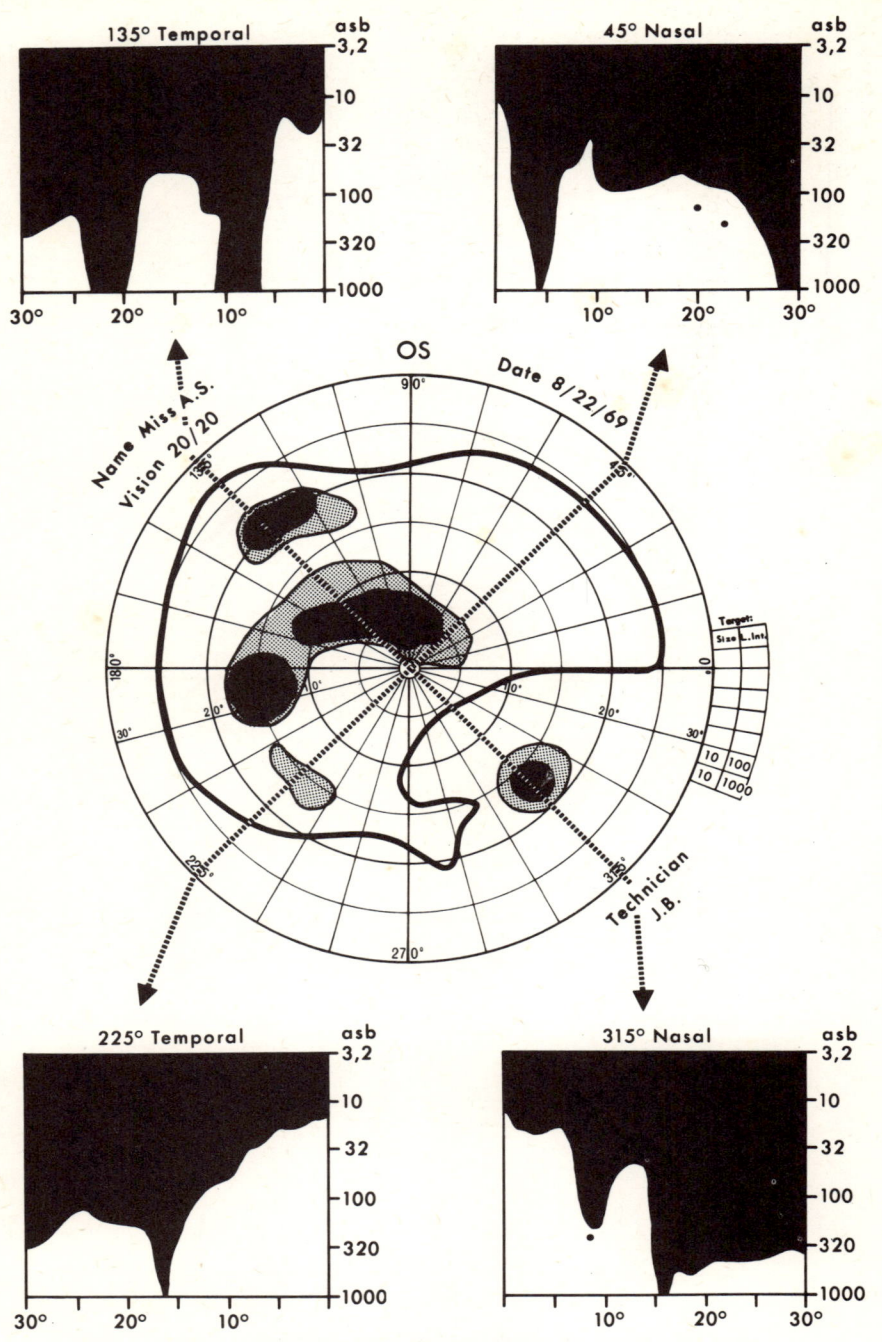

FIG. 101. Progression of the field defect shown in FIGS. 99 and 100. The superior arcuate scotoma is now absolute, longer and wider. There is a fresh absolute scotoma more peripherally, indicating involvement of a more peripheral nerve fibre bundle which was not involved before (135 degree profile).

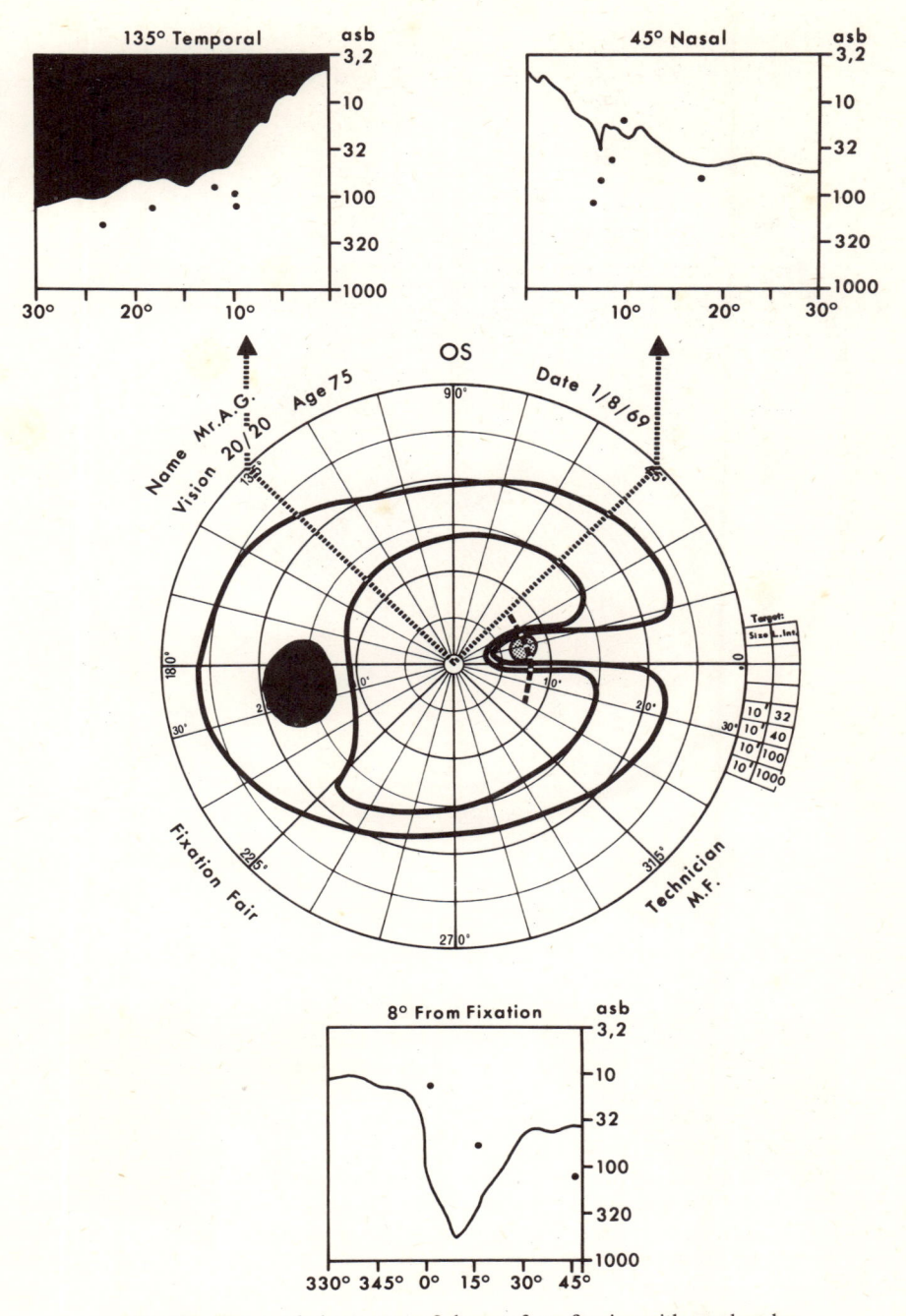

FIG. 102. Upper relative scotoma 8 degrees from fixation with nasal wedge.

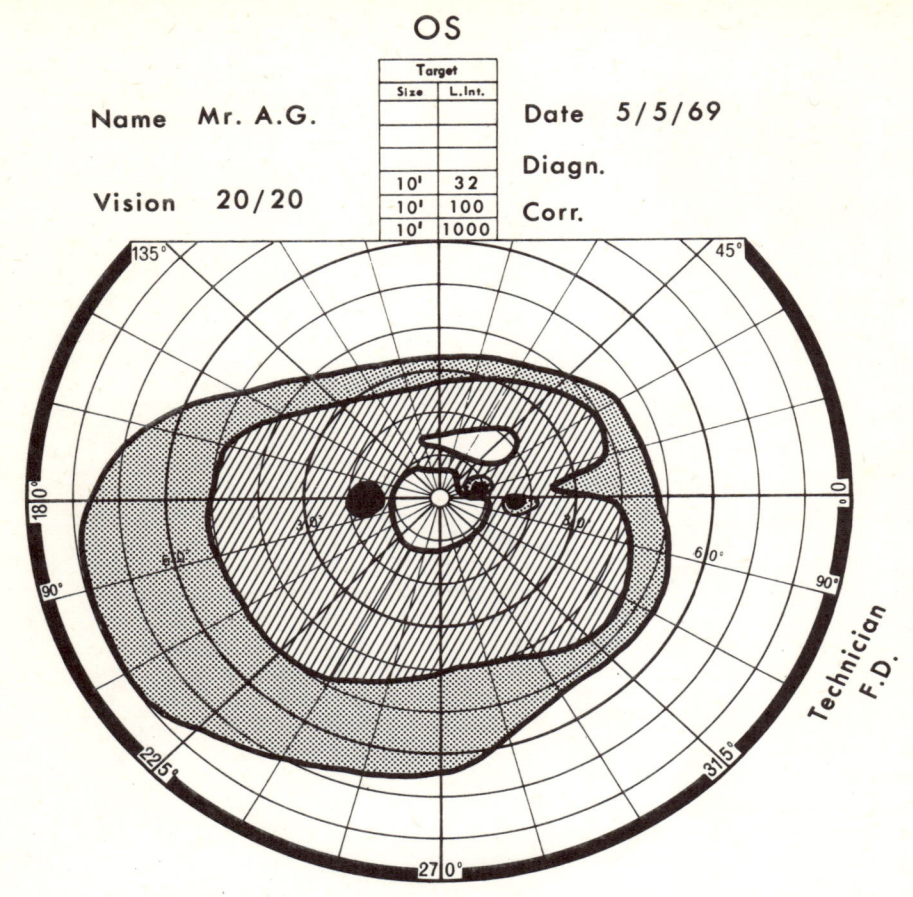

FIG. 103. Progression of field defect shown in FIG. 102. There is now a superior arcuate scotoma with an absolute nucleus producing a nasal step. There is a new inferior paracentral nucleus.

nutrition of nerve cells or fibres or because of fluctuations in the amount of oedema produced as a result of the ischaemic events.

The majority of visual field defects remain either unchanged or show progression. The progression may be related to poor intraocular pressure control due to failure of conservative or surgical management, to diurnal peaks of intraocular pressure, or to faulty estimation of intraocular pressure in those eyes in which unusual ocular rigidity factors make Schiotz tonometry inaccurate.

The progression is not related only to the levels of intraocular pressure. Many other factors should be taken into account. Visual field defects may occur or progress as a result of the medical reduction in systemic blood pressure or as a result of a reduction in blood pressure due to haemorrhage or myocardial infarction. If the blood pressure rises and remains at previous levels, progression in the visual field deficits may be halted. Further field loss may result from continued episodes of reduction in perfusion pressure. In other patients classical glaucomatous visual field defects develop with little intraocular pressure rise. In these patients other factors, usually small vessel disease, account for the ischaemia of the optic nerve head and they are likely to continue to lose visual field unless their intraocular pressures are so significantly changed as to improve the perfusion of the optic nerve head. Unfortunately, in these people, this is very difficult to achieve.

On the other hand, patients who lose nerve fibre bundles as a result of intraocular pres-

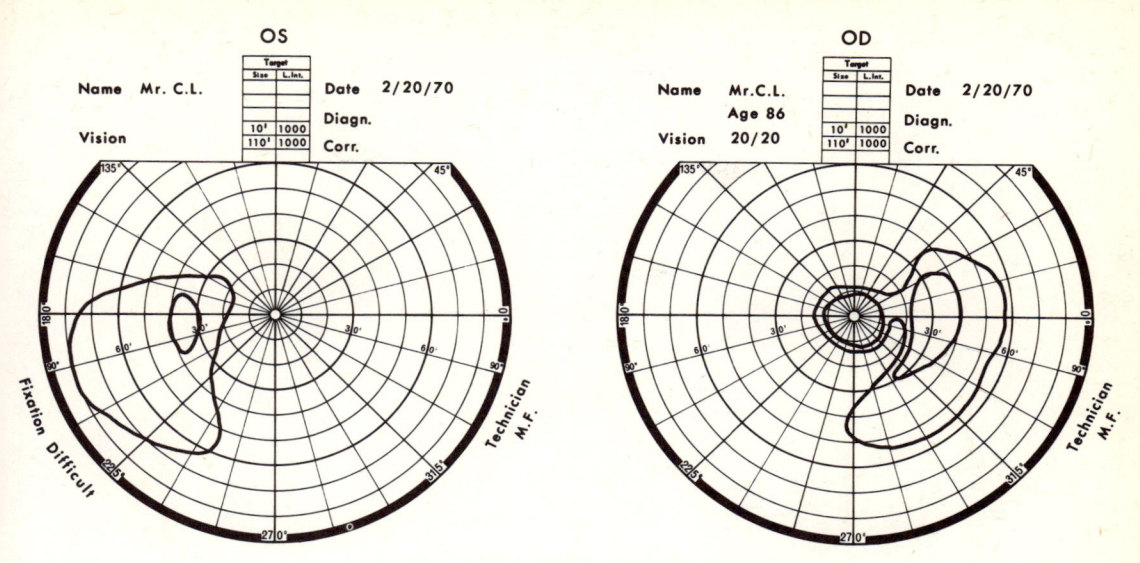

FIG. 104. Right eye: advanced glaucomatous field defect showing a change beyond a ring scotoma with remaining central and temporal field. Left eye: temporal island as the last remaining part of a glaucomatous field.

sures which are very high, e.g. 45 or 55 mm. Hg, and in whom the intraocular pressure can be reduced to the 'mid-twenties' may, because of the significant reduction in intraocular pressure, continue for many years without any further loss of visual field. This may occur despite the fact that the 'mid-twenties' is not normally accepted as adequate control in the presence of a visual field defect and a change at the optic nerve head. It is therefore important to evaluate each patient in terms of the components which make up the failure of perfusion at the optic nerve head and to try to modify those that lend themselves to medical or surgical manipulation. The intraocular pressure is the factor which lends itself most readily to modification. Thus the lower the intraocular pressure the better the perfusion at the nerve head is likely to be, and the more effective the treatment in preserving sight.

THE PLACE OF PERIMETRY IN MANAGEMENT OF CHRONIC SIMPLE GLAUCOMA

The patient with ocular hypertension and normal discs should have his visual fields studied on the tangent screen or on the Goldmann perimeter. Armaly's method has been

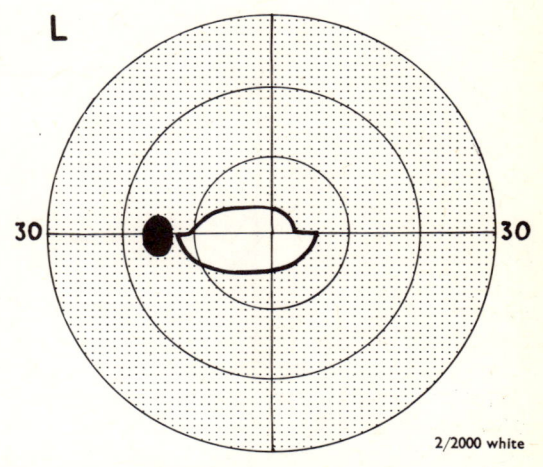

FIG. 105. Small residual field in glaucoma still showing a nasal step.

designed to search the most vulnerable areas of the visual field and can be highly recommended. If no field defect is demonstrated the examination should be repeated at periodic intervals varying from 4 to 12 months depending on the element of risk, i.e. the height of the intraocular pressure, the blood pressure, the presence of vascular or endocrine disease, the family history, etc.

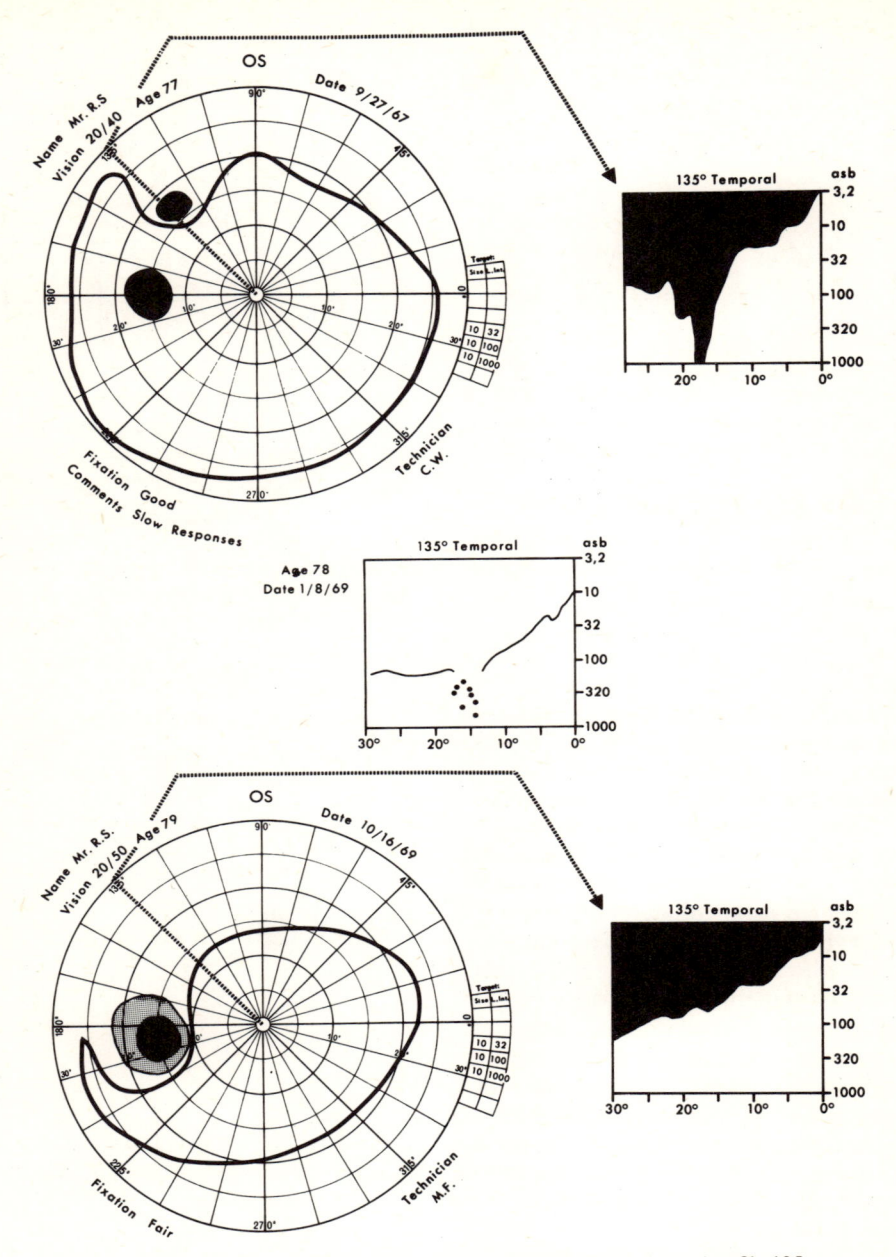

FIG. 106. Unusual sequence of an absolute paracentral scotoma (profile 135 degrees) gradually disappearing over a 2 year period. The upper baring of blind spot (lower left) is not accompanied by a scotoma (profile 135 degrees lower right).

The presence of a field defect or the suspicion of a field defect requires full analysis of the defective areas in terms of their extent and density. Quantitative kinetic perimetry or static perimetry lend themselves well to such an analysis. The tests under these circumstances should be repeated at 4–6 month intervals under the same conditions. Change of therapy which may lead to a different pupil size or a change of refraction should be followed by a fresh field analysis and any deterioration assessed from the new base line. If further field defects occur or there is an enlargement or increase in the density of field defects, the disease is out of control and changes in the medical management or surgery should be considered.

ANGLE CLOSURE GLAUCOMA

The events in chronic angle closure glaucoma are similar to those described for open angle, but the patients are younger, the intraocular pressures higher and the systemic factors fewer. After acute attacks of glaucoma optic atrophy may occur. The visual field defects are rather different, appearing as a rule as generalized contraction of the visual field with bizarre and irregular defects. Arcuate scotomata may occur but are not a constant feature. The involvement of centrocaecal fibres can lead to a severe reduction in visual acuity with a centrocaecal scotoma. More often, however, the central vision is spared with loss of the peripheral field.

APHAKIC GLAUCOMA

The field changes in aphakic glaucoma are identical to those found in chronic simple glaucoma but the pitfalls and artefacts are more pronounced. Attention must be paid to the adequacy of the refraction and the positioning of the correcting lens. Spherical aberration of the lens reduces the visual field to about 25 degrees. The blind spot is closer to fixation and defects will appear smaller than in the phakic eye. Contact lenses produce fewer anomalies, but even with these the blind spot appears slightly closer to fixation.

SECONDARY GLAUCOMA

The visual field loss in secondary glaucoma is more variable than in chronic simple glaucoma. If the pressure is markedly elevated for long periods of time, an optic atrophy not unlike that seen in unrelieved angle closure glaucoma may be found. There are, however, many cases of chronic secondary glaucoma which develop field and disc changes indistinguishable from chronic open angle glaucoma. In these cases the changes at the nerve head develop slowly. In cases of secondary glaucoma due to ischaemia there may be evidence of the occlusion of major retinal vessels in addition to the changes which occur in chronic simple glaucoma.

REFERENCES AND FURTHER READING

ARMALY, M. F. (1964) Effect of corticosteroids on intraocular pressure and fluid dynamics, *Arch. Ophthal.*, **71**, 636.

ARMALY, M. F. (1969) Ocular pressure and visual fields, *Arch. Ophthal.*, **81**, 25.

AULHORN, E., and HARMS, H. (1967) Early visual field defects in glaucoma, in *Glaucoma Symposium*, Tutzing Castle, 1966, p. 151, Basel.

DRANCE, S. M. (1962) Studies in the susceptibility of the eye to raised intraocular pressure, *Arch. Ophthal.*, **68**, 478.

DRANCE, S. M., and BEGG, I. S. (1970) Sector haemorrhage. Probable acute ischaemic disc change in chronic simple glaucoma, *Canad. J. Ophthal.*, **5**, 137.

HARRINGTON, D. O. (1965) The Bjerrum scotoma, *Amer. J. Ophthal.*, **59**, 646.

PETER, L. C. (1920) Visual fields in glaucoma, *Arch. Ophthal.*, **49**, 309.

TRAQUAIR, H. M. (1931) Perimetry in the study of glaucoma, *Trans. ophthal. Soc. U.K.*, **51**, 585.

10
RETINAL LESIONS

Most choroidal and retinal affections may be diagnosed from the ophthalmoscopic appearances alone. But, on occasions when the diagnosis is in doubt, it may be established by demonstrating a characteristic field defect.

RETINITIS PIGMENTOSA

This is a progressive disease in which the field defects advance steadily throughout a long period of time. Night blindness is the first symptom, but the onset and progress of the disease is so insidious that the condition is often fairly advanced before the patient seeks advice. The characteristic ophthalmoscopic appearances of peripheral bone corpuscle pigmentation, waxy pallor of the optic disc, and narrow retinal arteries are readily recognized.

In the early stages dark adaptation is markedly abnormal and later a ring scotoma may be demonstrated between the 10 and 40 degree meridians with the 3/330 white target [FIG. 107]. Since the outer circle on the Bjerrum screen is usually only 30 degrees, the perimeter is the best instrument for revealing the early field changes in this condition. The ring scotoma may be very patchy at first and become denser later. It is always more obvious if the illumination is reduced in intensity. It has a steep slope centrally and a shallow slope peripherally [FIG. 39]. As the disease progresses, the scotoma breaks through to the periphery, usually on the nasal side. The peripheral field gradually disappears. The central field decreases much more slowly than the peripheral field, and patients may retain a visual acuity of 20/20 for many years [FIG. 108]. Despite good central vision, the disability from loss of the peripheral field is great. Some develop macular degeneration and consequent poor visual acuity. The two eyes are usually equally affected, but occasionally the field change in one may be slightly in advance of the other.

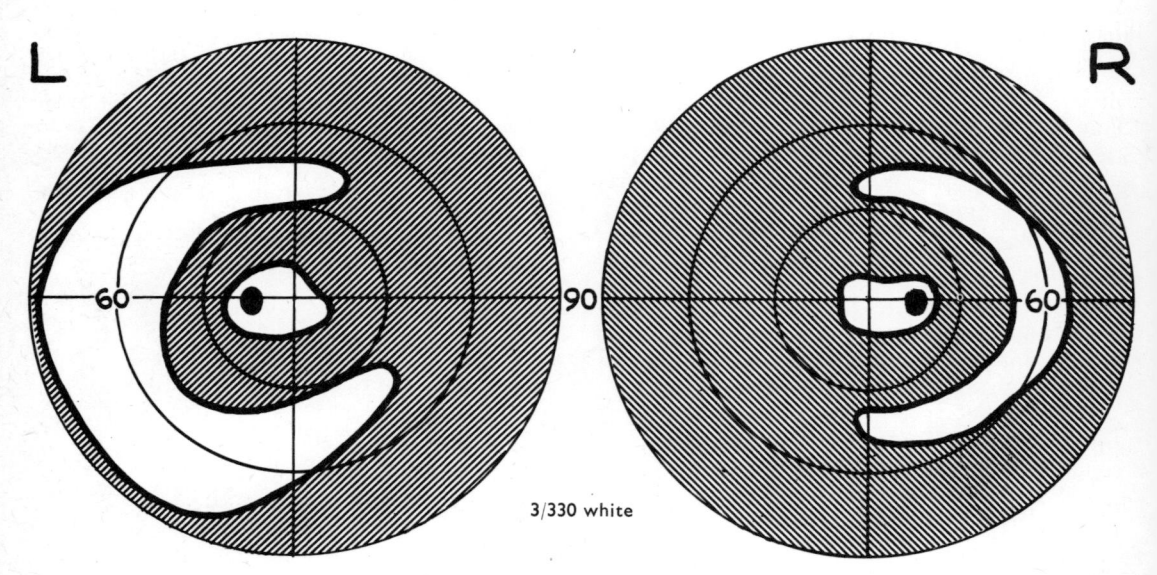

FIG. 107. Visual fields of early retinitis pigmentosa.

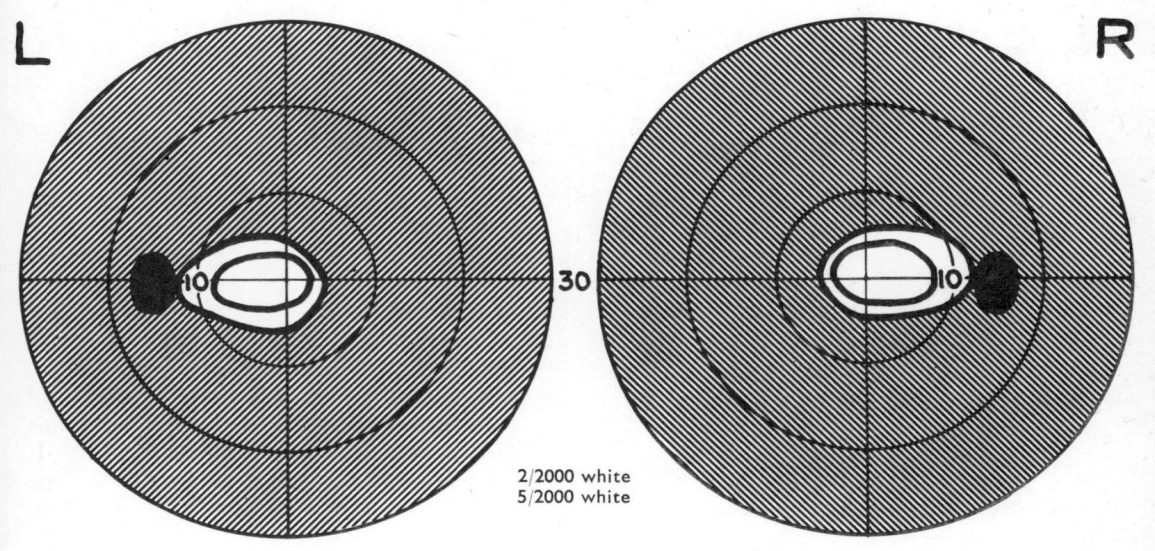

FIG. 108. Fields of retinitis pigmentosa in a late stage. Vision was still 20/30 in each eye.

2/2000 white
5/2000 white

The histological changes in eyes with advanced disease have been studied, but the early alterations have not been examined adequately because these eyes cannot be removed. No satisfactory explanation of the cause and progress of the field defects has yet been found.

In the Laurence-Moon-Biedl syndrome which consists of obesity, mental retardation, polydactyly, hypogenitalism, and occasional deafness, the associated retinitis pigmentosa is often atypical. Macular degeneration may occur and cause a central scotoma. In these cases the visual loss is severe even in early adult life.

VASCULAR OCCLUSION

It has been shown by histological studies that atherosclerosis at retinal arteriovenous crossings results in narrowing of the lumina of both vessels. When this happens either the vein or the artery may become occluded first, depending upon the relative degree of narrowing in each. Retinal artery occlusion causes an abrupt cessation of blood flow, so that the ganglion cells die rapidly. It is probable that a loss of blood supply and thus of oxygen of no more than four minutes results in death of retinal cells. The loss of vision is therefore sudden. When a venous branch is blocked, the visual failure is more gradual. Presumably a collateral venous circulation develops before the death of the ganglion cells. The vision in the whole area of supply is lost when a retinal artery is blocked. Retinal vein occlusion causes a central scotoma unless it is accompanied by a branch arterial occlusion. Occlusion of a retinal vein or artery is painless.

Whenever a vascular occlusion occurs several conditions which may be associated should always be considered. Atherosclerosis and hypertension are most commonly found. In the case of a central retinal vein occlusion the presence of chronic simple glaucoma should be suspected. In central retinal artery occlusion, conditions such as mitral stenosis which might cause an embolism should be sought. A complaint of headaches might suggest the presence of cranial arteritis which would need confirmation by the finding of a raised sedimentation rate and arteritis on biopsy of the superficial temporal artery. Inquiry should always be made regarding transient attacks of weakness or numbness on the opposite side of the body which would suggest an impending internal carotid occlusion.

RETINAL ARTERIAL OCCLUSION

Field defects due to arterial occlusion have a steep edge and are permanent. When the occlusion first occurs, its abrupt onset and the appearance of retinal oedema give rise to no

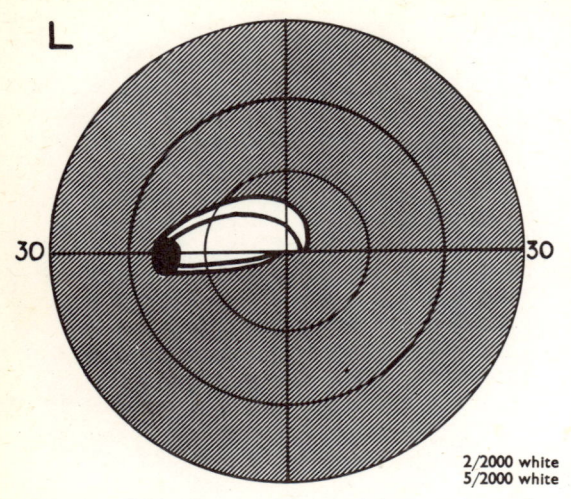

FIG. 109. Field defect in occlusion of the central retinal artery of the left eye with intact cilioretinal artery.

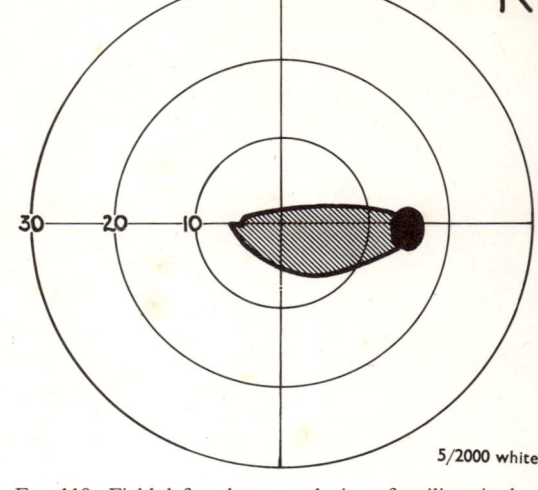

FIG. 110. Field defect due to occlusion of a cilioretinal artery.

difficulty in diagnosis. If the patient is first seen some time after an occlusion of the central artery, the pale disc and narrow arterial branches usually make the diagnosis obvious, but an old branch arterial occlusion may be difficult to recognize. It is in these cases that the shape of the field defect may establish the diagnosis.

Arterial occlusion usually occurs as a result of angiosclerotic narrowing of the lumen, combined with either spasm or thrombosis, or a combination of both. Embolism is probably an uncommon cause. If the *central retinal artery* is occluded, the eye becomes blind, but occasionally a small cuff of visual field remains around the blind spot, presumably due to the vascular anastomoses which occur about the optic nerve sheath. Occasionally a *cilioretinal artery* may supply the macular area. In these patients a small centrocaecal field of vision remains intact, and they may retain visual acuity of 20/20 [FIG. 109]. If a cilioretinal artery supplying the macular area becomes blocked, an absolute central scotoma with a normal peripheral field results [FIG. 110].

Any branch of the central retinal artery may become occluded, usually at an arteriovenous crossing. The *superior temporal* [FIGS. 72 and 111] is the branch which is most commonly affected. A sector field defect occurs, the characteristic feature of which is the horizontal edge bisecting the macula. This feature is absent if there is an intact cilioretinal artery.

RETINAL VENOUS OCCLUSION

At its onset the diagnosis of occlusion of the *central retinal vein* is seldom in doubt. The story of gradual painless loss of vision or of blurred vision on waking in the morning, the appearance of the oedematous disc, the dilated tortuous veins, and the haemorrhages extending to the periphery, present a clinical entity which is easily recognized. All degrees of severity of occlusion are seen, varying from cases in which vision is little more than perception of light, to those in which vision is as good as 20/60 or even 20/20. The loss of vision varies with the duration and severity of the ischaemia before circulation is restored. This in turn depends upon such factors as the rate of retraction of the clot occluding the vein, recanalization, the presence of alternative channels, and the development of collateral circulation. Absence of perception of light suggests the retinal artery is also occluded.

In most cases central vision is affected. A central scotoma occurs which may vary from a small one, 5–10 degrees in diameter, to a large dense one breaking through to the periphery [FIG. 112]. Some contraction of peripheral isopters is usual but the presence of a sector-shaped defect should suggest concomitant arteriolar involvement. A few patients, particularly those under 45 years of age, show a

VASCULAR OCCLUSION

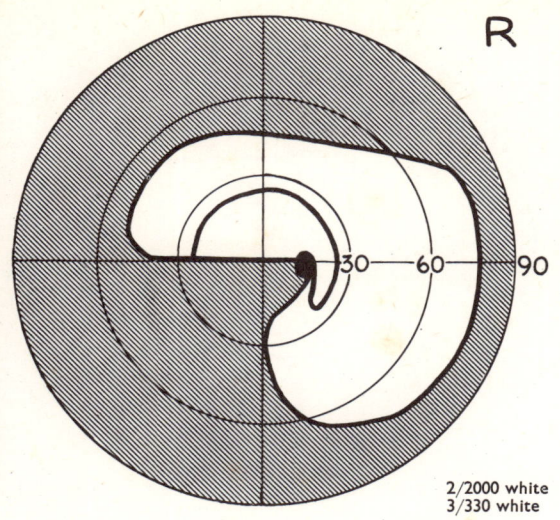

FIG. 111. Field defect due to occlusion of the right superior temporal artery.
2/2000 white
3/330 white

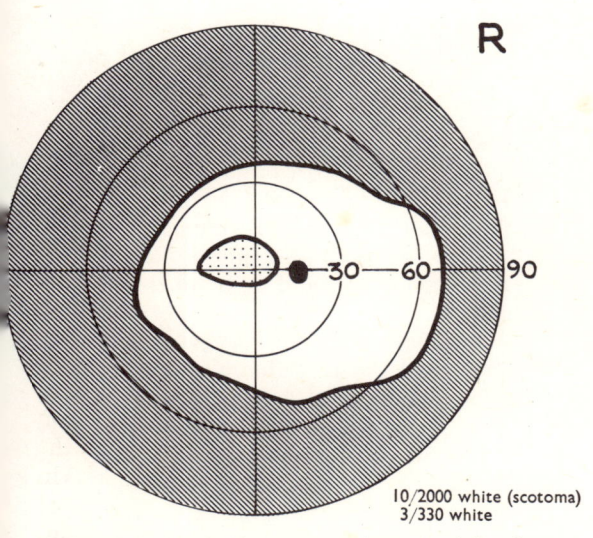

FIG. 112. A central scotoma and some peripheral contraction due to occlusion of the central retinal vein.
10/2000 white (scotoma)
3/330 white

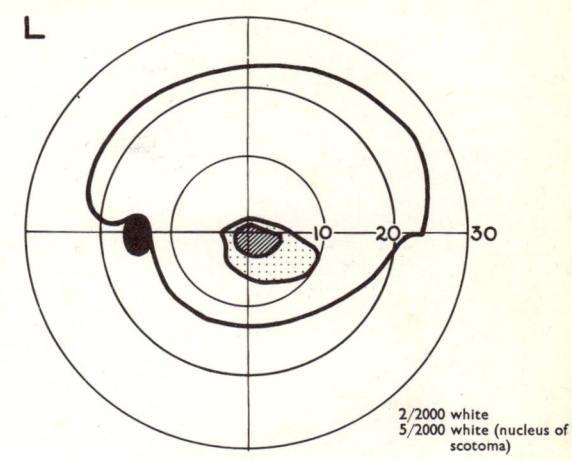

FIG. 113. Field defect due to occlusion of the superior temporal vein.
2/2000 white
5/2000 white (nucleus of scotoma)

surprising restoration of vision, even to 20/20. In the great majority, however, there is little or no recovery, and about 15 per cent of these later develop haemorrhagic thrombotic glaucoma.

Since about 20 per cent of patients who suffer central retinal vein occlusion have glaucoma, the other eye should always be investigated for this condition.

If occlusion of the superior or inferior temporal vein occurs it is usually where it is crossed by the corresponding artery.

The *superior temporal vein* is the branch which is most commonly affected. When the haemorrhages and oedema have subsided, in most cases only a small scotoma remains, situated below the macula. The peripheral field remains intact [FIG. 113].

Sometimes the oedema and haemorrhages involve the macular area so severely that the visual acuity is greatly reduced. This is more likely to occur in occlusion of the superior temporal vein than of any other branch. This may be due to the effect of gravity, which causes the oedema and haemorrhage to spread downwards and damage the macular cones.

RETINAL DETACHMENT

The outer neurones of the retina are dependent upon the choriocapillaris for nutrition. They are therefore deprived of nutrition when the retina is detached. The resulting field defect will depend upon the site, size, and degree of separation, and the length of time that it has been present.

Perimetry is used little in the diagnosis of retinal detachment, but it is of value for the following purposes:

1. The extent of a detachment, and its encroachment upon the central area, may be estimated with great accuracy by plotting the 2/2000 white isopter. A 10 mm. blue target

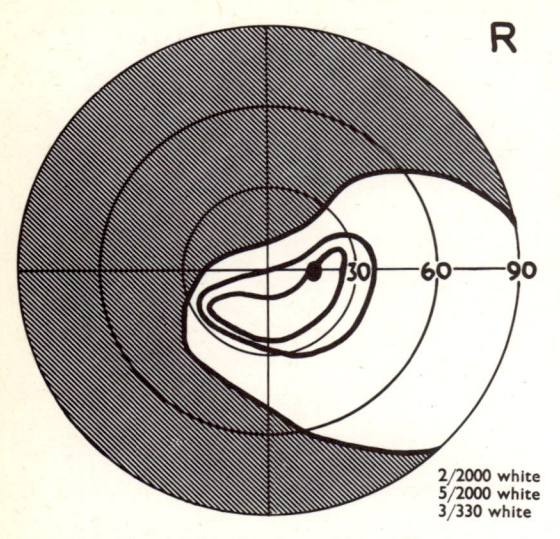

FIG. 114. Visual field of patient with an inferotemporal retinal detachment, before operation.

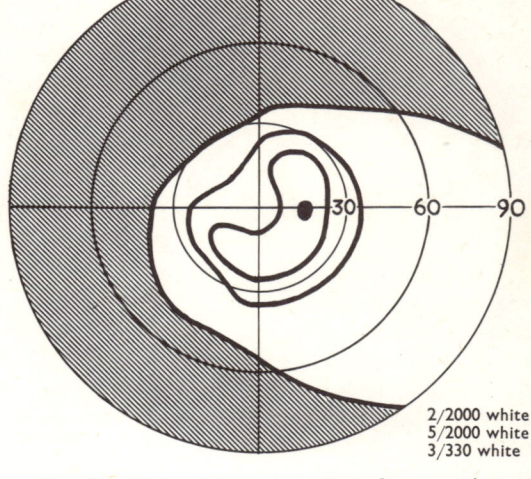

FIG. 115. Field of the same patient after operation.

often reveals a much larger defect than was suspected on ophthalmoscopic examination. Reduced illumination may also be of value in charting the affected area.

2. The functional impairment of the detached retina may be estimated in some measure by the 'slope' of the margin of the field defect. If a 5 mm. white target cannot be seen in the central area, and the history suggests that the macula has been detached for some time, there is little hope for recovery of good central vision.

3. A record of the residual field defect, taken 4–6 weeks after operation, is valuable [FIGS. 114 and 115]. If a recurrence of the detachment is suspected at a later date, the visual field may be plotted and compared with the post-operative chart. A contraction suggests that the retina is detached.

RETINAL DETACHMENT DUE TO NEOPLASMS OF THE CHOROID

Perimetry is of little assistance in the differential diagnosis of simple retinal detachment from a detachment due to a choroidal tumour, but there are two features which may be of occasional value:

1. When a neoplasm is in the central area, it will usually cause a defect with no break-through to the periphery—a feature which is most unlike a simple detachment. Such a break-through will occur only if there is a secondary inferior serous detachment.

2. The slope of the edge of a defect caused by a neoplastic detachment is steep compared with the shallow slope of the simple detachment, unless a secondary fluid detachment has developed.

Examination of the visual fields may sometimes be of value in differentiating an early malignant melanoma from a benign one. In malignant lesions the field defect is usually larger than the neoplasm and in most cases the defect extends towards the periphery. In benign naevi a scotoma can sometimes be demonstrated by kinetic perimetry but it is always smaller than the lesion. With static perimetry depressions in the photopic threshold over the site of the naevus can almost always be found.

FURTHER READING

FLINDALL, R. J., and DRANCE, S. M. (1969) Visual field studies of benign choroidal melanomata, *Arch. Ophthal.*, **81**, 41.

11
THE TOXIC AMBLYOPIAS

The action of the various toxins which affect the visual pathway is incompletely understood. Sight is seldom completely destroyed, so it is not possible to remove and examine the eyes to determine the pathological changes. Animal experiments have been carried out with many of the toxic substances, but it cannot be assumed that the same changes occur in man. It appears, however, that each toxin picks out a characteristic group of ganglion cells or nerve fibre bundles. Degeneration in these groups of conduction units causes the visual disturbances. Some of the toxins, especially arsenic, ethyl alcohol, and lead, also cause peripheral neuritis.

The toxins may be divided into three groups by the field changes which they produce. It must not be assumed, however, that because a drug is listed as causing central scotomata it does not cause peripheral contraction. For example, whilst the early and most characteristic changes produced by chloroquine are in the central area, in advanced cases there is almost always some peripheral contraction. Similarly, drugs which characteristically cause peripheral contraction may also, in advanced cases, lead to loss of central vision. The development of central scotomata indicates the involvement of the macular neurones and the maculopapillary bundle which crosses the temporal margin of the optic disc to occupy the central area of the optic nerve. In peripheral contraction the peripheral neurones and the axons situated peripherally in the optic nerve are affected. Some refer to these two conditions as axial retrobulbar neuritis and periaxial retrobulbar neuritis respectively, but it is not really known whether the action of the toxin produces an active inflammation or a nutritional defect. It is therefore probably better to call these lesions either toxic amblyopias or ocular neuropathies.

The three groups of toxins are:

Group 1. Toxins causing bilateral central scotomata.
Group 2. Toxins causing bilateral peripheral contraction.
Group 3. Toxins causing both central scotomata and peripheral contraction.

TOXINS CAUSING BILATERAL CENTRAL SCOTOMATA
TOBACCO

Tobacco is usually cited as the characteristic example of this group. Although earlier studies suggested that vitamin B_1 or thiamine deficiency was responsible for the sensitivity to tobacco resulting in tobacco amblyopia, recent evidence shows that lack of vitamin B_{12} is more likely to be the cause of the condition. Heaton and his colleagues investigated a group of patients with tobacco amblyopia. All had abnormally low serum vitamin B_{12} levels, more than half had histamine-fast achlorhydria and a few had glossitis and macrocytic anaemia. These investigators emphasize the close correlation of these findings with those occurring in pernicious anaemia. Some patients were allowed to continue smoking and were treated with cyanocobalamin. All recovered more rapidly than those who merely stopped smoking. A later paper by Chisholm and his co-workers showed that hydroxocobalamin was more effective in treatment than cyanocobalamin. There is therefore good evidence for the opinion that deficiency of vitamin B_{12} is the essential cause of tobacco amblyopia. Further evidence suggests that the lack of this vitamin may prevent the conversion of cyanide to thiocyanate. (See Leber's optic atrophy and pernicious anaemia for further discussion, pages 108 and 109.)

Patients who develop tobacco amblyopia are usually past middle age, and have smoked ½ oz. or more of pipe tobacco daily for at least 15 years. Cigarette smoking rarely causes the condition. The occasional case due to cigar smoking, tobacco chewing, or snuff, may be encountered. There are a number of factors which appear to play an important part in reducing resistance and increasing susceptibility to the disease. Most patients are heavy drinkers. All are somewhat arteriosclerotic. Many have severe dental caries and pyorrhoea alveolaris. A few have diabetes mellitus or pernicious anaemia.

Clinical Features

Tobacco amblyopia is always bilateral, although one eye is usually affected more severely than the other. The onset is very gradual. The scotomata are negative, so loss of vision is seldom noticed until the central area is involved. Occasionally a patient will complain that he has suddenly lost the sight of one eye. This seemingly abrupt loss of vision occurs when the centrocaecal scotoma invades the fixation area. There is an early failure to recognize red, and occasionally a patient may say that he has noticed that his wife has become paler in the last few months.

The Field Defect

The peripheral field is normal, so that the perimeter is of no value in diagnosis. The field defect is centrocaecal in situation, and is best demonstrated with a 2 mm. white target on a 2 metre Bjerrum screen [FIG. 116]. On plotting this isopter an indentation is found opposite the blind spot. Careful examination of the centrocaecal area with a 2 mm. target may show one or two small oval absolute scotomata lying between the blind spot and the fixation point. These defects have sloping margins. In the early stages it may be difficult to plot exactly because the patient's answers are indefinite. The red isopter is best demonstrated with a 15 mm. red target. It shows an indentation temporally and, in the better eye, this may be the only defect.

As the amblyopia progresses the centrocaecal scotomata increase in size [FIG. 117]. They spread temporally to join the blind spot, and medially to involve the fixation area. Their growth is slow, but the loss of the central vision may seem to the patient to be rapid. If these characteristic field changes are found, the diagnosis may be made with confidence, but it

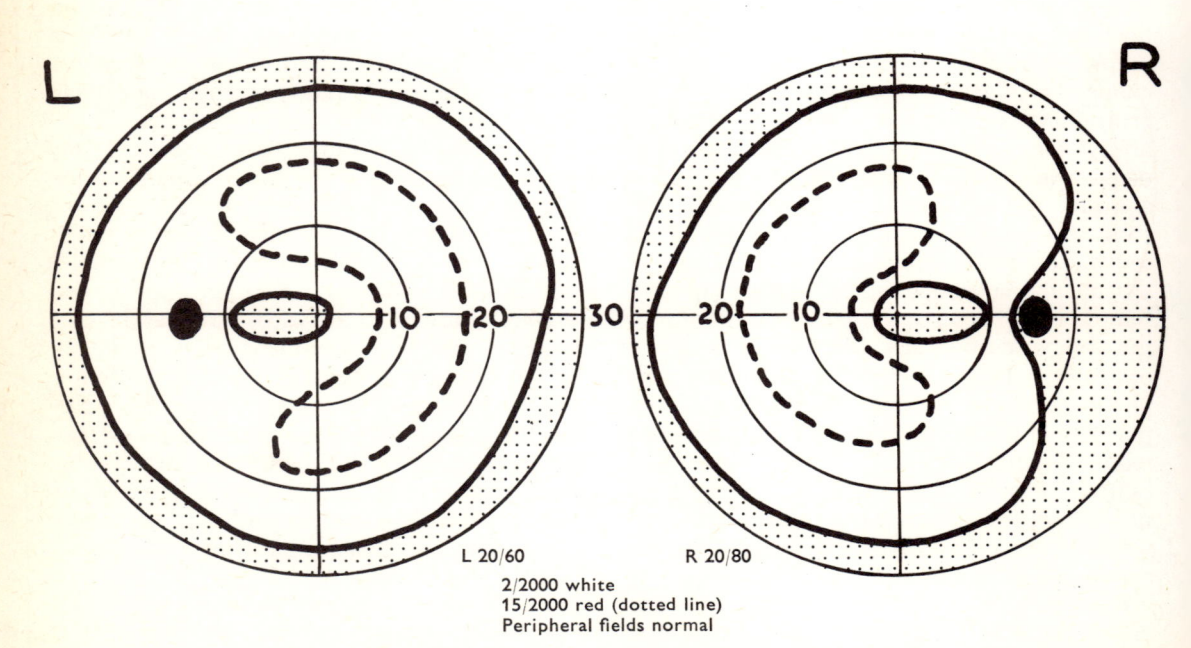

L 20/60   R 20/80
2/2000 white
15/2000 red (dotted line)
Peripheral fields normal

FIG. 116. Visual fields in a patient with tobacco amblyopia.

TOBACCO AMBLYOPIA

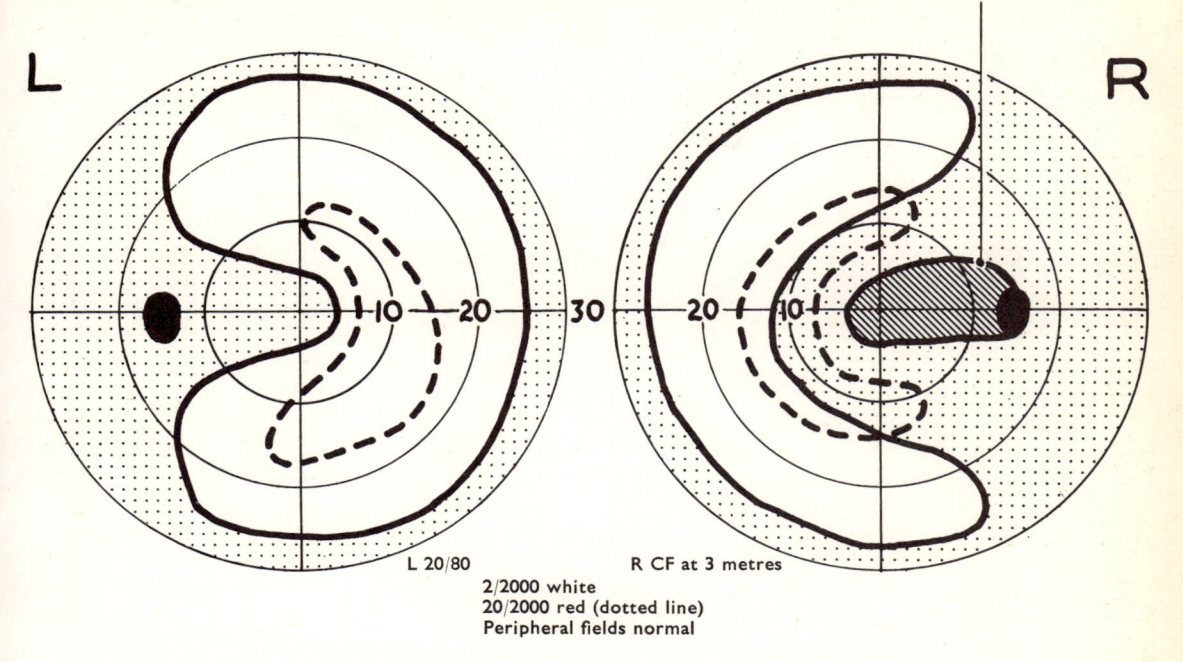

L 20/80 R CF at 3 metres
2/2000 white
20/2000 red (dotted line)
Peripheral fields normal

FIG. 117. Visual fields of a patient with tobacco amblyopia (first visit).

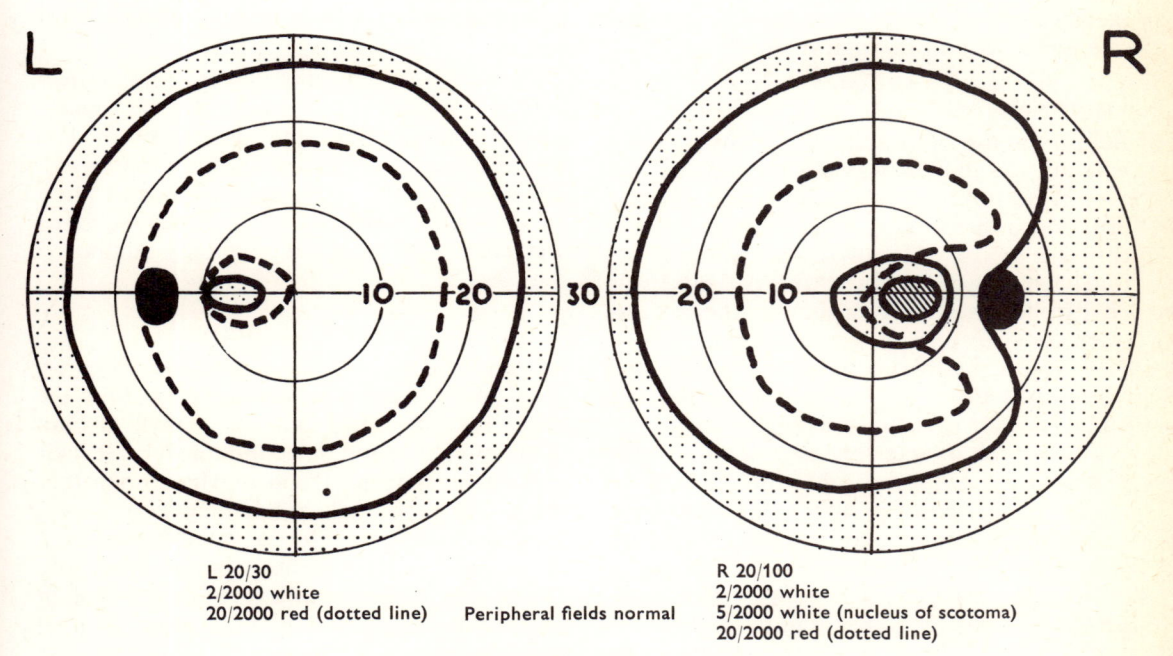

L 20/30 R 20/100
2/2000 white 2/2000 white
20/2000 red (dotted line) Peripheral fields normal 5/2000 white (nucleus of scotoma)
20/2000 red (dotted line)

FIG. 118. Fields of same patient one month later.

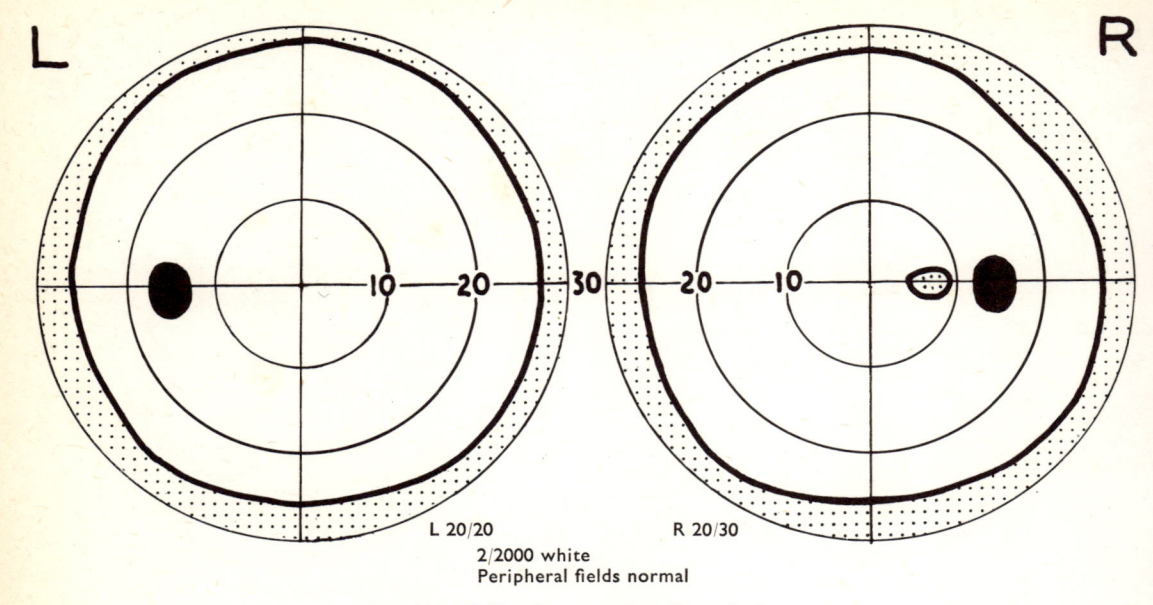

L 20/20   R 20/30
2/2000 white
Peripheral fields normal

Fig. 119. Fields of same patient 5 months later.

is now known that in view of the multiple factors involved, smoking need not be excessive for the condition to develop.

Prognosis

Before the use of vitamin B_{12} or hydroxocobalamin the patient was always warned that even if he followed instructions and stopped drinking and smoking, the condition might continue to worsen for two or more months before beginning to improve. Most patients made an excellent recovery, although the process often took up to 2 or 3 years [Figs. 118 and 119]. With hydroxocobalamin therapy recovery is relatively rapid and it seems patients do not need to give up smoking.

The degree of recovery depends upon the severity of the optic atrophy at the time at which the disease is first diagnosed and hydroxocobalamin therapy commenced. Thus, in a few cases, a field defect persists. The pallor of the optic disc gives some indication of the permanent damage to nerve fibres and the recovery that may be expected. It is interesting to follow the improvement in the visual fields and to note that the field defects disappear in exactly the reverse order to their development. When recovery is complete patients may resume moderate smoking with safety, particularly if their diet and vitamin B_{12} requirements are met.

Since it is rarely possible to remove eyes affected with tobacco amblyopia for microscopic examination, the pathology of this condition is not well understood. It is believed, however, that the toxin causes a degeneration of the retinal ganglion cells and the associated nerve fibres of the maculopapillary bundle.

ETHYL ALCOHOL

Chronic alcoholism may sometimes give rise to bilateral central scotomata even without the associated use of tobacco. Ethyl alcohol amblyopia is found in alcoholics who get their calorie intake from alcohol and have no further desire for food. As a result they lack protein and vitamins and are severely undernourished. A chronic gastritis causes severe anorexia. There may be polyneuritis. Patients complain of increasing haziness of vision and even of positive central scotomata. Examination on the Bjerrum screen may reveal scotomata of 5 degrees or more in diameter [Fig. 120]. Recovery from ethyl alcohol amblyopia is seldom complete.

ALCOHOL AMBLYOPIA

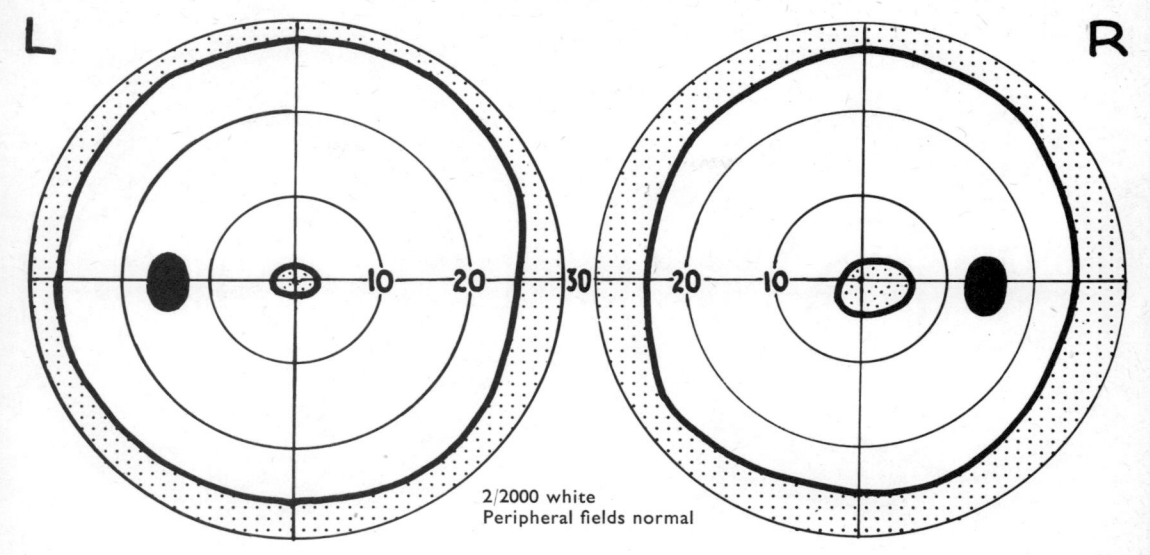

Fig. 120. Visual fields of an alcoholic. 2/2000 white. Peripheral fields normal.

Some observers have considered that impurities in the alcoholic beverages are the cause of the visual failure. But it would appear that the excessive alcoholic intake causes a chronic gastritis which in turn leads to poor appetite, anorexia, and defective absorption. Most alcoholics eat a very inadequate diet and these factors combine to lead to protein and vitamin B complex deficiency. The fact that there is so little recovery of sight also suggests a closer resemblance to nutritional amblyopia than to tobacco amblyopia.

METHYL ALCOHOL

Methyl alcohol or wood alcohol is sometimes used to lace a drink and add to its potency. Innocent victims may sometimes drink methyl alcohol in error. During the Second World War, groups of service men occasionally raided stores and obtained supplies of methyl alcohol, thinking it was ethyl alcohol. The parties that followed provided material for careful studies of methyl alcohol poisoning and amblyopia.

Susceptibility to its effects varies considerably from person to person. Some may ingest small quantities over a long period without harm. On the other hand, a teaspoonful has been reported to cause total permanent blindness. Ethyl alcohol appears to give some protection. If both forms of alcohol are imbibed together, the toxic effects of the methyl alcohol appear to be moderated.

Clinical Features

Methyl alcohol is metabolized more slowly than ethyl alcohol and it may be several days before it is fully excreted. When it is ingested there is usually a latent period of 18–48 hours. In mild cases the vision becomes hazy and there is headache, nausea, and vomiting. In more seriously affected patients, abdominal cramps and drowsiness may progress to coma and cyanosis. Fixed dilated pupils suggest a poor prognosis and, if persistent, herald approaching death.

Examination of the fundi during the early phase reveals hyperaemic optic discs. This is soon followed by oedema of the disc margins and adjacent retina and some venous congestion and dilatation. In mild cases the retinal oedema gradually subsides and the vision returns to normal.

The primary failure of vision which occurs at the onset persists a variable length of time. If sight returns within a few days the outlook is good, but if there is no improvement at the end of a week, the prognosis is poor. Secondary visual failure, which is common, may begin after a few weeks, and progress for 6–12 weeks, with increasing pallor of the optic disc

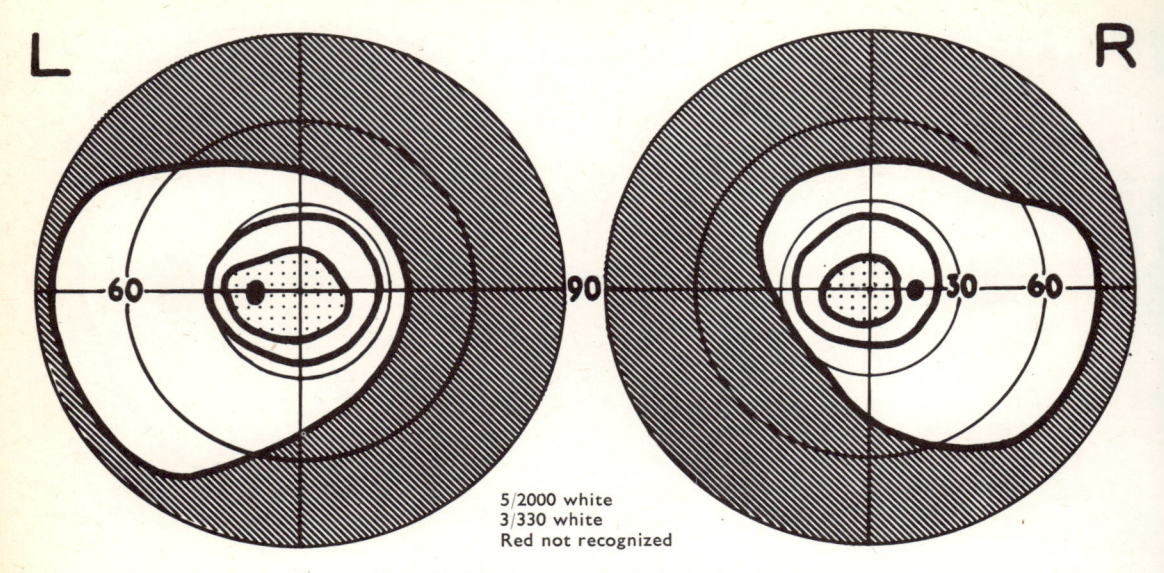

FIG. 121. Fields in methyl alcohol poisoning.

5/2000 white
3/330 white
Red not recognized

and narrowing of the blood vessels. An interesting phenomenon is that, in the more seriously affected patients, there may be cupping of the optic discs like that which is seen in ischaemia of the optic nerve resulting in cavernous atrophy.

Eyes which have been removed from persons who have died in the first 2 days have revealed almost normal retinal ganglion cells and optic nerve fibres apart from oedema of these structures which might be due to post-mortem changes. But in the late stages of the condition degeneration of the retinal ganglion cells and optic nerve fibres is apparent.

Field Changes

During the primary visual failure there is a marked loss of colour vision, particularly to green and red. Dense bilateral central scotomata appear [FIG. 121]. The peripheral field usually remains normal, but sometimes there is a break-through to the periphery.

In mild cases, there may be complete recovery of vision and disappearance of scotomata. More severely affected patients may be left with permanent central scotomata. When secondary visual failure occurs, the central scotomata become progressively larger and denser, and complete blindness may result.

Prognosis should be guarded, because the secondary visual failure may be delayed for several weeks, and may continue for several months.

Pathogenesis

The exact mechanism of the action of methyl alcohol is unknown. It is believed that it is oxidized through formaldehyde to formate and thence to carbon dioxide and water. But it is still not known whether formaldehyde, formate or formic acid is the main toxic element. The most striking action of methyl alcohol is the production of acidosis, the severity of which appears to be closely related to the severity of the poisoning and the visual failure.

CHLOROQUINE AND HYDROXYCHLOROQUINE

These drugs were originally introduced for the prophylaxis and treatment of malaria. For this purpose they are effective in relatively small doses of 500 mg. weekly and appear to cause no toxic changes. However, in higher doses of 250–500 mg. daily, they have been found to be of value in such conditions as rheumatoid arthritis, actinic dermatitis, lupus erythematosus and other collagenous diseases. About one third of the patients who are maintained

CHLOROQUINE AND HYDROXYCHLOROQUINE AMBLYOPIA

on this high dosage develop a keratopathy after 6 months. The lesions are bilateral and are situated in the lower half of the cornea. They begin as minute, intraepithelial, yellowish, punctate dots and may progress to become denser and darker to a brownish coloration. The corneal epithelium may become oedematous so that the visual acuity is defective. Later the opacities may coalesce to form lines. If the drug is stopped these corneal changes rapidly disappear.

A much more serious lesion is the retinopathy which occasionally develops. Chloroquine appears to be bound to desoxyribonucleic acid and is concentrated in the pigmented tissues of the eye. In certain individuals it causes destruction of the ganglion cells and rods and cones and dispersal of the retinal pigment.

These pathological changes are sometimes preceded by complaints of blurred vision, photopsia and colour hallucinations. In the early stages no fundal changes may be observed but there is a gradual loss of the foveal reflex followed by the deposition of fine pigment dots in the macular area round the fovea with the later development of the typical 'bull's eye' appearance. Unfortunately, loss of foveal reflex and fine pigment changes in the macular area occur quite commonly in the older age group so that their relation to chloroquine toxicity in a given case may be difficult to determine. With time, however, the pigmentary changes become more obvious, the field defects more definite and there is narrowing of the retinal arteries and optic atrophy.

Once toxic changes begin to develop they usually progress even though the administration of chloroquine is stopped immediately. In fact, cases have been recorded in which loss of central vision occurred months or even a few years after the use of the drug was discontinued.

For a long time attempts were made to discover a method of detecting those patients who might develop toxic changes in the retina, so that chloroquine could be stopped in time to prevent loss of vision. These attempts at first were unsuccessful, but in a large series of cases Percival and Behrman showed that in a small group of patients arcuate scotomata could be demonstrated with a 7·5 mm. red target 4–9 degrees from fixation [FIG. 122] before any defects could be found with a 1/1000 white target, and before any loss of visual acuity occurred. They termed this condition 'premaculopathy' and showed that if the chloroquine was stopped immediately these changes were observed, there was no loss of vision, and the arcuate scotomata to red disappeared.

Patients who are not discovered in this early stage progress to more serious loss of vision. The arcuate scotomata become denser and

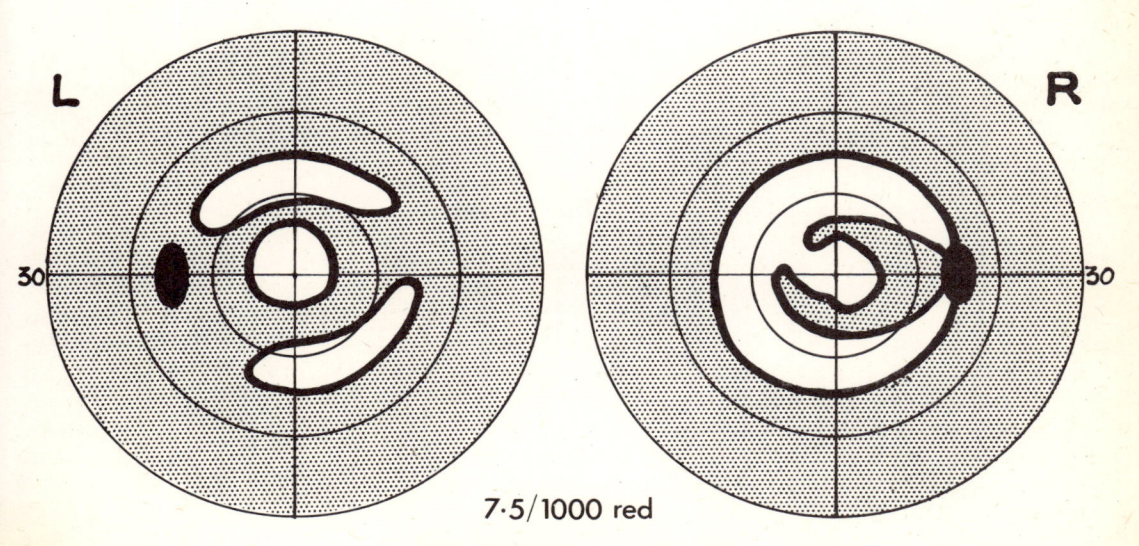

FIG. 122. Chloroquine 'premaculopathy'.

2/2000 white
V.A. 20/20 R and L

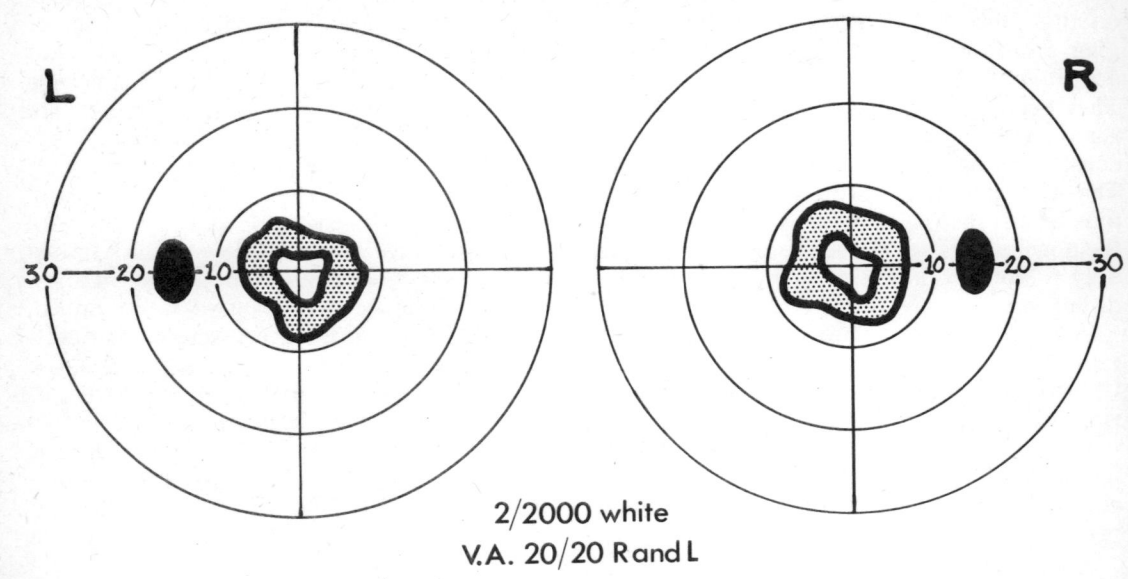

FIG. 123. Early chloroquine amblyopia.

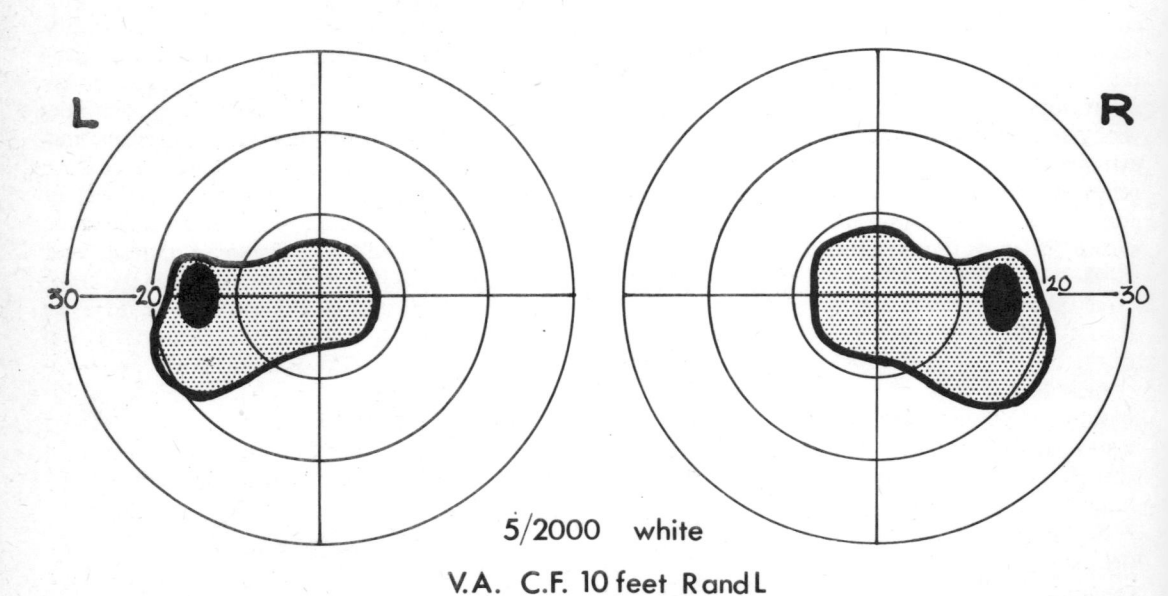

5/2000 white
V.A. C.F. 10 feet R and L

FIG. 124. Late chloroquine amblyopia.

3/330 white
V.A. R.C.F. at 5 feet
L.C.F. at 2 feet

FIG. 125. Late chloroquine retinopathy.

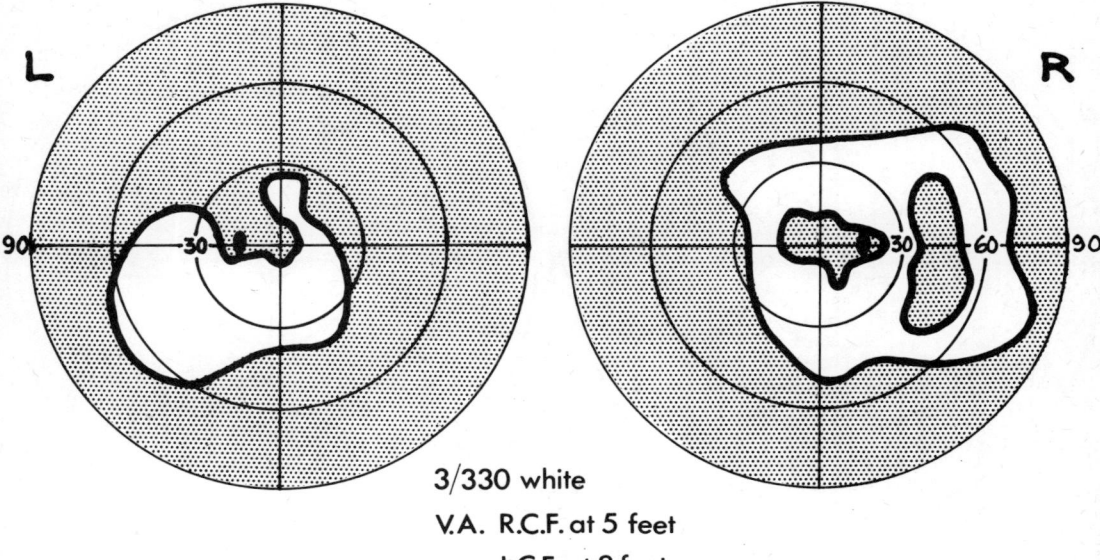

larger and can be plotted with white targets. They arch around the fovea to form a complete ring scotoma, often leaving a small central island of vision [FIG. 123]. This island eventually disappears and a dense central scotoma develops so that vision is reduced to less than 20/200 [FIG. 124]. If the patient is first discovered at this stage, stopping the administration of chloroquine does not halt the progress of the disease. The central scotoma usually becomes denser and spreads to involve the area within 10 degrees from the fixation. Peripheral vision usually persists though there may be some contraction of the peripheral field in the late stages [FIG. 125].

Some cases have been reported in which the drug was stopped because of the corneal changes but loss of vision nevertheless developed months later. Unfortunately the visual fields in these cases were not studied at the time the administration was stopped. It is not known, therefore, whether scotomata to 7·5/1000 red would have been demonstrated at that time. It is obvious that patients taking large doses of chloroquine for long periods require very careful, regular monitoring to prevent the development of chloroquine retinopathy.

DIGITALIS

Visual illusions or hallucinations are not uncommon when patients take an excessive dose of this drug. Objects may appear brilliant or scintillating, and flashes of light may be seen. Green, blue, or yellow vision may be described. It often occurs about two weeks after the commencement of treatment and, in susceptible patients, even a normal dosage may cause these symptoms. Persistence with excessive dosage may lead to the development of bilateral central scotomata, usually within the 5 degree isopter [FIG. 126]. Recovery occurs in about 3 weeks when the dosage is reduced.

SULPHONAMIDES

A few cases have been reported in which sulphonamide intoxication caused optic neuropathy with central scotomata. Withdrawal of the drug resulted in recovery.

THALLIUM

Depilatory creams used to contain this ingredient but do so no longer. This very toxic heavy metal is still used as a poison for rodents and insects, especially rats and cockroaches. It produces nausea, vomiting, abdominal cramps

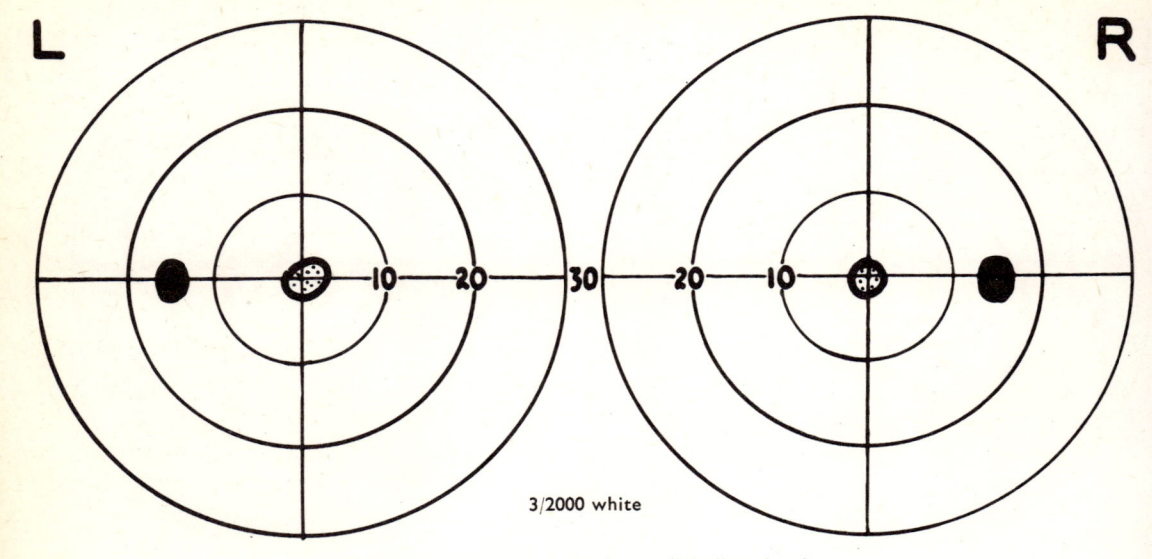

FIG. 126. Central scotomata due to digitalis poisoning.

and polyneuritis of feet and legs with painful weakness and paralysis. There may be difficulty in breathing and psychic anomalies such as depression and insomnia.

After 2 or 3 weeks the hair may loosen and fall out, including the outer one third of the eyebrows.

Optic neuropathy may occur, giving rise to central scotomata. Thallium is rapidly excreted, and stopping the ingestion of the drug usually results in speedy recovery from the general symptoms, but although some visual improvement may occur the central scotomata usually persist.

IODOFORM

Formerly iodoform was in frequent use for dressing wounds. It is rarely used today and intoxication by this drug is therefore extremely rare. Bilateral central scotomata may result from its excessive use.

TOXINS CAUSING BILATERAL PERIPHERAL CONTRACTION

QUININE

People with an idiosyncrasy to this drug may develop cinchonism or symptoms of overdosage with small doses, but this is rare. It is more commonly the result of excessive administration. Until its displacement by newer and more effective remedies, quinine was the most popular antimalarial drug. It was then not uncommon for overdosage to occur as a result of a mistaken belief that the greater the intake the more rapid the cure. It is still used at times in an attempt to end an undesired pregnancy.

Clinical Features

Cinchonism causes deafness and tinnitus, and these symptoms always precede the visual disturbances. Contraction of the visual field occurs abruptly. In the acute stage the pupils are dilated and fixed and do not react to light. If the fundi are examined at this time, the picture is that of generalized retinal arterial spasm, with blurring of the disc margins and retinal oedema. In severe cases, the ophthalmoscopic appearance may resemble a central retinal artery occlusion.

If the administration of quinine is stopped at once, the patient may recover. Improvement is slow and it may continue for several months. Recovery may be slight or complete.

Many methods of treatment have been recommended but it appears that repeated blocks of the stellate ganglion on each side to combat the retinal vasospasm offers the best hope of visual recovery. One case is reported in which full recovery from complete blindness

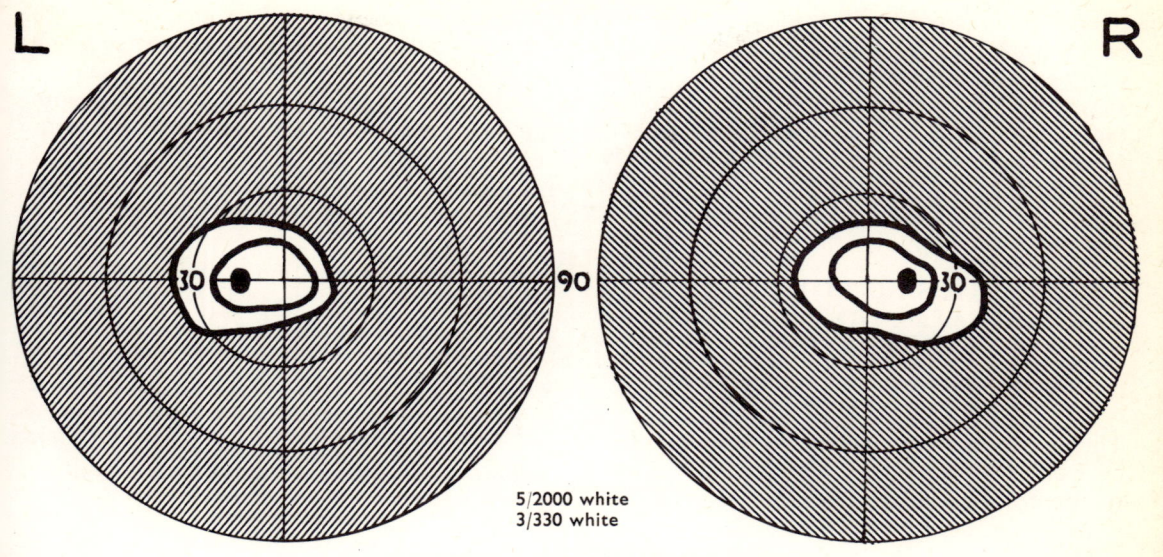

FIG. 127. Visual fields of a patient 3 years after she took 90 grains of quinine in one dose to cause abortion.

5/2000 white
3/330 white

followed stellate ganglion block repeated 19 times during 7 days, each injection being given when the patient noticed any deterioration of vision.

Field Changes

The field changes are best demonstrated by perimetry [FIG. 127]. This reveals bilateral 'telescopic' fields. The contraction is seldom circular. It is usually oval in shape with the long axis horizontal. The vision may remain surprisingly good, e.g. 20/30, despite marked field contraction and pale optic discs.

The patient is left with bilateral central islands of vision with steep edges. She complains of night blindness and has difficulty in locating objects outside her telescopic view. The end result thus resembles retinitis pigmentosa from the functional point of view though not in fundal appearance.

SALICYLATES

As in the case of quinine, large doses of salicylates are usually required to produce toxic symptoms. These may occasionally follow the administration of a small dose in patients with idiosyncrasy. Deafness and tinnitus precede the visual symptoms. The visual changes are similar to those caused by quinine, but less severe. Withdrawal of the drug always results in complete recovery.

ARSENIC

In earlier days, tryparsamide was used a great deal in the treatment of general paralysis of the insane. It was the custom for venereologists to send patients who were receiving this drug to the ophthalmic department at monthly intervals for checking of the peripheral fields. At the first sign of peripheral contraction, the tryparsamide was stopped. If the condition was not recognized at once, the vision deteriorated rapidly and little recovery could be expected.

Other arsenical compounds like *Acetylarsan*, atoxyl, *Stovarsol*, and *Soamin* may all produce progressive peripheral contraction leading to severe visual failure from which there is no recovery (Igersheimer). Dimercaprol (B.A.L.) has been shown to be a valuable antidote. Several cases with severely contracted fields due to arsenicals have made remarkable recoveries following its use.

FILIX MAS (ASPIDIUM)

This drug is used as a vermifuge. Tapeworms are sometimes very difficult to dislodge, and filix mas is one of the most useful remedies in stubborn cases. It resembles quinine in its effects, and it may cause temporary or permanent contraction of the fields. Idiosyncrasy appears to play a large part in the severity of symptoms. A strange feature of this drug is that the visual loss may sometimes be confined to one eye. This has not been satisfactorily explained.

TOXINS CAUSING BOTH CENTRAL SCOTOMATA AND PERIPHERAL CONTRACTION

QUINOLINE AND PHENOTHIAZINE DERIVATIVES

This group of drugs includes a large number of medications used in high dosage in the treatment of psychiatric patients, e.g. NP 207, thioridazine, chlorpromazine.

These patients may develop pigmentation of skin, cornea, and conjunctiva, which appears to result from exposure to light. Light brown, dusty pigmentation may appear in the pupillary area of the lens and progress to form an anterior capsular and subcapsular stellate cataract. Scattered retinal pigmentation may develop through the fundus.

The visual acuity is severely depressed. The visual fields are constricted and exhibit central scotomata. Most of these patients are difficult or impossible to examine adequately for visual fields because of their mental state. When the drug is stopped vision often deteriorates further for about 2 months before improvement occurs, but full recovery is seldom obtained and retinal pigmentation usually persists.

ETHAMBUTOL

This drug has proved of value in the treatment of advanced tuberculosis. It has been found that when a dosage greater than 35 mg. per kg. per day is administered for about 6 months, some 15 per cent of patients develop ocular toxicity. A dosage of 25 mg. per kg. per day appears to be relatively safe. The ocular neuropathy which develops may affect either the central or peripheral vision. When the axial nerve fibres are involved the patient complains of blurring of vision. A central or paracentral scotoma may be found. The optic discs and fundi appear normal. An unusual feature which has been reported is the inability to recognize green, which is thought to be white or grey.

When the drug is stopped the vision may continue to deteriorate for a few weeks but then recovery occurs. In most patients vision is restored to normal in 6 months. The administration of vitamins does not hasten recovery.

An unusual observation is that ocular toxicity is almost confined to males. There appears to be no explanation of this sexual incidence.

It is essential that all patients being treated with ethambutol or any related drug should have visual acuity and visual fields examined before therapy and at regular monthly intervals while it is being administered.

CHLORAMPHENICOL

A few patients who have been on prolonged courses of chloramphenicol have developed optic neuropathy. These patients have usually been severely ill and debilitated. The suggestion has been made that the condition may really be a nutritional optic neuropathy due to malabsorption of vitamins. Both eyes are affected and vision fails rapidly. The optic discs may or may not be swollen and in a few of the reported cases retinal haemorrhages and exudates have been observed.

Some improvement following the administration of vitamin B complex has been reported in a few cases, but in most there is little or no recovery.

The field changes which occur are not well documented but central scotomata and peripheral constriction have both been described.

LEAD

Lead intoxication is rarely seen today because precautions are enforced by law in factories where it is used in industrial processes. It may occur in painters or plumbers. Young children may be affected by sucking lead paint off toys.

Acute intoxication causes abrupt loss of sight, but recovery is usually complete. Chronic intoxication is more serious. There is a history of long exposure. In patients with pyorrhoea, a blue 'lead' line may appear on the gums. There is anaemia, and the red cells may show basophilic stippling. Colic may be severe. Lead is found in the urine. Bilateral diffuse central scotomata occur most commonly, and there is often an associated peripheral field loss. In severe intoxication, optic atrophy ensues and there may be little or no recovery.

ANILINE DYES

These are much used in industry and may be inhaled or absorbed through the skin. Methaemoglobinaemia and cyanosis precede the loss of vision. Bilateral central scotomata occur, but there may also be some peripheral field loss.

CARBON BISULPHIDE

This chemical is used in vulcanizing rubber, and in the rayon industry. Like the aniline dyes it may be absorbed through the skin or inhaled. It, too, causes central scotomata and associated peripheral field loss.

OPTOCHIN

Before the introduction of the antibiotics, this drug was used in the treatment of pneumonia. It is interesting that, although it is a derivative of quinine, it tended to cause bilateral central scotomata. Peripheral contraction sometimes occurred, but the central defects were more pronounced.

ERGOT

Serious outbreaks of ergot poisoning have occurred in poor communities, especially in Russia. It is due to a fungus growing on stored damp rye. In acute intoxication, peripheral contraction and central scotomata may develop. There may be some recovery, but it is seldom complete.

In all these intoxications there appears to be much variation in susceptibility from person to person. The state of nutrition is also an important factor. Lack of protein and deficiency of the vitamin B complex reduce resistance to these toxins. Diabetes also reduces resistance considerably.

Numerous new drugs and chemical substances are constantly being produced. It is inevitable that some of these will cause toxic amblyopia. One must therefore be on the alert for new preparations which may be the cause of unexplained loss of vision.

Other substances which have been reported to cause toxic amblyopia are:

Barbital
Benzene
Carbon monoxide
Carbon tetrachloride
Disulfiram
Some hair dyes (coal-tar derivatives)
Isoniazid
Mepacrine
Methyl bromide (used in fire extinguishers)
Methyl chloride (used in refrigerators)
Methyl iodide
Pamaquin
Para-aminosalicylic acid
Phenytoin
Streptomycin

REFERENCES AND FURTHER READING

BENTON, C. D., and CALHOUN, F. P. (1953) The ocular effects of methyl alcohol poisoning (Report of a catastrophe involving 320 persons), *Amer. J. Ophthal.*, **36**, 1677.

CARROLL, FRANK D. (1956) Toxic amblyopia, *Trans. Amer. Acad. Ophthal. Otolaryng.*, **60**, 74.

CHISHOLM, I. A., BRONTE-STEWART, J., and FOULDS, W. S. (1967) Hydroxocobalamin versus cyanocobalamin in the treatment of tobacco amblyopia, *Lancet*, ii, 450.

HEATON, J. M., MCCORMICK, A. J. A., and FREEMAN, A. G. (1958) Tobacco amblyopia: A clinical manifestation of vitamin B_{12} deficiency, *Lancet*, ii, 286.

HOBBS, H. E., EADIE, S. P., and SOMERVILLE, F. (1961) Ocular lesions after treatment with chloroquine, *Brit. J. Ophthal.*, **45**, 284.

LAMBA, P. A., SOOD, N. N., and MOORTHY, S. S. (1968) Retinopathy due to chloramphenicol, *Scot. med. J.*, **13**, 166.

LEIBOLD, J. E. (1963) in *Transactions of Lederle's 3rd Ethambutol Conference*, p. 52, Denver.

OEHNINGER, C., BARRIOS, R. R., and HAEDO, C. A. G. (1955) Optic neuritis caused by arsenicals; treatment with B.A.L., *Brit. J. Ophthal.*, **39**, 422.

PERCIVAL, S. P. B., and BEHRMAN, J. (1969) Ophthalmological safety of chloroquine, *Brit. J. Ophthal.*, **53**, 101.

REED, H., and KARLINSKY, W. L. (1967) Delayed onset of chloroquine retinopathy, *Canad. med. Ass. J.*, **97**, 1408.

SHIRLEY, S. Y. (1963) Ocular complications of chloroquine therapy, *Trans. Canad. ophthal. Soc.*, **26**, 153.

12
OPTIC NERVE LESIONS

The optic nerve is the beginning of the visual pathway. Only its nerve head in the eye can be examined directly with the ophthalmoscope. This may show, among other changes, oedema, inflammation, or atrophy. Without the aid of perimetric examination it is sometimes difficult, or even impossible, to distinguish with certainty between oedema and inflammation, or between a pale but normal disc and early atrophy. In the majority of optic nerve lesions the appearance of the optic disc contributes little to the diagnosis. Most information about the nature of the lesion is gained by a study of the visual fields.

The various affections will be considered in the following order: Hereditary affections, deficiency disorders, inflammatory lesions, compression, traumatic and vascular lesions.

HEREDITARY AFFECTIONS
HEREDITARY OPTIC ATROPHY

During recent years it has become clear that a number of separate clinical entities have been included under this one heading. The best-known type was described by Leber. It was formerly assumed that Leber's disease followed a simple sex-linked recessive mode of inheritance. This cannot be accepted because, although it affects males chiefly, females often develop it. Moreover, in sibships, the sisters of affected men are usually carriers, but it seems that an affected man does not pass the condition to a son, nor cause a carrier state in a daughter. Transmission appears to be by continuous descent through female carriers. Thus, Leber's disease cannot be adequately explained by our present knowledge of sex chromosomes.

There appear to be at least four other types of hereditary optic atrophy.
1. A dominant congenital type in which the optic atrophy is present at birth. This is probably better termed hereditary agenesis.
2. A recessive congenital optic atrophy or agenesis.
3. A dominant juvenile optic atrophy commencing at any age from two to adolescence.
4. A dominant optic atrophy beginning either during or after adolescence and in many cases slowly progressive throughout life.

It will thus be seen that there is a great variation in the age of onset of hereditary optic atrophy. The recorded pedigrees show that most of the known modes of inheritance have been represented. In any given family the visual acuity of some members may be worse than others. Nystagmus and mental defects may also occur.

Field Changes

The typical case of Leber's disease occurs abruptly in the late teens, develops over a period of a few months, and shows little tendency to recover. The second eye is affected a few weeks or months after the first. Occasionally, this condition occurs in childhood or even in adult life.

Each eye develops a central scotoma [FIG. 128]. The central area of the scotoma is absolute and it has fairly steep margins. The peripheral vision normally remains intact, but occasionally a break-through to the periphery can be found with small targets. The field changes resemble those of retrobulbar neuritis in development, but differ in that they remain stationary throughout life. Scotometry is difficult, because steady central fixation is not possible. Vision is usually reduced to counting fingers at 3 or 4 metres, but occasionally it does not deteriorate beyond 20/80.

These cases may cause difficulty in diagnosis at their onset. If other members of the family show signs of the disease, the diagnosis is clear, but occasionally no other member of the family is affected. The appearance in a male at or just after puberty of bilateral central scoto-

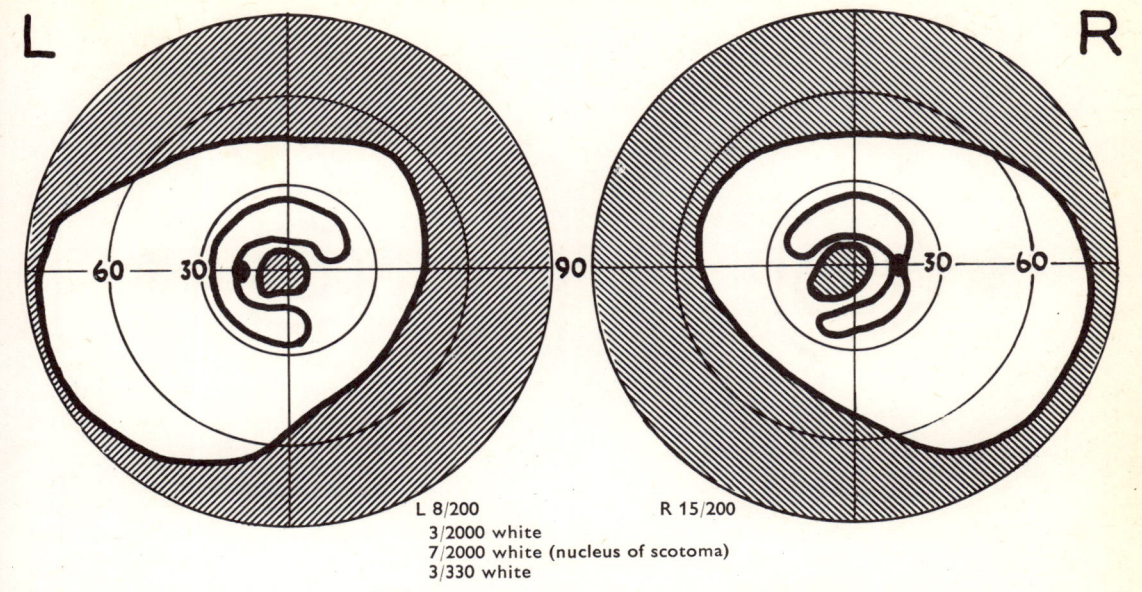

FIG. 128. Visual fields of a patient with hereditary optic atrophy.

L 8/200
R 15/200
3/2000 white
7/2000 white (nucleus of scotoma)
3/330 white

mata, which develop fairly rapidly, show little tendency to improve, and then remain stationary without any other associated neurological sign, is adequate evidence of Leber's disease. If the condition occurs in a female or in a young child careful investigations to eliminate a demyelinating disease, and a period of observation are required before the diagnosis of hereditary optic atrophy should be accepted.

Wilson found that the plasma thiocyanate level was significantly lower in smokers with Leber's optic atrophy than in normal cigarette smokers. He suggested that this indicated a block in the conversion of cyanide to thiocyanate. It appears that thiamine or cyanocobalamin or perhaps both are required for this conversion to occur. It seems possible that a breakdown of the conversion is responsible for the central scotomata which occur in tobacco amblyopia, pernicious anaemia, nutritional amblyopia, and even Leber's optic atrophy.

DEFICIENCY DISORDERS
NUTRITIONAL AMBLYOPIA

Defective vision developed in many prisoners in Japanese camps during the Second World War. They were grossly undernourished and it appeared that lack of vitamin B and an inadequate protein intake were the chief causes of the amblyopia (see Leber's optic atrophy).

Visual failure was the chief manifestation of this condition. But many prisoners developed manifestations of pellagra and beriberi. Ataxia and paraesthesiae in the legs and feet resulted from posterior column loss, and were accompanied by paraplegia. Diarrhoea was common, and some had nerve deafness and vocal cord paralysis.

In most of these patients the vision of each eye was reduced to 20/200 by a dense central scotoma [FIG. 129]. Temporal pallor was marked, and little recovery occurred on return to a normal diet. The peripheral field was normal.

OPTIC NEUROPATHY DUE TO PERNICIOUS ANAEMIA

Centrocaecal scotomata, more obvious with red targets and indistinguishable from defects found in tobacco amblyopia, may occur in pernicious anaemia. The peculiar susceptibility to tobacco amblyopia of patients with pernicious anaemia has been noted by several earlier authors but the fact that the optic neuropathy of pernicious anaemia and tobacco amblyopia

OPTIC NERVE LESIONS

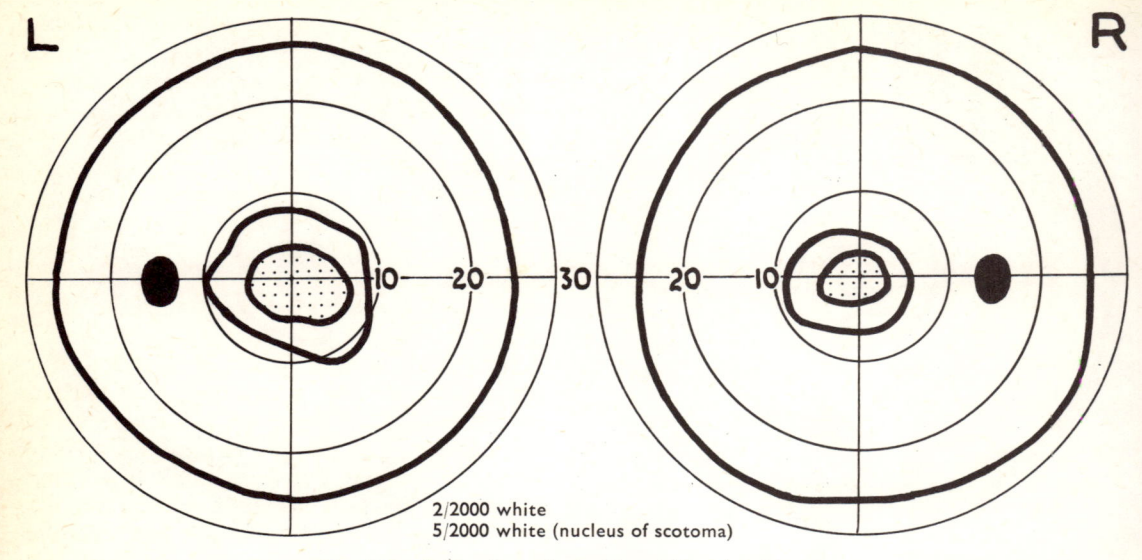

2/2000 white
5/2000 white (nucleus of scotoma)

Fig. 129. Fields of a patient with nutritional amblyopia.

are probably the same lesions has only recently been emphasized by Foulds and his co-workers.

They have shown that whilst the haemopoietic abnormality in pernicious anaemia may be cured rapidly with cyanocobalamin, in some cases the visual defect does not recover until treatment is changed and hydroxocobalamin is given. In tobacco amblyopia hydroxocobalamin has also been found to be more effective in treatment than cyanocobalamin (see tobacco amblyopia).

It has been suggested that both these conditions are a manifestation of a failure to detoxify cyanide. There is also some evidence that Leber's optic atrophy may be due to a related defect.

INFLAMMATORY LESIONS
RETROBULBAR NEURITIS AND PAPILLITIS

No useful purpose is served by separating these two conditions. Both are types of optic neuritis with the same aetiology and visual field changes. The only difference is the site of the inflammation: If the inflammation of the optic nerve is close enough to the globe to cause an inflammatory swelling of the disc which can be seen with the ophthalmoscope, it is called papillitis. If the inflammation is farther back, so that no swelling can be seen, it is termed retrobulbar neuritis.

It should be noted that retrobulbar neuritis is more common than papillitis.

Clinical Features

Retrobulbar neuritis occurs most commonly in young women. It is usually unilateral. The loss of vision is rapid, reaching a maximum in a few hours or days. It may be associated with pain behind the eye, which is made worse by ocular movements or by pressure upon the eye. The insertion of the superior rectus muscle is sometimes especially tender. The pupil shows a lack of sustained constriction to direct light, and the fundus appears normal.

In *papillitis*, involvement of the optic disc is indicated by oedema, and perhaps a few adjacent haemorrhages. The field defect is usually more extensive than in cases of retrobulbar neuritis.

The ophthalmoscopic appearance of papillitis may resemble that of papilloedema. Papillitis is usually associated with rapid visual failure, whilst in papilloedema the vision is relatively unaffected until a late stage. In papillitis, inflammatory cells can sometimes be seen in the posterior vitreous but they do not normally occur in papilloedema.

The pupil reaction to direct light is especially

INFLAMMATORY LESIONS

clude the diagnosis but its presence is highly significant.

The characteristic field defect of both retrobulbar neuritis and papillitis is a central scotoma [FIGS. 130 and 131]. It may be only 2 or 3 degrees in diameter, but more often it is larger and can be 40 or 50 degrees in diameter. The peripheral field is usually intact, but there may be a break-through from the centre to the periphery, particularly on the nasal side. In some cases the vision may be reduced to mere perception of light.

The central scotoma is usually absolute, but occasionally it may be relative. It is seldom exactly central and circular, and it may be of any shape or size. Rarely, it may not involve the fixation area. It may be arcuate, arching around the fixation point. In these cases the visual acuity may be unaffected. The scotoma usually has steep margins, but the steepness tends to vary in different areas. Sector and arcuate defects, though not usual, tend to occur more frequently in papillitis than in retrobulbar neuritis.

Plotting the isopter for recognition of the red 15/2000 target is often of value in assessing disproportion. At first, red may not be recognized in any part of the field. With recovery, its hue is first recognized about 20 degrees from the fixation point. Gradually the area in which the colour can be identified increases.

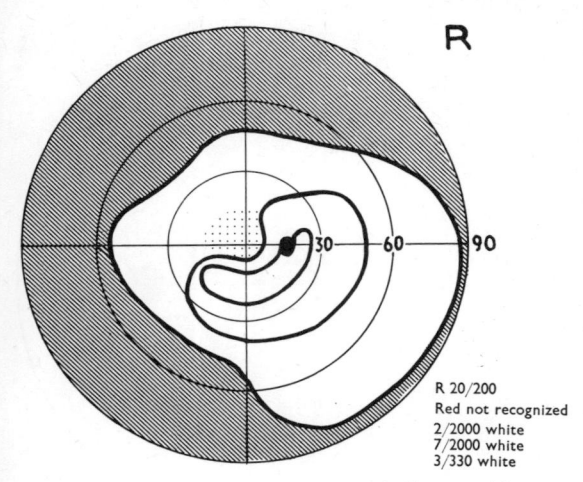

FIG. 130. Visual field defect in retrobulbar neuritis.

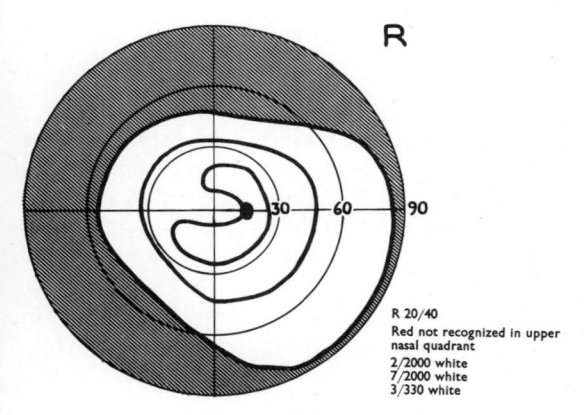

FIG. 131. Retrobulbar neuritis; the field 8 days later (cf. FIG. 130).

important in diagnosis. If one eye is covered to exclude light and a bright light is shone into the other eye and then the cover and light alternated between the two eyes, the pupil of the eye with the optic neuritis will dilate when illuminated in contrast with the pupil of the normal eye which constricts. This phenomenon occurs because the dilatation produced by withdrawal of light from the normal eye outweighs the constriction produced by the light on the affected eye.

Pain behind the eye aggravated by movement or pressure on the eye is an important symptom in both papillitis and retrobulbar neuritis. It occurs in less than half the patients with this condition. Its absence therefore does not ex-

Prognosis

Recovery usually occurs and may take from 3 weeks to 3 months. The more rapid the recovery, the more complete it is likely to be [FIGS. 132 and 133]. Slow recovery usually indicates that there will be severe residual visual impairment.

Some improvement may take place even after 3 months. The presence of disproportion is an indication of activity, and, as long as this sign remains, further recovery may be hoped for. Even when recovery appears to be complete and vision has returned to 20/20 a relative scotoma may be found with a 10/2000 red target. If this is analysed carefully it may be found to have a dense paracentral nucleus.

Pallor of the disc usually begins to develop about one month after the onset of the disease. The vision may return to 20/20 even whilst the disc is developing the pallor.

OPTIC NERVE LESIONS

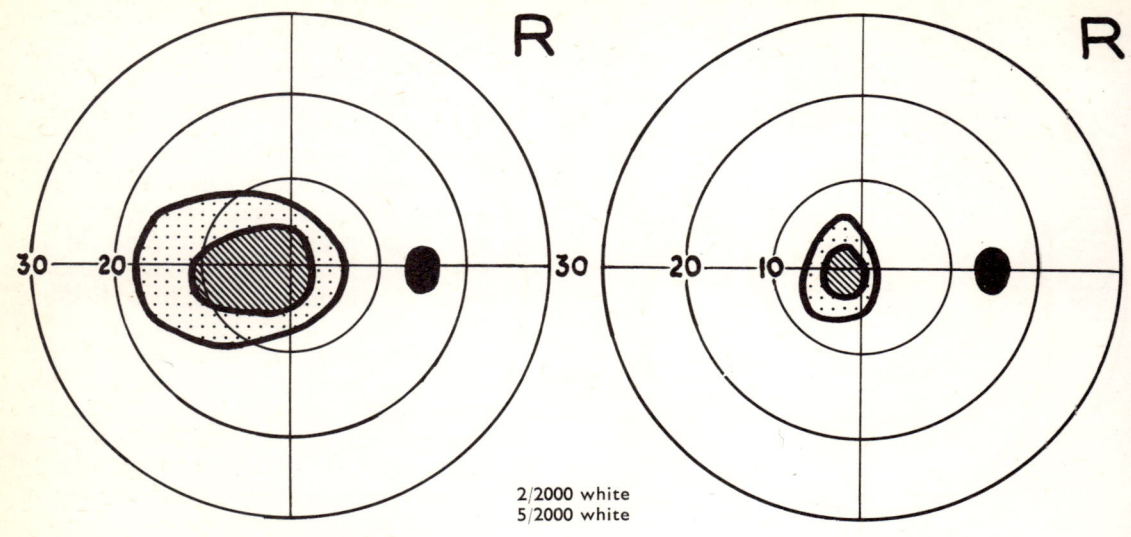

FIG. 132. Central scotoma in retrobulbar neuritis.

2/2000 white
5/2000 white

FIG. 133. Two weeks later.

In disseminated sclerosis the patient may be able to read 20/20 in spite of apparently advanced optic atrophy. If the visual fields of these patients are examined with small targets they are usually found to have relative scotomata with small dense nuclei close to the fixation point, and some contraction of peripheral isopters.

If recovery is not almost complete after 2 or 3 months the diagnosis should be reviewed. The possibility of an intracranial tumour such as a meningioma of the olfactory groove or sphenoid ridge, or an aneurysm compressing the optic nerve should always be borne in mind. These tumours may even permit partial recovery followed by further loss of vision after a few weeks or months. All cases of retrobulbar neuritis should be followed at regular intervals for checks of vision and field to eliminate the possibility of intracranial tumours.

Investigations

It is seldom possible to determine the site of a patch of inflammation in the optic nerve by the characters of the field defect. When a scotoma has been discovered, it should always be analysed in an attempt to determine which group of nerve fibres is involved. Only one field pattern gives a clear indication of the site of the lesion.

A characteristic junction defect [FIG. 134] is produced by a lesion of the optic nerve at its union with the optic chiasma. In all cases of retrobulbar neuritis the field of the apparently normal eye must therefore be examined to eliminate a hemianopic defect or junction scotoma which would indicate chiasmal interference.

BILATERAL RETROBULBAR NEURITIS

When the disease is bilateral, the visual loss is usually more severe, and it develops with greater rapidity [FIG. 135]. As a rule, one eye is affected before the other. There is often an accompanying inflammatory swelling of the optic discs, and in these cases the term papillitis is more correct.

Myelitis of the spinal cord may precede or follow bilateral retrobulbar neuritis, a combination known as Devic's disease or neuromyelitis optica. A number of these patients later develop disseminated sclerosis, but others show no further signs of neurological disease. The aetiology of Devic's disease and of disseminated sclerosis is not understood, but it seems likely that they are closely related.

Aetiology of Retrobulbar Neuritis

In the majority of cases exhaustive investiga-

INFLAMMATORY LESIONS

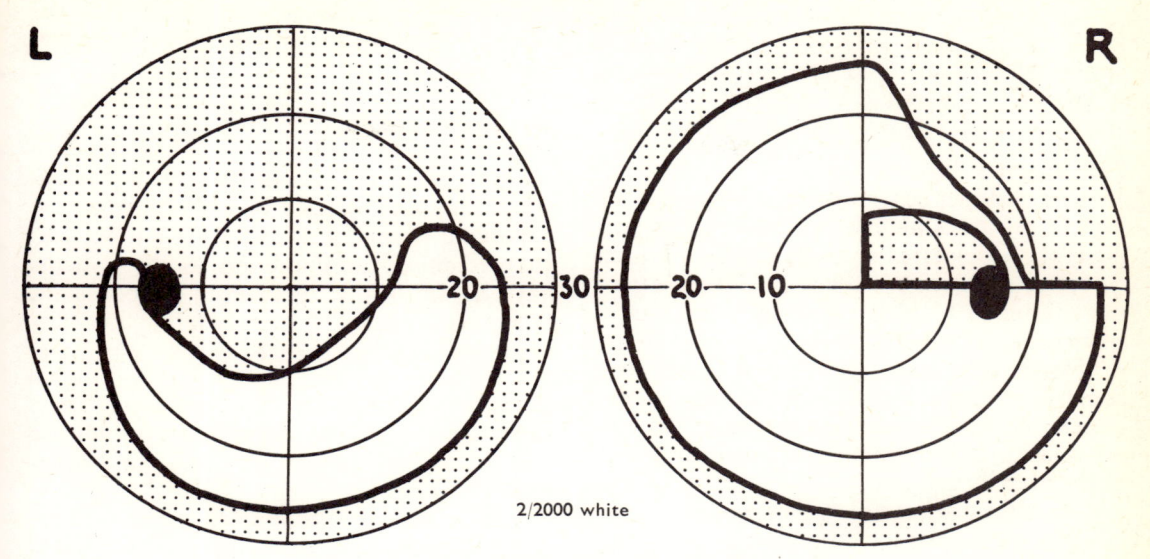

2/2000 white

FIG. 134. A junctional scotoma in the visual field of the right eye.

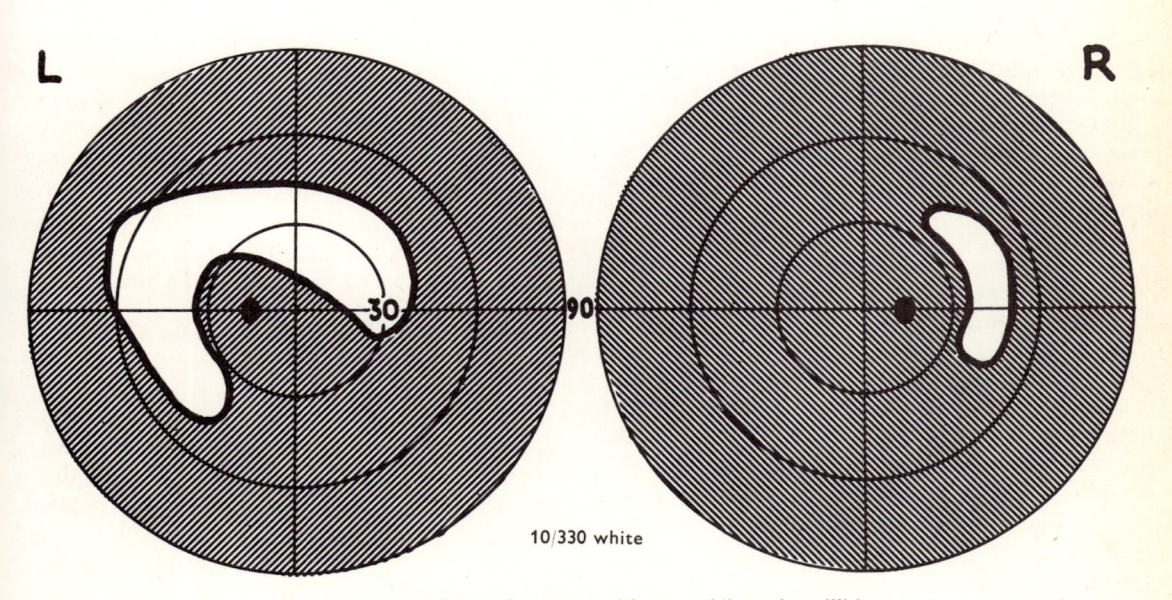

10/330 white

FIG. 135. Visual fields of a patient with severe bilateral papillitis.

tions reveal no definite evidence of the cause of optic neuritis. It belongs to the demyelinating group of diseases, and the nature of these affections is imperfectly understood.

Disseminated Sclerosis
Less than 50 per cent of patients who have an attack of optic neuritis eventually develop signs of disseminated sclerosis in other parts of the central nervous system. This disease frequently makes its debut with an acute attack of retrobulbar neuritis. It is this manifestation of disseminated sclerosis which is most often seen by ophthalmologists. Not infrequently the attack of retrobulbar neuritis may precede other symptoms of multiple sclerosis by many years, even 20 or more.

Late in the disease, a slowly progressive optic atrophy may cause increasing peripheral contraction and visual depression. Ophthalmologists see these patients less frequently, because at this stage they are usually under the care of a neurologist.

The optic nerve is most commonly attacked in disseminated sclerosis, but, occasionally, the chiasma or the optic tract and even the optic radiations [FIG. 167] may also be involved. A characteristic feature of retrobulbar neuritis due to disseminated sclerosis is the changing nature of the field defects which may vary from day to day. Occasionally, homonymous scotomata may appear and disappear like those of the more anterior demyelinating lesions.

It may be stated in general terms that disseminated sclerosis may attack any part of the visual pathway, but that the more posterior the area the less frequently it is affected.

Sinusitis
It was once thought that sinusitis was a common cause of retrobulbar neuritis. It had been found that drainage of the sinuses at the onset of the condition was followed by rapid recovery of sight. It was therefore argued that this must be cause and effect. But the great majority of cases of retrobulbar neuritis recover without treatment, and they are rarely associated with frank sinusitis. Authentic cases secondary to sinusitis do occur, but in these the signs of the purulent sinusitis are likely to be more obvious than the visual defects. It is wise, however, in all cases of retrobulbar neuritis, to investigate the possibility of an associated or causative sinusitis.

Other Associations
Retrobulbar neuritis may be associated with puberty, pregnancy, lactation, and the menopause. In these cases it is possible that the metabolic change may reduce resistance and so precipitate the condition. Some patients have no further demyelinating episodes, but others later develop manifestations of disseminated sclerosis. There is also good evidence that the metabolic and hormonal changes occurring in these conditions may activate meningiomas and pituitary tumours so that visual field changes may occur and simulate optic neuritis.

Rare causes of retrobulbar neuritis are sub-acute combined degeneration of the spinal cord, diabetes mellitus, syphilis, arachnoiditis, and acute viral infections.

SYPHILITIC OPTIC ATROPHY
Tabetic optic atrophy occurs about 15 years after the primary infection with syphilis. It is progressive and bilateral. One eye is usually more severely affected than the other.

In the early stages the visual field may show general depression [FIG. 136]. It is best demonstrated with the 3/330 and 5/2000 white targets. The depression may be most irregular.

Gross disproportion is a characteristic finding. The red target isopters contract rapidly, and after the disease has been present for a time the patient may be unable to recognize red at all.

Localized areas of depression cause sector defects. Binasal or even bitemporal defects may occur, so that chiasmal lesions may be simulated. Altitudinal hemianopia may be seen in which either the upper or the lower halves of the fields of both eyes may be affected [FIG. 137].

Central vision may remain relatively unimpaired, e.g. 20/30, for a long time, but very rarely central scotomata occur.

Pallor of the optic disc occurs early, but it is an unreliable sign, unless accompanied by characteristic field changes.

Only after a full investigation and careful observation over a period of time should a

INFLAMMATORY LESIONS

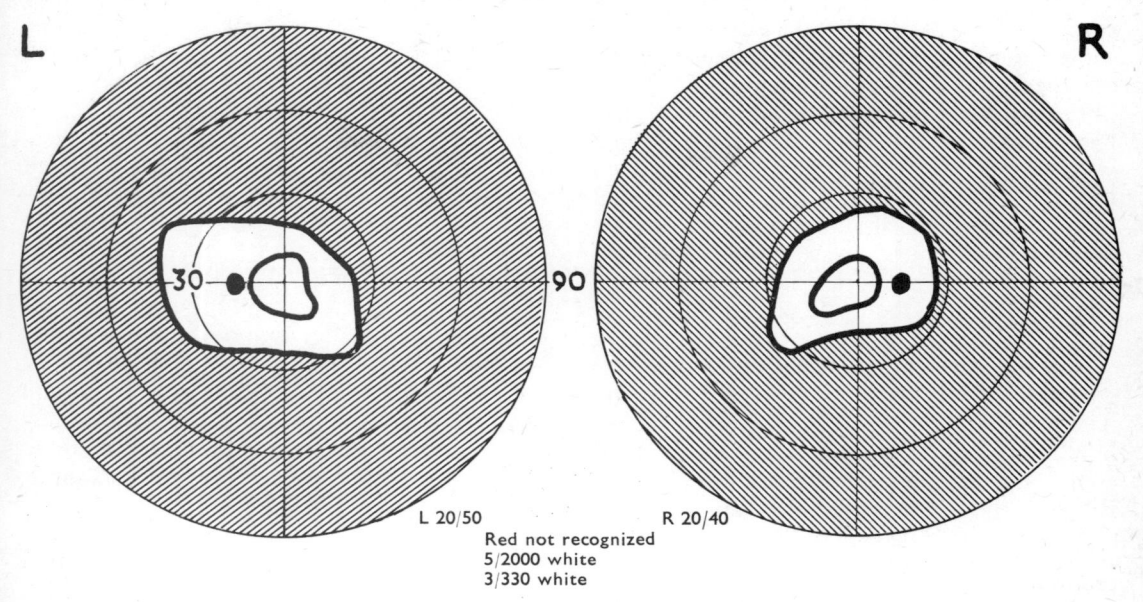

L 20/50   R 20/40
Red not recognized
5/2000 white
3/330 white

FIG. 136. Visual fields in a patient with syphilitic optic atrophy.

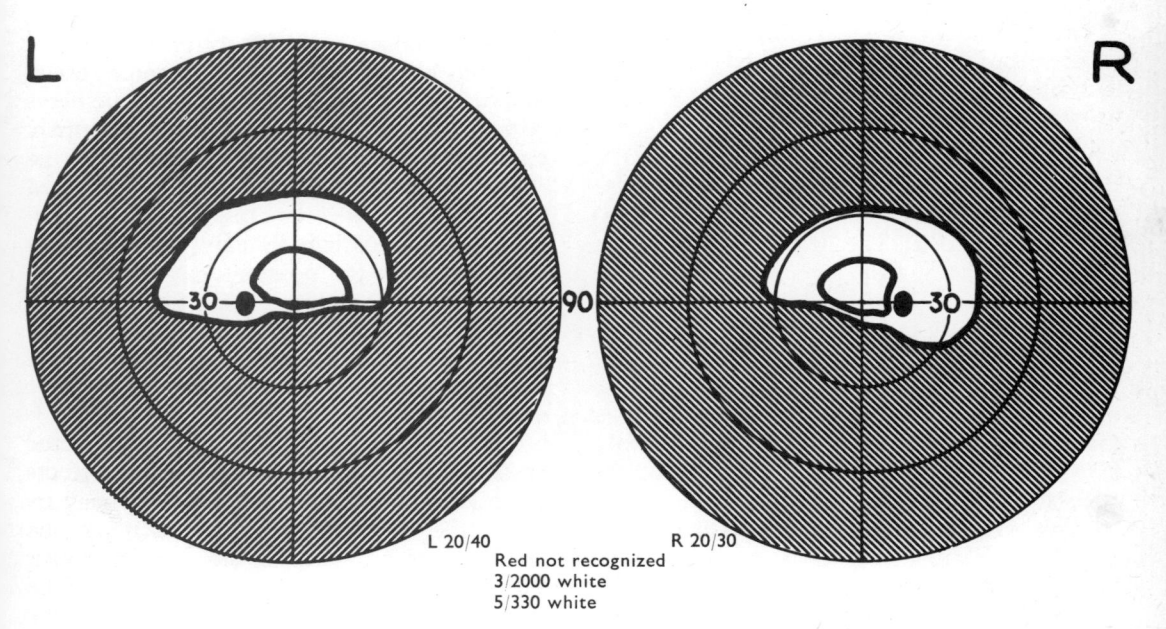

L 20/40   R 20/30
Red not recognized
3/2000 white
5/330 white

FIG. 137. Altitudinal hemianopia in a patient with syphilitic optic atrophy.

diagnosis of syphilitic optic atrophy be accepted in cases with bizarre field defects. They may be due to a cerebral tumour.

The loss of vision is due to syphilitic inflammation of the connective tissue septa within the optic nerve. The ensuing gliosis causes gradual obliteration of interstitial blood vessels, which in turn produces ischaemic degeneration of the nerve fibres. The disappearance of capillaries accounts for the marked pallor of the optic disc in this condition.

This disease is rare nowadays because of the effective early treatment of syphilis. Formerly, it tended to progress inexorably towards blindness, and treatment with neoarsphenamine and bismuth often failed to arrest it. Bruetsch showed that prolonged and intensive administration of penicillin offers the best hope of arrest, and even of some recovery of vision in early syphilitic optic atrophy. In late inactive cases penicillin offers little hope of recovery and in some patients vision continues to deteriorate despite intensive therapy.

COMPRESSION
OPTIC NERVE COMPRESSION

Compression of the optic nerve is usually due to slow-growing tumours, which may arise from the nerve itself, its coverings, or neighbouring structures. The field defects advance slowly, and they may be severe before the patient is aware of any disability. Pallor of the optic disc occurs early.

In optic nerve compression the visual acuity usually deteriorates slowly but there may be rapid loss of vision when the area of fixation is invaded or if the tumour is enlarging rapidly [FIG. 138]. In these cases field examination reveals scotomata in the central area often with a break-through to the periphery. The internal isopters may show early contraction, and they are the last to recover when pressure is relieved. The more rapid the advance of the compression, the more dense the scotoma. The slope of its margin may vary in different areas.

The scotomata are best demonstrated with the 2/2000 and 5/2000 white targets. The discovery of disproportion with the 15/2000 red target may give a valuable hint as to the chances of recovery if the tumour can be removed successfully.

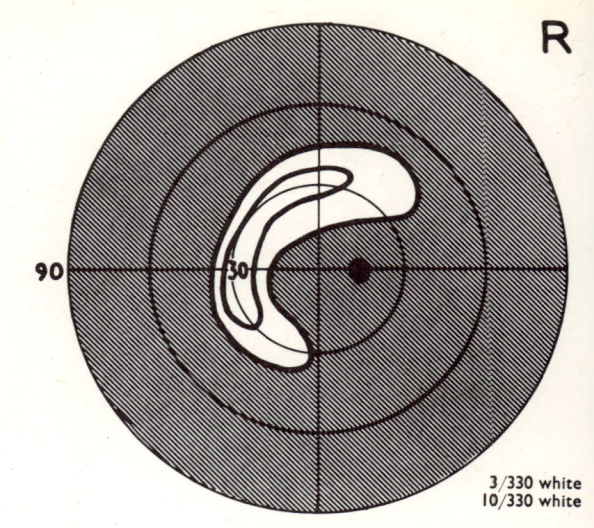

FIG. 138. Right visual field of a patient with a meningioma of the right sphenoid ridge. The left field was normal.

Occasionally arcuate defects are seen because the nerve fibre bundles of the retina remain as separate units in the optic nerve.

It will be noted that there is some resemblance between the field defects in optic nerve compression and those in retrobulbar neuritis, particularly if the visual loss has occurred rapidly. This often leads to errors of diagnosis, but if after 3 or 4 weeks there is no improvement in vision in a patient thought to have retrobulbar neuritis the possibility of optic nerve compression should be considered. The reason for the vulnerability of the central fibres is not known. It will be remembered, however, that the macular bundle is in the centre of the optic nerve, and that posteriorly the optic nerve is nourished by branches from external blood vessels penetrating the nerve. It may be that the central axial blood vessel system is particularly susceptible to pressure because it represents the terminal branches of the arterial system derived from the blood vessels supplying the optic nerve sheath and then passing into the substance of the nerve along the pial connective tissue network.

Compression of the optic nerve may occur:
1. In the orbit.
2. In the optic foramen. This occurs comparatively rarely in bony diseases such as osteopetrosis and will not be discussed further.
3. In the cranial cavity. This is usually due to

COMPRESSION

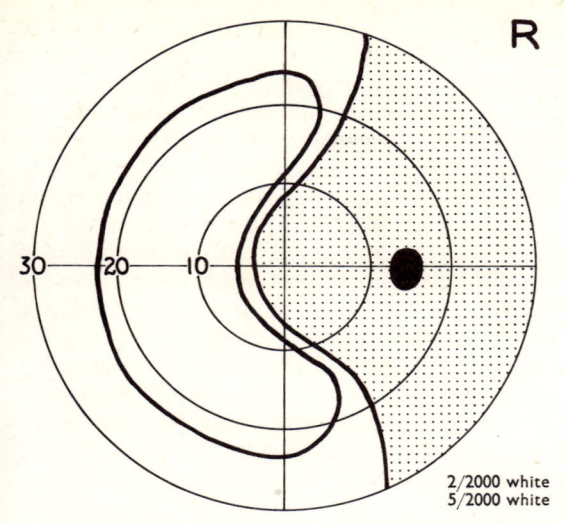

FIG. 139. Central field of a patient with a tumour at the apex of the orbit on the medial side of the optic nerve.

targets should be used in varying intensities of illumination. If the recognition of colour is still present the richness of hue should be compared in each of the four quadrants [FIG. 140]. Any difference in intensity is of significance and may afford valuable information about the site of the tumour.

As the compression increases the area of depression extends to the blind spot, but a break-through to the periphery occurs late.

The changes in the visual field do not always correspond to the site of the tumour. This lack of correspondence cannot always be explained. The field defects are due to interference with the blood supply to the optic nerve, and to stretching of the nerve fibres. Sometimes the tumour forces the nerve against a more rigid structure, such as a bony ridge or an artery, which causes more interference than the tumour itself.

TUMOURS OF THE OPTIC NERVE

These are not very common. They may occur both in the orbit and in the intracranial cavity. Those arising in the orbit have fairly characteristic features and will be described in this section. They are of two types, intrinsic and extrinsic.

tumours, but occasionally a dilated arteriosclerotic internal carotid artery will cause optic nerve compression.

ORBITAL COMPRESSION OF THE OPTIC NERVE

The orbit is pyramidal in shape with the apex placed posteriorly.

A tumour in the anterior part of the orbit is less likely to compress the optic nerve than one at the apex. When the tumour is anterior in situation, there may be marked proptosis and displacement of the eye, so that diplopia is often the chief symptom.

The closer the tumour is to the apex of the orbit, the less space there is for expansion. At the apex the optic nerve is relatively fixed, and thus more readily compressed. Tumours of the apex of the orbit are most commonly situated medial to the nerve [FIG. 139].

The field defects caused by a tumour at the apex of the orbit usually correspond to the site of the tumour. If it is nasal, the scotoma tends to be temporal. If the compression is from above, the scotoma usually involves a greater area below the horizontal meridian.

Hughes has pointed out that if the four quadrants of the central scotoma are analysed and compared, differences in density may often be demonstrated. Different sizes of small white

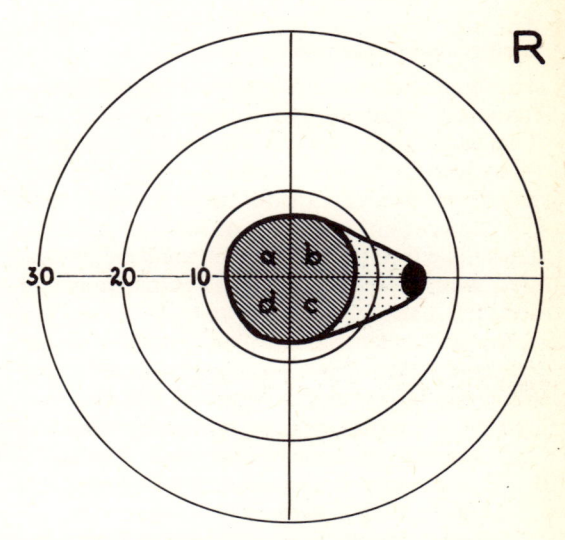

FIG. 140. To show the four quadrants of a central scotoma which should be compared for density, especially in optic nerve compression (after Hughes).

Intrinsic Tumours

These are usually gliomata, which occur most commonly during the first decade of life. A glioma of the optic nerve causes a slowly developing proptosis, loss of central vision, limitation of ocular movements, and optic atrophy. A unilateral optic atrophy in a child should always give rise to a suspicion of a glioma of the optic nerve.

A central scotoma occurs, its shape and extent depending upon the nerve fibres which have been destroyed. Not infrequently the glioma spreads backwards and involves the chiasma. If this occurs, the eye on the affected side will be blind and have optic atrophy. The visual field of the other eye may show temporal hemianopia due to chiasmal interference.

Extrinsic Tumours

The most common extrinsic tumour is the meningioma of the nerve sheath. It usually occurs in adults between the ages of 20 and 40. The tumour fills out the rectus muscle cone, so that proptosis and restriction of ocular movements are early symptoms. Deterioration of vision and optic atrophy occur relatively later than in glioma of the optic nerve.

EXOPHTHALMIC OPHTHALMOPLEGIA (ENDOCRINE OR PITUITARY EXOPHTHALMOS)

Endocrine Exophthalmos

This condition may follow treatment of thyrotoxicosis by radioactive isotopes or by surgery. The patient may be hyperthyroid, euthyroid, or hypothyroid. The contents of the orbit are increased by oedema, additional fat and round cell infiltration of the extra-ocular muscles. There is exophthalmos which may be associated with severe conjunctival congestion and oedema, tearing, and blurring of vision. The upper lids are retracted and elevation of the eyes and convergence are invariably defective. Fibrosis of the inferior rectus muscle may cause vertical diplopia. Extreme exophthalmos and infrequent blinking may cause drying of the cornea and superficial keratitis leading to corneal scarring and loss of vision.

The gross orbital congestion may cause elevation of the intra-ocular pressure presumably by impeding drainage. The ocular tension should always be measured with the eyes depressed because attempts to elevate the eye against a fibrotic inferior rectus muscle tend to give falsely high readings. Papilloedema may occur and ocular neuropathy may develop. Central, paracentral and arcuate scotomata and large sector defects may result [FIG. 141]. If the visual acuity begins to fail or scotomata can be demonstrated, active measures are indicated. Some patients appear to be helped by thyroid therapy, particularly those who are hypothyroid. Others gain relief from large doses of prednisone. If medications fail, decompression of the orbit may be indicated but even this does not save the sight in every case.

All cases of endocrine exophthalmos should have regular central field studies to detect any early development of visual loss. The rapidity of visual deterioration is very variable. In some it may be gradual over a period of months. In others severe loss may occur in a few days. Some patients may show slow, spontaneous visual recovery months or years after active therapy failed to arrest visual deterioration.

INTRACRANIAL COMPRESSION OF THE OPTIC NERVE

The optic nerve may be compressed by meningiomata of the sphenoid ridge, aneurysms of the anterior part of the circle of Willis, craniopharyngiomata, pituitary tumours, and, occasionally, gliomata of the frontal lobe. These tumours may spread and become quite large before causing serious visual loss.

The field changes resulting from compression of the optic nerve by an intracranial tumour are similar to those produced by one of the apex of the orbit. If, however, the tumour involves the anterior angle of the chiasma, the anterior knee of Wilbrand may be damaged, thus producing a corresponding defect in the upper temporal quadrant of the field of the other eye. In all cases where optic nerve compression is suspected, the upper temporal field of the opposite eye should be examined carefully with small targets. The 10/2000 red target occasionally reveals a defect not discoverable with a 2/2000 white target. If a 'junction scotoma' is present or the small target isopters of the upper temporal quadrant are contracted, the anterior knee of Wilbrand at the anterolateral angle of the chiasma is involved [FIG. 134].

COMPRESSION

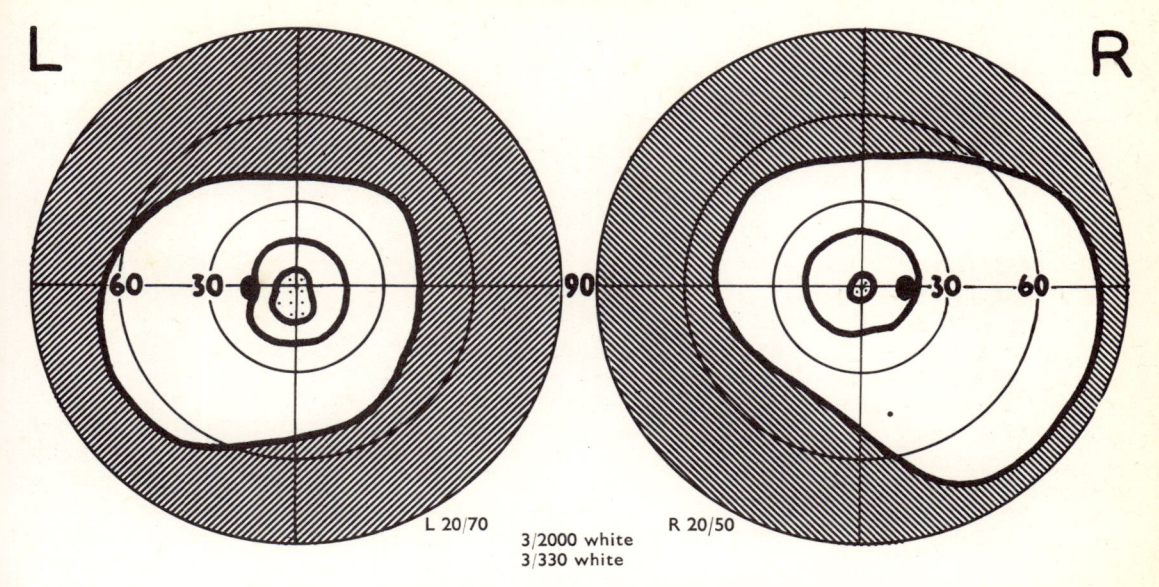

FIG. 141. Visual fields of a patient with exophthalmic ophthalmoplegia, showing central scotomata and slight peripheral contraction.

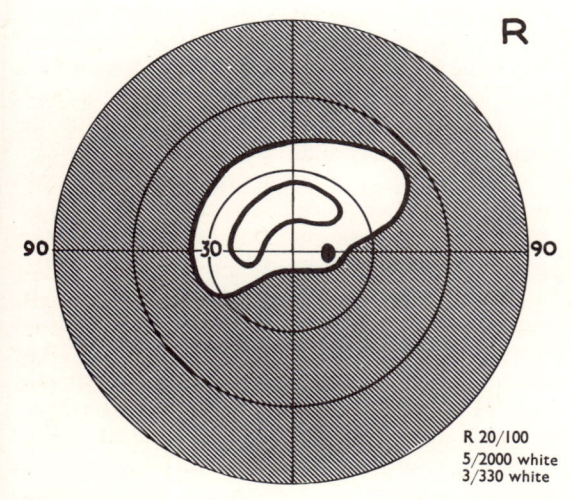

FIG. 142. Field defect caused by an intracranial tumour elevating the right optic nerve and compressing it against the upper margin of the optic foramen.

Radiography is of value in the diagnosis of these cases. Hyperostosis of the lesser wing of the sphenoid is characteristic of a meningioma. Erosion of the lesser wing of the sphenoid, widening of the sphenoidal fissure, or erosion of the anterior clinoid processes, are all signs of an expanding space-occupying lesion, such as an aneurysm of the circle of Willis. Calcification may occur within the tumour in craniopharyngiomata. It should be remembered that a normal X-ray does not exclude an intracranial tumour.

FOSTER KENNEDY SYNDROME

Primary optic atrophy in one eye associated with papilloedema in the other is known as the Foster Kennedy syndrome [FIG. 143]. It may be caused by any frontobasal tumour, such as meningiomata of the olfactory groove or sphenoidal ridge, frontal lobe tumours, and aneurysms. The lesion is on the same side as the eye with the optic atrophy and central scotoma, which are caused by compression. The papilloedema in the other eye is caused by the secondary rise in intracranial pressure. The full syndrome usually indicates the presence of a large intracranial growth or aneurysm.

If the optic nerve is raised by a tumour growing beneath it, an inferior field defect may occur due to compression of the optic nerve against the upper margin of the optic foramen [FIG. 142]. Cases have been described in which a tumour caused such a defect in both eyes.

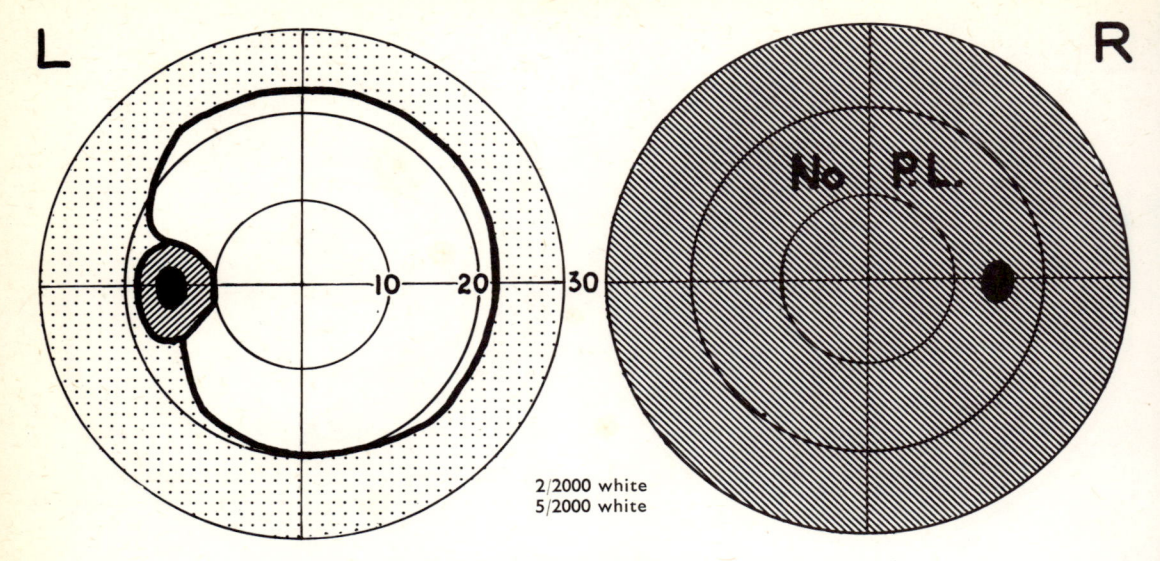

FIG. 143. Visual fields of a patient with the Foster Kennedy syndrome due to a large meningioma occupying the right anterior cranial fossa.

PROGNOSIS

When the pressure upon the optic nerve is relieved by removal of the tumour, considerable recovery may be expected, provided the optic atrophy is not severe. The presence of disproportion on analysis of the field defects suggests the possibility of such improvement.

TRAUMA

TRAUMATIC LESIONS OF THE OPTIC NERVE

Injuries due to high-velocity bullets or fragments of shell occurred frequently in both world wars. The passage of the missile at high speed close to the optic nerve was often sufficient to damage it and cause partial loss of sight. Direct injury to the nerve usually caused total loss of vision, but was less common.

Cases seen in civilian practice often result from a blow upon the temple from a car accident. The blow may be severe enough to cause a fracture of the skull, but sometimes there is no demonstrable bony injury.

The patient may be unconscious when first seen, so that it is difficult to assess loss of vision. On recovering consciousness, he may state that he is unable to see with one eye. On examination, the pupil of the affected eye may react sluggishly or not at all to direct light, while the consensual light reaction is preserved. The fundus may appear normal, or there may be some oedema of the disc, with or without adjacent haemorrhages.

Some recovery of vision may occur up to one month, but after this period further recovery is unlikely. The optic disc begins to pale after a period of about one month.

The popularity of the small motor cycle in Japan has resulted in many accidents of this nature and ophthalmologists there have had a considerable experience of this condition. Several series have been recorded in which prompt decompression of the optic canal by the transethmoidal route has resulted in considerable recovery of vision. These workers have been able to demonstrate radiologically the fractures in the wall of the optic canal and show, by visual field studies before and after decompression, marked reduction in the visual field defects.

Field Changes

No particular defect is characteristic in these traumatic cases. A sector defect with a steep edge is the commonest type of field loss caused

TRAUMA

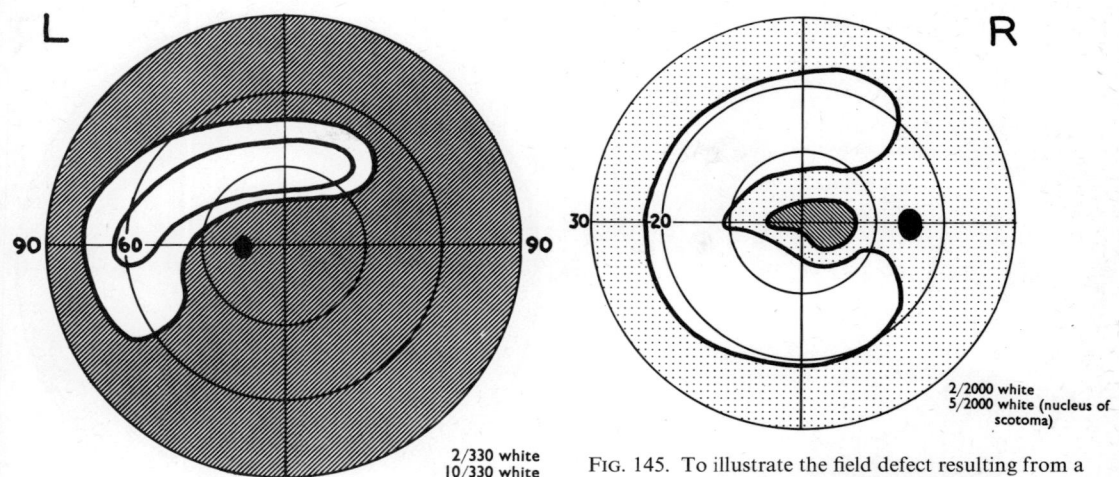

FIG. 144. Visual field of the left eye following a car accident.

FIG. 145. To illustrate the field defect resulting from a tear of the temporal fibres of the optic nerve.

by trauma to the optic nerve. It may occur in any part of the field, but the lower field is most commonly involved [FIG. 144]. A central scotoma may be found but this is usually due to traumatic oedema of the retina following a non-penetrating blow on the eye rather than to damage to the optic nerve.

It will be recalled that the meninges of the optic nerve are adherent to the roof of the optic foramen. It is thought that trauma often ruptures the blood vessels passing from the sheath of the optic nerve into its substance in this situation. This may account for the frequency of inferior field defects.

If a temporal defect with a vertical edge occurs, it suggests that the nasal retinal fibres have been damaged in the region of the septum near the junction of the optic nerve with the chiasma.

A relatively uncommon injury is one in which the eye is forcibly rotated, so that the optic nerve is partially avulsed from the eyeball. External rotation is the commoner injury. When this occurs the nasal fibres are torn, and a retinal haemorrhage is usually seen adjacent to the optic disc. The haemorrhage is gradually absorbed and replaced by an area of pigmentation. A sector defect in the temporal field usually results.

If the eye is internally rotated, the temporal fibres of the optic nerve and the maculopapillary bundle are torn. Hughes has stated that this may lead to a central scotoma with some field remaining between the blind spot and the fixation point [FIG. 145].

VASCULAR LESIONS OF THE OPTIC NERVE

OPTIC ATROPHY FOLLOWING SEVERE SYSTEMIC HAEMORRHAGE

Visual failure is usually caused by severe recurrent losses of blood from the gastro-intestinal tract or uterus, or a single gross haemorrhage in an elderly patient.

The vision may fail at any time up to 3 weeks after a haemorrhage. Both eyes are usually affected, but in 15 per cent of patients only one is involved. The pupils are dilated, and sluggish or fixed. The fundus picture varies. It may be normal, but more commonly the retinal arteries are constricted. There is a slight oedema of the disc and macular area, and there may be a few scattered soft exudates and haemorrhages.

The outlook is grave. About half the patients become blind, and very few regain normal vision. In some, sight may partially return, only to deteriorate a few weeks later. Optic atrophy begins to develop after about one month.

Field Changes

These are variable. One eye is usually affected more severely than the other. There may be peripheral field loss, sector defects, or even an

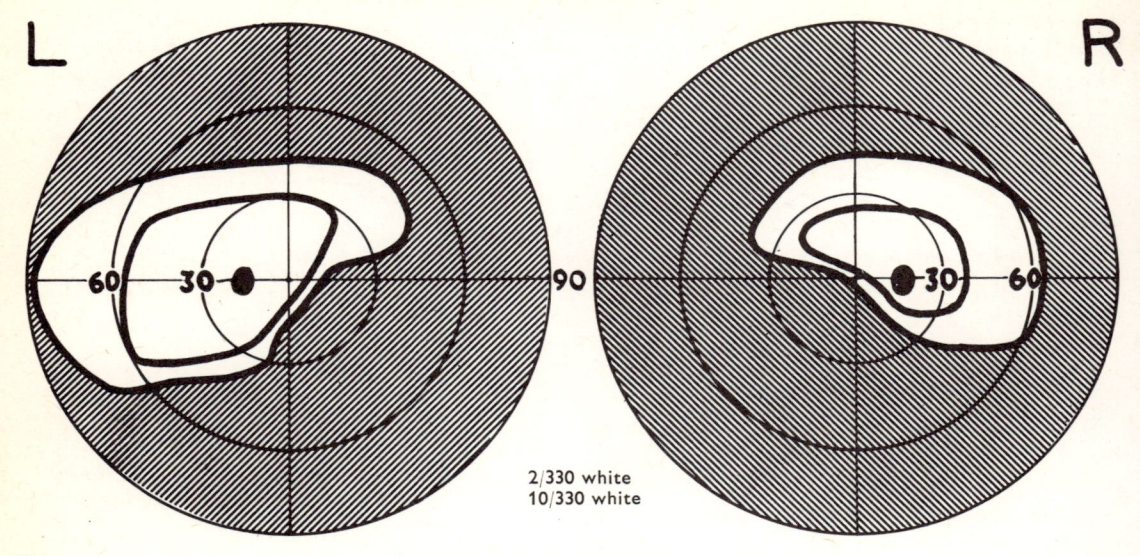

FIG. 146. Visual fields 3 weeks after a severe haematemesis from a gastric ulcer.

arcuate scotoma. Big sector defects affecting the lower field occur most commonly [FIG. 146]. Wolff suggested that this is due to gravity causing more blood to reach the lower half of the retina than the upper half. Less frequently scotomata are found.

The optic atrophy is due to the sudden fall in blood volume in a patient who is already anaemic from repeated bleeding or whose cardiovascular system is abnormal. The retinal neurones appear to be particularly vulnerable to anoxia and, once devitalized, they are unable to regenerate. In such patients, the head should be kept low, and the blood lost should be replaced by transfusion as rapidly as possible.

VASCULAR LESIONS WITHIN THE OPTIC NERVE

These cases occur occasionally and may cause some difficulty in diagnosis. Two types of vascular lesions may be encountered.

Acute Occlusion

Acute occlusion of blood vessels within the nerve near the optic disc results in sudden loss of vision. This may, on rare occasions, be associated with oedema of the disc, and a few scattered haemorrhages, so that the condition resembles papillitis. Sometimes a segment of the disc is particularly oedematous. In this case there is usually a corresponding field defect related to the nerve fibres passing through this affected area. It might be argued that these cases are in fact a true papillitis. Some may well be, but when loss of sight occurs suddenly in an elderly arteriosclerotic, and there is little

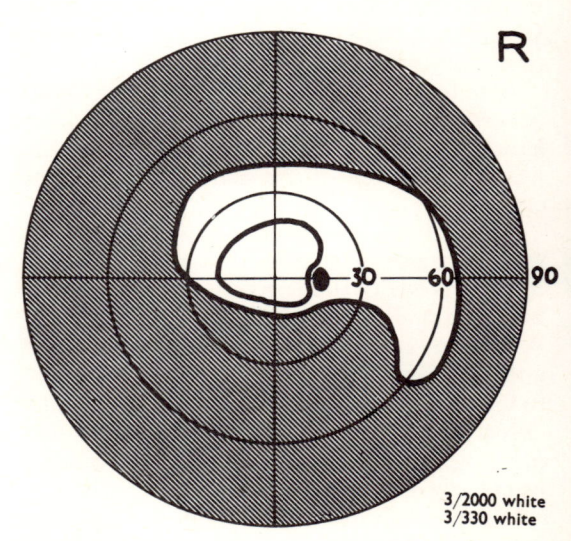

FIG. 147. Sudden loss of the lower half of the visual field in an elderly patient. There were no fundus changes to account for the field loss.

or no recovery, it seems that occlusion of small blood vessels within the nerve is the more likely explanation.

Large sector defects occur, particularly in the lower field [FIG. 147], corresponding to the nerve fibres deprived of blood supply.

Gradual Occlusion

Gradual occlusion of small vessels in the optic nerve, leading to optic atrophy and shallow cupping, may be indistinguishable from low-tension glaucoma. It may also be confused with syphilitic optic atrophy but in this case the other signs of syphilis will be absent.

The visual acuity is usually well maintained but it may fail gradually. Contraction of the peripheral isopters of the field occurs [FIG. 148]. Occlusion of small blood vessels in the region of the optic disc may sometimes cause nerve bundle defects such as arcuate scotomata. It is difficult, and perhaps no more than an academic exercise, to distinguish between arteriosclerotic atrophy and low-tension glaucoma.

In cranial arteritis or temporal arteritis, the retinal arteries may be involved and 50 per cent of patients develop field defects which progress to blindness if untreated. The field defects may be sector-shaped, arcuate, or central scotomata. Massive infiltration of the retinal arteries may lead to very severe loss of vision at the outset. The patients are usually 65 or more years of age and complain of severe headaches and pain and tenderness in the scalp. There may be malaise, anorexia, and insomnia. The sedimentation rate is high, usually about 100. Immediate treatment with steroids is essential because if untreated about one-third of these patients become blind in both eyes. There is usually a rapid response to steroid therapy which prevents blindness if started in time, but is valueless in restoring sight to a blind eye.

REFERENCES AND FURTHER READING

BRUETSCH, W. L. (1953) *Syphilitic Optic Atrophy*, Springfield, Ill.

DAY, R. M., and CARROLL, F. D. (1962) Optic nerve involvement with thyroid dysfunction, *Arch. Ophthal.*, **67**, 289.

FOULDS, W. S. (1969) in *Ischaemic Optic Neuropathy in the Ocular Circulation in Health and Disease*, ed. Cant, J. S., p. 136, London.

FOULDS, W. S., CHISHOLM, I. A., STEWART, J. B., and WILSON, T. M. (1969) The optic neuropathy of pernicious anaemia, *Arch. Ophthal.*, **82**, 427.

HAYREH, S. (1970) Pathogenesis of visual field defects, *Brit. J. Ophthal.*, **54**, 289.

JOSEPH, R., and DAVEY, J. B. (1958) Dominantly inherited optic atrophy, *Brit. J. Ophthal.*, **42**, 413.

NIHO, S., NIHO, M., and NIHO, K. (1970) Decompression of the optic canal by the transethmoidal route and decompression of the superior orbital fissure, *Canad. J. Ophthal.*, **5**, 22.

SORSBY, A. (1970) *Ophthalmic Genetics*, London.

WILSON, J. (1965) Leber's hereditary optic atrophy. Possible defect of cyanide metabolism, *Clin. Sci.*, **29**, 505.

13
CHIASMAL LESIONS

CAUSES OF CHIASMAL INTERFERENCE

Chiasmal interference is usually due to compression by tumours. The chiasma may be compressed from any direction, depending upon the site of the tumour. Tumours which cause chiasmatic compression may be grouped into intrasellar and extrasellar neoplasms. The intrasellar neoplasms are pituitary adenomata. The commonest tumour of this group is the chromophobe adenoma. The eosinophilic adenoma occurs less frequently, and the basophilic type is rare.

The extrasellar tumours form a large group of which craniopharyngiomata, meningiomata, aneurysms, and frontal gliomata are probably the commonest.

In children, gliomata of the chiasma may occur either as a primary tumour, or as an extension of the growth from an optic nerve.

Occasionally, distension of the third ventricle, in cases of internal hydrocephalus, acts as an extrasellar tumour and causes bitemporal hemianopia.

CLINICAL FEATURES

Chiasmal compression is usually due to a slowly-growing tumour. The field loss therefore progresses slowly and a large peripheral defect may develop before involvement of the central area arrests the patient's attention. The nerve fibres degenerate and optic atrophy occurs but the field defect is often advanced before optic atrophy is obvious.

If the tumour is in the midline the atrophy develops in each eye simultaneously, so that if it is not marked its recognition may be difficult. When the discs are only slightly pale, the demonstration of the field defects is essential to confirm the diagnosis of optic atrophy. An asymmetrical tumour may compress an optic nerve and cause unilateral optic atrophy, making it possible to compare the two optic discs and to recognize the difference in the degree of pallor. Sometimes the sight of one eye may be lost, unbeknown to the patient.

Both bitemporal hemianopia and optic atrophy may be advanced before an intracranial tumour in the region of the chiasma is diagnosed. But if a patient has had visual symptoms for 2 years or more, optic atrophy in some degree is usually present and recognizable. About 50 per cent of patients with chiasmal compression are found to have optic atrophy by the time the diagnosis is made.

Neoplasms usually cause slow but steady field loss but there may sometimes be periods of rapid progression interspersed with periods of apparent arrest or even of slight recovery. This may lead to a mistaken diagnosis of retrobulbar neuritis.

Sudden enlargements of the field defect may also result from a rapid increase in the size of the neoplasm due to haemorrhage, necrosis, or degenerative changes leading to cyst formation. The term 'pituitary apoplexy' is sometimes applied to the state resulting from a sudden infarction, cystic degeneration or haemorrhage into a chromophobe adenoma of the pituitary. This may cause severe headache, loss of vision, bilateral ophthalmoplegia, collapse, and even coma. The increase in the size of the tumour compresses and inhibits the function of the remaining glandular tissue, thus causing an abrupt depletion of pituitary hormones.

Carotid aneurysms may enlarge suddenly, causing sudden visual loss and paralysis of the extraocular muscles, associated with deep seated pain behind the eyes.

Chromophobe adenomata of the pituitary cause features of hypopituitarism such as mental apathy, dry scaly skin, increased sensitivity to cold, amenorrhoea, loss of libido, hypothyroidism, and increased sugar tolerance. Eosinophilic adenomata give rise to gigantism if they develop before union of the epiphyses, and to acromegaly after the union of the epiphyses. When large, they also cause hypopituitarism by compressing functioning pituitary tissue. The rare basophilic adenoma is associated with Cushing's syndrome of hirsuties, obesity, reversal of secondary sexual characters, hypertension, and diabetes. Cushing's syndrome may also occur in association with chromophobe adenomata or with pituitary carcinomata. After adrenalectomy for Cushing's syndrome it is particularly important to follow the patient with regular visual acuity and field studies because associated chromophobe adenomata may enlarge rapidly causing the characteristic signs and symptoms of chiasmal compression. The commonest of these pituitary adenomata is the chromophobe. This type of adenoma tends to grow large. Thus, it causes visual loss and optic atrophy early, whilst the eosinophilic type gives rise to these ocular features late in its course. The basophilic adenoma is small and never causes chiasmal compression.

Tumours in the region of the chiasma cause an increase of intracranial pressure less frequently than those arising in the posterior cranial fossa, because the latter tend to obstruct the flow of cerebrospinal fluid from the fourth ventricle to the basal cisterns. Severe morning headaches due to a rise of intracranial pressure are therefore not very common in cases of chiasmal compression.

Pregnancy may provoke or accelerate chiasmal compression in pituitary tumours, suprasellar meningiomata and craniopharyngiomata. These patients are difficult problem cases and their visual fields need to be checked at weekly intervals. Their management involves the services of ophthalmologist, neurosurgeon, obstetrician, radiologist, and radiotherapist. If visual loss is not too severe no active measures should be undertaken until after the birth of the baby because reports of cases indicate that there is usually considerable post-partum visual recovery.

When an internal carotid aneurysm expands, it produces a severe pain which may seem to be maximal behind the eye or at the root of the nose. Headache may also occur in a pituitary adenoma, particularly in the early stage before it has burst through the diaphragma sellae. A meningioma may cause aching in the temporal region, but more often it is painless.

Any parasellar tumour may compress the oculomotor, abducens, trochlear, or trigeminal nerves, causing ocular palsies and pain or numbness in the distribution of the ophthalmic, maxillary, and mandibular divisions of the trigeminal nerve. Subclinoid

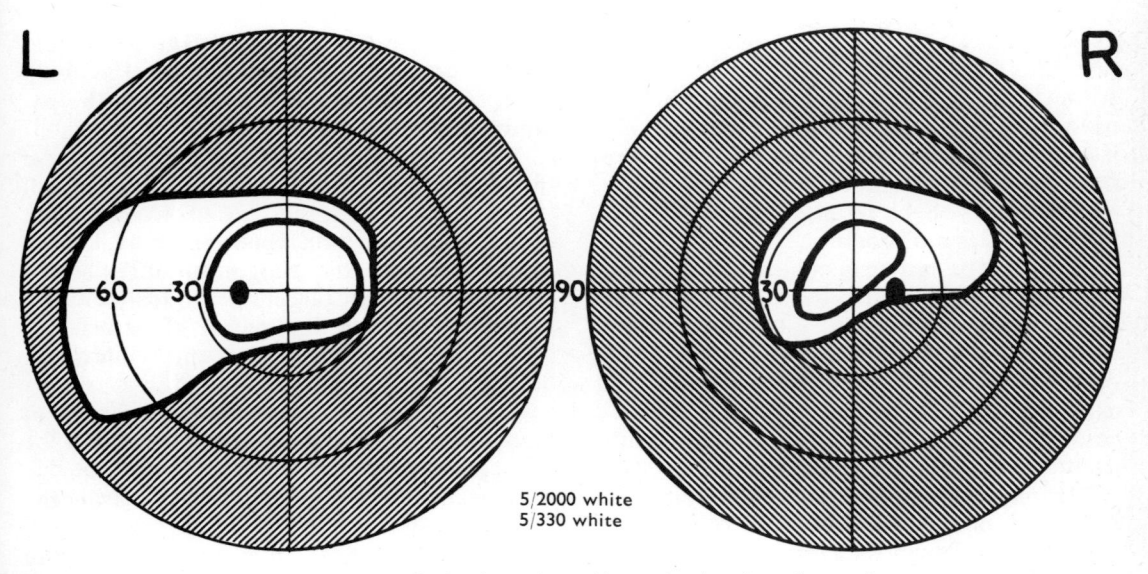

FIG. 148. Visual fields of a patient with arteriosclerotic optic atrophy.

2/2000 white
5/2000 white
Red not recognized

2/2000 white
10/2000 red (dotted line)

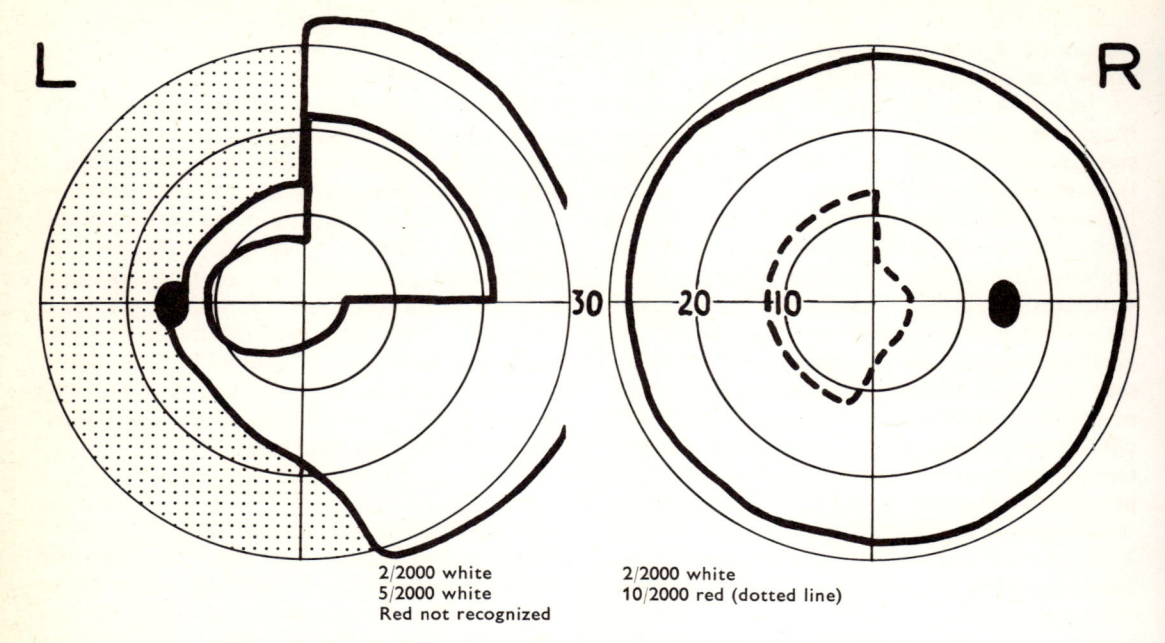

Fig. 149. Central fields of a patient with a chromophobe adenoma of the pituitary. The bitemporal nature of the defects was demonstrated with a red target in the right eye.

aneurysms and other lesions within the cavernous sinus are especially prone to do this. A pituitary adenoma may extend beyond the pituitary fossa and produce the same symptoms.

EXAMINATION

About half the patients with chiasmal compression seek advice for visual symptoms and it is all too easy in busy practice to overlook these cases. Visual field studies and radiograph studies of the pituitary area should be done in all cases of doubt.

It should be borne in mind that a patient may still be able to read the 20/20 or 6/6 line despite optic atrophy [Fig. 148]. Thus, even if the patient is able to read 20/20, pallor of the optic disc indicates the need for a visual field examination. If any optic atrophy is present, contraction of the peripheral and central isopters will always be found.

Atrophy of the optic disc is not a diagnosis. It is a sign of degeneration of the optic nerve, and it always demands an immediate and complete investigation of its cause.

In the diagnosis of cases of chiasmal compression, the perimeter should not be used by itself. All early field defects are best demonstrated with the Bjerrum screen because the central fields show the earliest changes. If bitemporal hemianopia is suspected, a 2 mm. white target and a 15 mm. red target should first be used on the Bjerrum screen [Fig. 149]. The perimeter should be used after the examination of the central field.

Since the lesion affects the retinal nerve fibres passing from the retina to the lateral geniculate bodies, it is essentially a conduction defect. Disproportion therefore occurs. Hence, if the isopter for the recognition of the hue of the 15 mm. red target is plotted in these patients, the bitemporal nature of the defect is often more obvious than if a 2 mm. white target is used.

An early chiasmal compression defect in an apparently normal field may sometimes be detected by:
1. Darkening the room slightly and using the 2/2000 white target again.
2. Using the 1/2000 or even 0·5/2000 white target (Chamlin).

3. Asking the patient to compare the brightness and hue of a 10 mm. or 15 mm. red target in the four quadrants about 5–10 degrees from the fixation point. Provided the illumination of the screen is even, any difference may be of significance. He may say it appears greyish in the upper temporal quadrant, orange in the lower temporal quadrant, and a definite red nasally. This is a most valuable and rapid test in doubtful cases [see FIG. 140, p. 117].

4. Demonstrating a step in the midline between the two upper quadrants. The method is similar to that used to demonstrate a nasal step in glaucoma. The upper lid must be fully raised to prevent false contraction. The 2 mm. white target is moved downwards in the upper temporal quadrant near the midline until it is just visible. It is then moved up until the patient is just unable to see it, and then across to the nasal quadrant at the same level. If a step is present, the target will at once be seen [FIG. 150].

Once a field defect is found it must be analysed with targets of different sizes to determine its slope. A sloping edge and marked disproportion indicate that the lesion is progressive, and that, if the cause of the compression can be removed, recovery may be expected.

An expanding tumour is rarely exactly in the midline, so one should not expect to find symmetrical field defects.

When fixation is good in each eye, the demonstration of bitemporal hemianopia is not difficult. But if the vision of one eye is reduced to bare perception of light, or vision is so poor that steady fixation is not possible, accurate assessment of the field is difficult. Nevertheless, it is usually possible in most cases to recognize a temporal hemianopia in such a defective eye by using pieces of white paper of varying sizes [FIGS. 151 and 152]. Sometimes, if a flashlight is moved from quadrant to quadrant in the visual field, the patient will be unable to see it on the temporal side.

FIELD CHANGES

The textbooks upon this subject show a bewildering variety of field defects which are liable to confuse the student. It is possible to understand these varied patterns only if the essential facts of the anatomy of this area are borne in mind. The defects depend upon the anatomy of the chiasma which was outlined in an earlier chapter, and the site of the lesion.

Four basic patterns will be described, but many cases are met which do not fit neatly into any one of these groups.

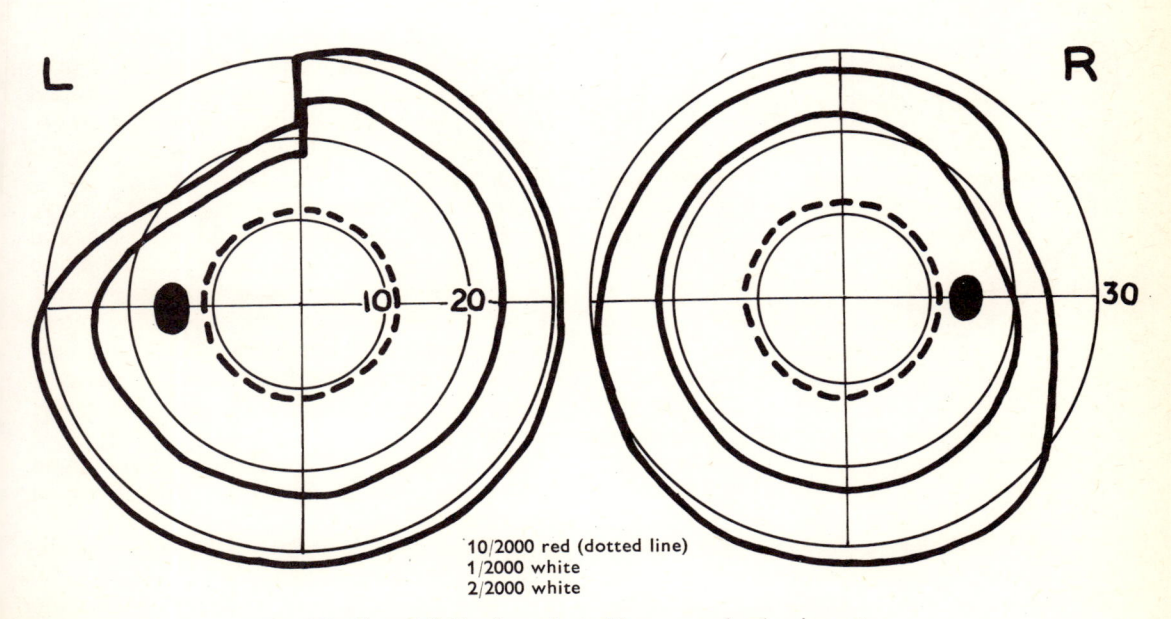

10/2000 red (dotted line)
1/2000 white
2/2000 white

FIG. 150. Central fields of a patient with acromegaly, showing a step in the left field.

CHIASMAL LESIONS

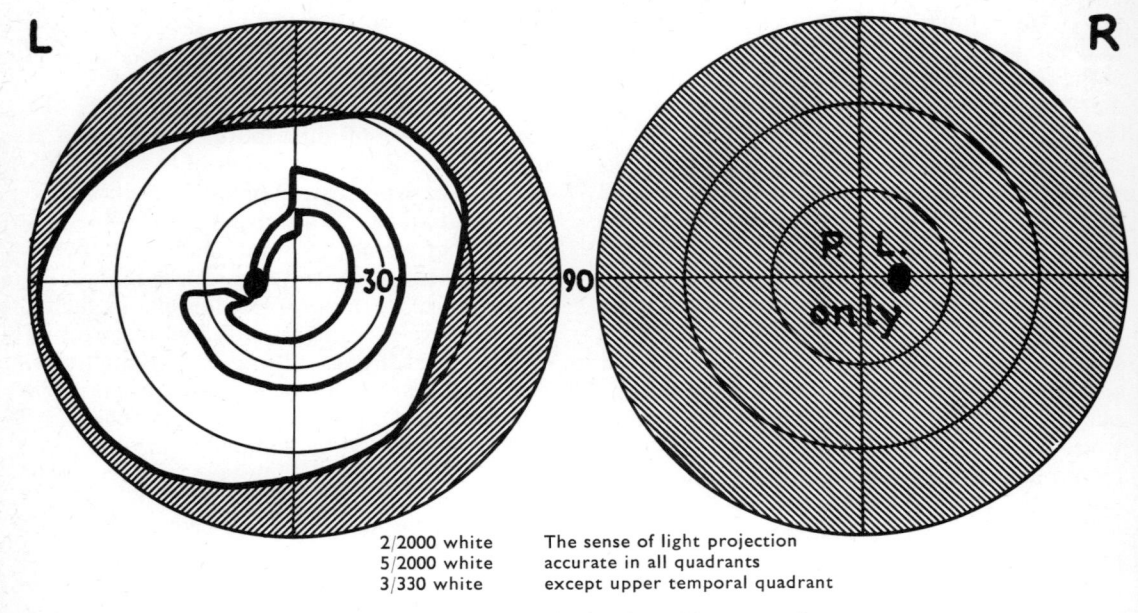

2/2000 white
5/2000 white
3/330 white

The sense of light projection accurate in all quadrants except upper temporal quadrant

FIG. 151. Visual field changes in a patient with a suprasellar cyst.

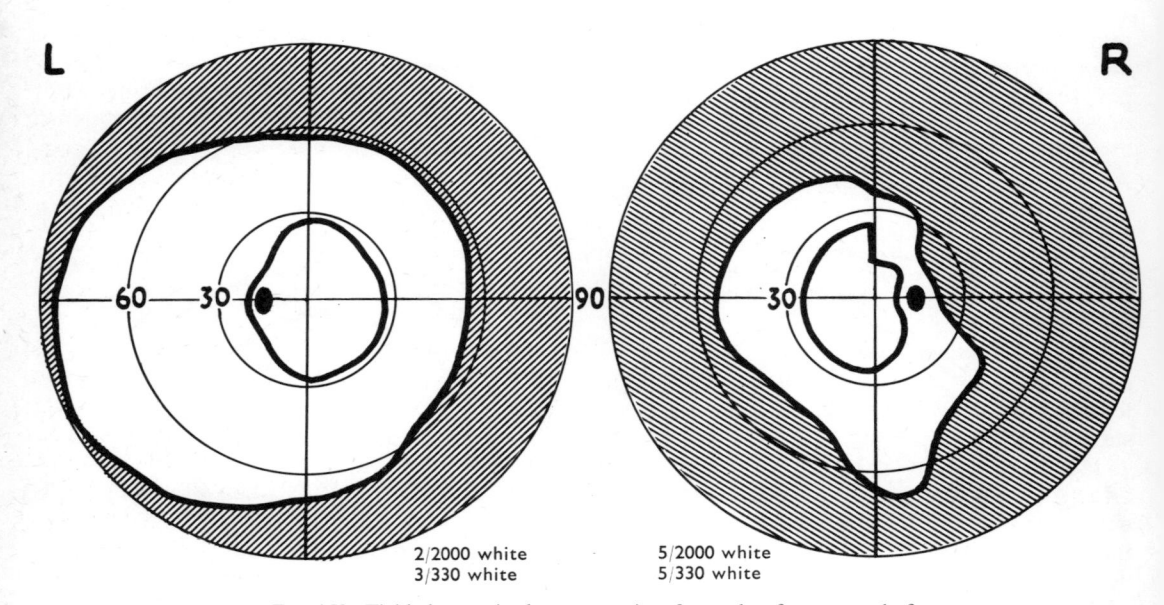

2/2000 white
3/330 white

5/2000 white
5/330 white

FIG. 152. Field changes in the same patient 3 months after removal of the suprasellar cyst.

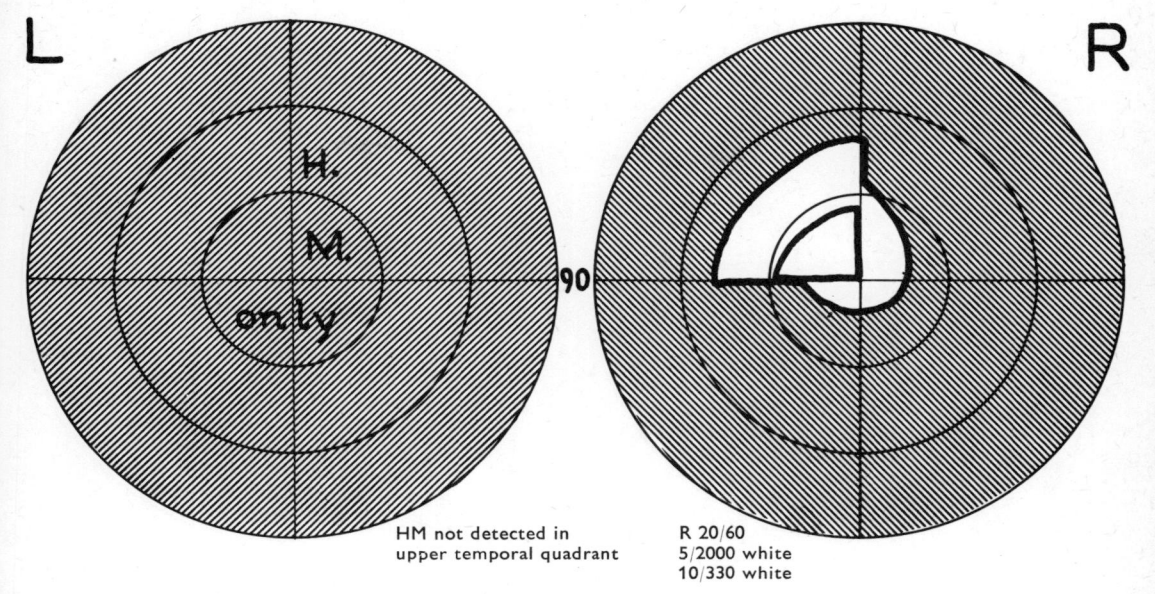

FIG. 153. Advanced chiasmal compression, showing persistence of the upper nasal quadrant of the right visual field.

HM not detected in upper temporal quadrant

R 20/60
5/2000 white
10/330 white

MIDLINE PRESSURE FROM BELOW

A chromophobe adenoma of the pituitary gland is the best example of a lesion which causes pressure upon the chiasma in the midline from below. It usually produces first a field defect in the upper temporal quadrant. As the compression increases in severity, the defect extends downwards into the inferior temporal quadrant, passes across the midline to the inferior nasal quadrant, and finally invades the superior nasal quadrant.

The lower nasal quadrant of the field is affected before the upper nasal quadrant because the upper temporal fibres are medial to the lower temporal fibres in the chiasma. It will be recalled [p. 5] that it was formerly accepted that there was a nasal rotation of nerve fibres which began in the optic nerves, and was continued through the chiasma and tracts, to complete its rotation of 90 degrees in the lateral geniculate bodies. There is now some doubt about this but in practice it does appear that the superior temporal retinal fibres are more exposed to damage from tumours in the midline whether the compression is from above or below the chiasma. The extreme lateral situation of the lower temporal fibres explains why the upper nasal fields remain unaffected for so long [FIG. 153].

A pituitary tumour usually stretches the anterior part of the chiasma first so that contraction of the 2/2000 white isopter in the upper temporal quadrant of each eye is often the earliest field change [FIG. 154]. It is obvious that much variation may occur, depending on the degree of pre- or post-fixation of the chiasma, and the direction in which a tumour is enlarging. Pressure on the posterior part of the chiasma may occasionally cause bitemporal scotomata.

MIDLINE PRESSURE FROM ABOVE

If the pressure is from above, as may occur in some cases of craniopharyngioma or aneurysm of the anterior cerebral artery, the field loss proceeds differently. The quadrants tend to be affected in the following order: the inferior temporal, the upper temporal, the lower nasal, and finally the upper nasal [FIG. 155]. It will be noted that the upper nasal quadrant is again the last to be lost.

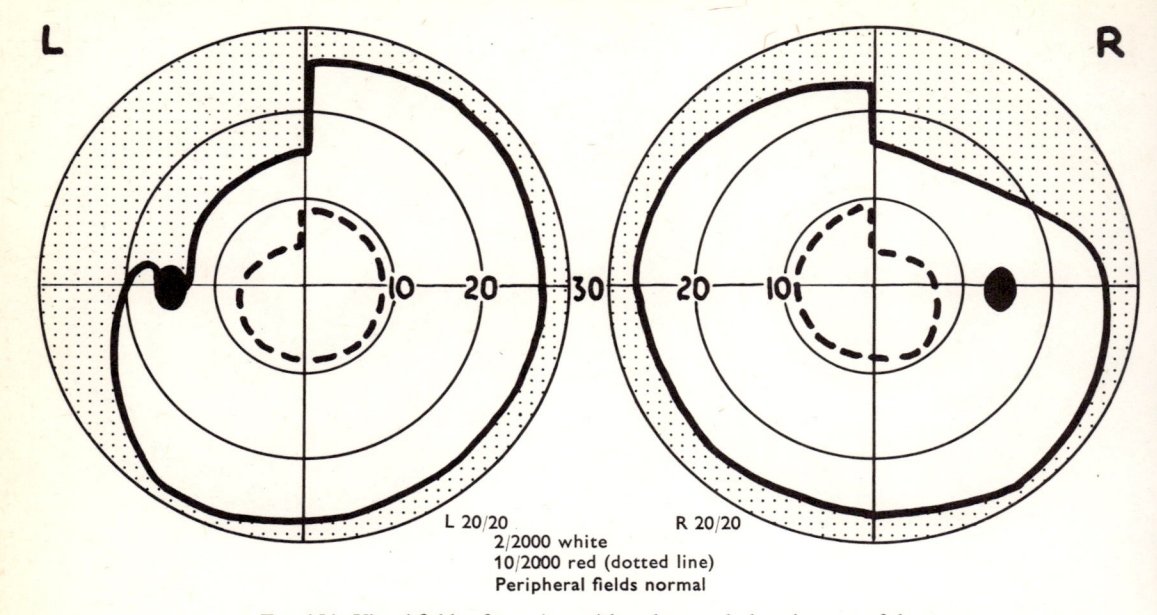

FIG. 154. Visual fields of a patient with a chromophobe adenoma of the pituitary, showing early changes in the upper temporal quadrants.

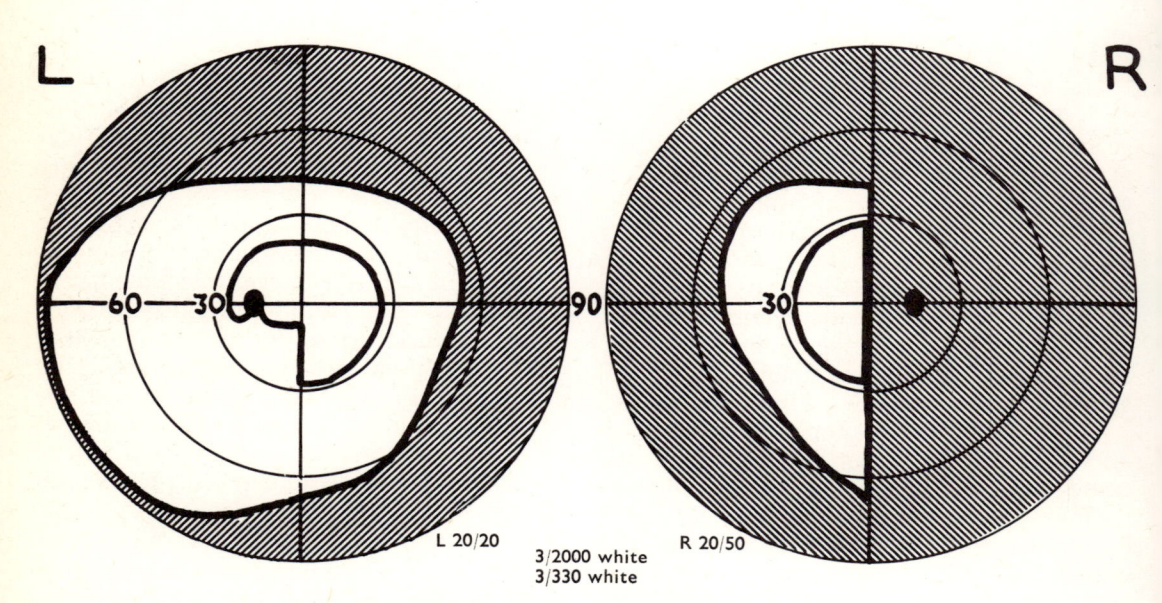

FIG. 155. Left visual field, illustrating the effect of midline pressure from above. Hand movements only were seen in the right temporal field.

FIELD CHANGES

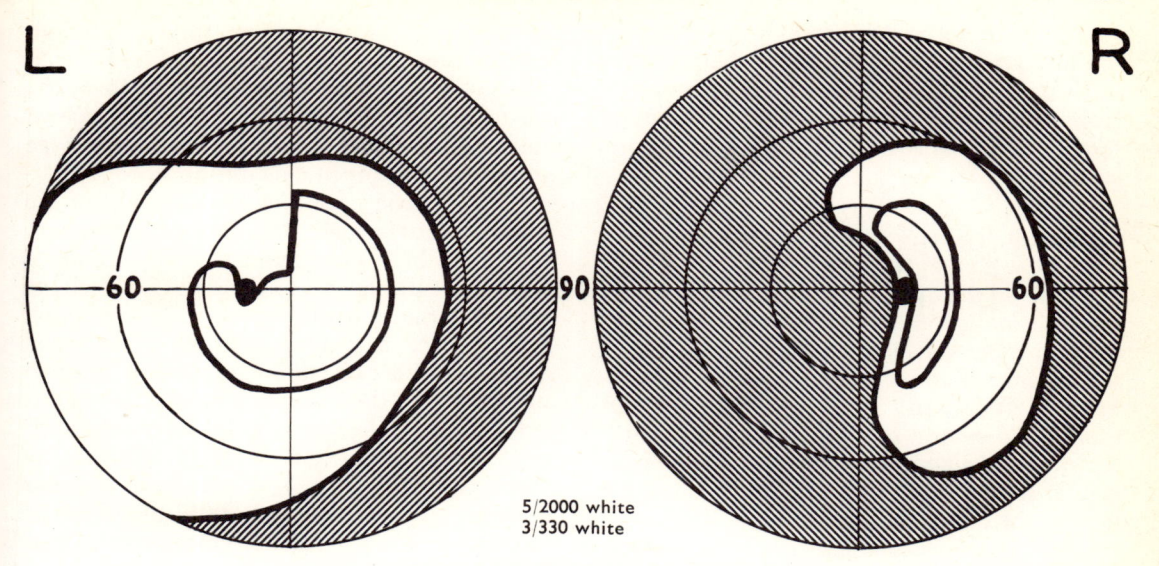

5/2000 white
3/330 white

Fig. 156. Right optic nerve compression with a junction defect in the left visual field.

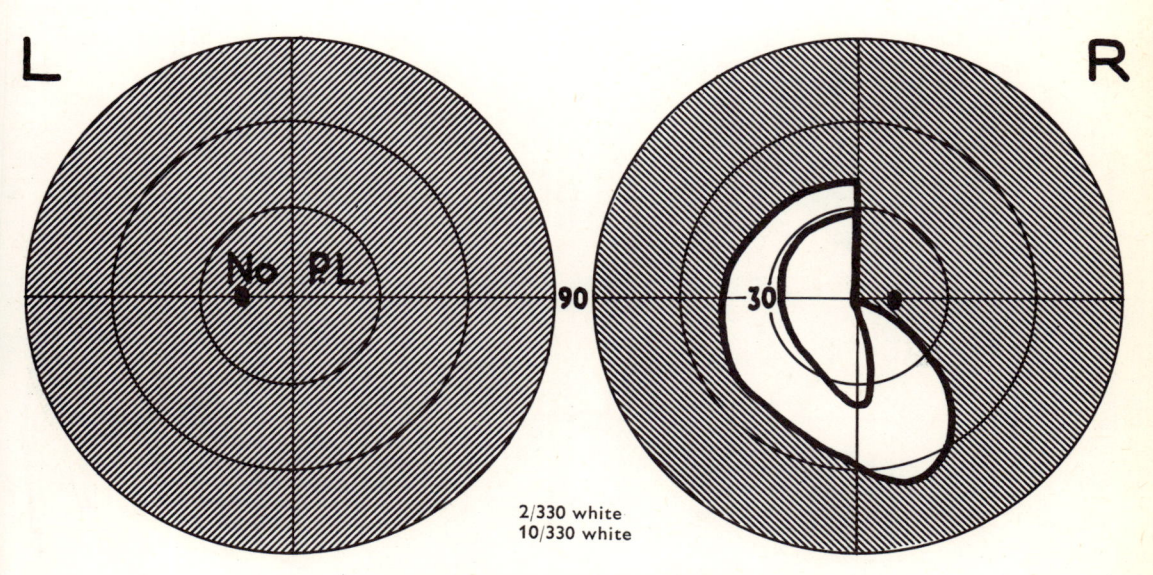

No P.L.

2/330 white
10/330 white

Fig. 157. Visual fields of a patient with a chromophobe adenoma of the pituitary. The left eye was blind when the patient was first seen.

A contraction of the 2/2000 white isopter in the lower temporal quadrant is therefore the most usual early change if the interference is from above. Less commonly posterior interference from above may cause bitemporal scotomata.

PRESSURE ON THE ANTEROLATERAL ANGLE OF THE CHIASMA

Pressure on the optic nerve at its junction with the chiasma is a fairly common form of compression. The visual fields show signs of optic nerve compression plus damage to the anterior knee of Wilbrand. The typical changes are therefore a central scotoma on the side of the tumour, and a contraction of the 2/2000 white isopter in the upper temporal quadrant of the field of the other eye [FIG. 156].

As the compression increases, the eye on the side of the lesion becomes blind, optic atrophy develops, and the field defect on the opposite side becomes a more complete temporal hemianopia [FIG. 157].

This pattern of the field defect may result from such causes as a meningioma of the inner one-third of the sphenoid ridge, a chromophobe adenoma of the pituitary, or an aneurysm of the anterior cerebral or internal carotid arteries.

The tumour may exert pressure from the medial or lateral side, or from above or below, thus displacing the optic nerve, so that the edge of the optic foramen cuts into it.

Compression upon the lateral aspect of the optic nerve at its junction with the chiasma may be caused by a meningioma arising from the sphenoid ridge lateral to the optic foramen, or by an internal carotid aneurysm. The resulting field defects may simulate those of an optic tract lesion, because the nasal field of the eye on the side of the lesion is first affected, and it is followed by the upper temporal quadrant of the field of the opposite eye [FIG. 156]. But, as the compression increases, a central scotoma develops and progresses to total blindness of the eye on the side of the compression. The other eye develops temporal hemianopia.

PRESSURE ON THE POSTEROLATERAL ANGLE OF THE CHIASMA

A lesion in this situation is much less common than one affecting the anterolateral angle of the chiasma or its body [FIG. 158].

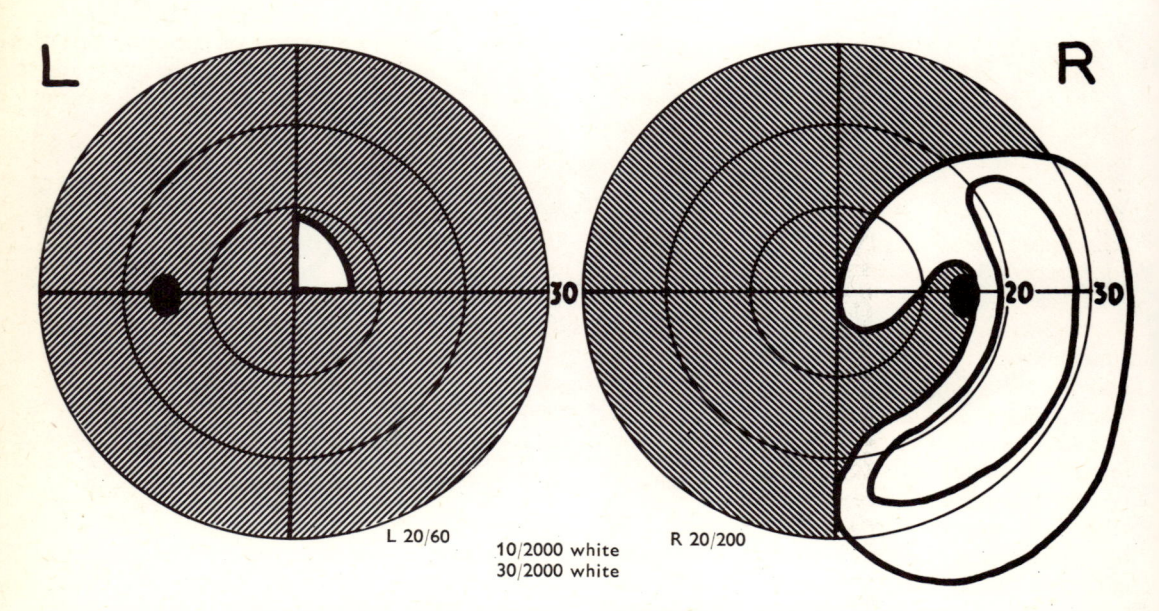

FIG. 158. Central fields of a patient with a large chromophobe adenoma. At operation it was found that the tumour had spread to compress the right optic tract.

It will combine the features of a chiasmal and a tract lesion. Theoretically, pressure on the junction of the optic tract and the chiasma will damage the posterior knee of Wilbrand, and cause a lower temporal defect in the field on the same side. But this is seldom seen.

The field defects depend upon whether the tract, or the chiasma, has suffered the greater damage. If the tract is more severely involved, the fields will exhibit the characteristics of a tract lesion. Sometimes the macular crossing fibres are damaged, and a scotoma on the temporal side of the midline will appear in the visual fields of one or both eyes.

BITEMPORAL SCOTOMATA

The earlier perimetrists considered that the presence of bitemporal scotomata indicated a rapidly growing tumour, and that bitemporal contraction of the isopters for the smaller targets suggested slow growth. Whilst there is no doubt this is so in many cases, interference with the nasal macular fibres which cross in the posterior part of the chiasma is the more usual cause of such scotomata.

It has usually been accepted that chromophobe pituitary tumours which compress the chiasma most commonly cause bilateral contraction of the isopters for smaller targets in the upper temporal quadrants but this may not be true [FIGS. 159 and 160].

The degree of pre-fixation or post-fixation of the chiasma is important in this connexion [see FIG. 12, p. 11]. The much quoted findings of de Schweinitz gave support to the commonly accepted view that chromophobe adenomata most frequently cause bitemporal contraction of the 2/2000 isopter by pressure on the anterior chiasma and that bitemporal scotomata due to pressure on the posterior chiasma are rare. But the findings of Wilson and Falconer challenge this traditional belief. They studied 50 patients with chromophobe pituitary tumours and found that 24 had bitemporal scotomata compared to 18 with typical bitemporal hemianopia. Their studies with air encephalography confirmed the orthodox view that bitemporal scotomata occurred when the pituitary tumour compressed the posterior part of the chiasma, whilst the classical pattern of field loss occurred when the pressure was anterior. They also confirmed that whilst steady and rather slow progression was the rule in the classical type of field defect, progression tended to be rapid in patients with scotomatous defects.

According to the usual anatomical description and illustration [FIG. 10] the anterior cerebral artery crosses just above the junction of the optic nerve and chiasma. Jefferson has pointed out that it frequently crosses above and just posterior to the middle of the chiasma. Thus, in his cases of anterior cerebral aneurysms, bitemporal scotomata usually occurred as the result of damage to the posterior macular crossing fibres.

Gliomata and craniopharyngiomata involving the posterior part of the chiasma, especially from above and behind, are also likely to cause bitemporal scotomata.

The bitemporal nature of refraction defects in myopia [p. 164] must always be borne in mind as a possible source of confusion.

FACTORS AFFECTING THE NATURE AND THE EXTENT OF FIELD DEFECTS

The chiasma is a relatively small structure measuring only 12 mm. by 8 mm. It is suspended above the diaphragma sellae in the cerebrospinal fluid of the cisterna basalis. It has been mentioned in the anatomical section that the intracranial length of the optic nerves may be from 10 mm. to 24 mm. Moreover, the optic nerves and chiasma may pass upwards and backwards from the optic foramina, making an angle of from 15 to 60 degrees with the horizontal. The importance of pre-fixation and post-fixation of the chiasma has already been emphasized. Its relation to surrounding structures is thus very variable.

Operative findings show that the chiasma may be markedly displaced without interference with the conduction of nerve impulses. A tumour must, therefore, reach a considerable size and cause much displacement before damaging the nerve fibres and causing field defects.

Cases occur in which the field defects do not indicate the site of the lesion clearly [FIG. 161]. A space-occupying tumour may displace the chiasma in any direction. There may be less damage at the site where it compresses the chiasma than occurs in other situations. Several factors may be responsible for this. It

134   CHIASMAL LESIONS

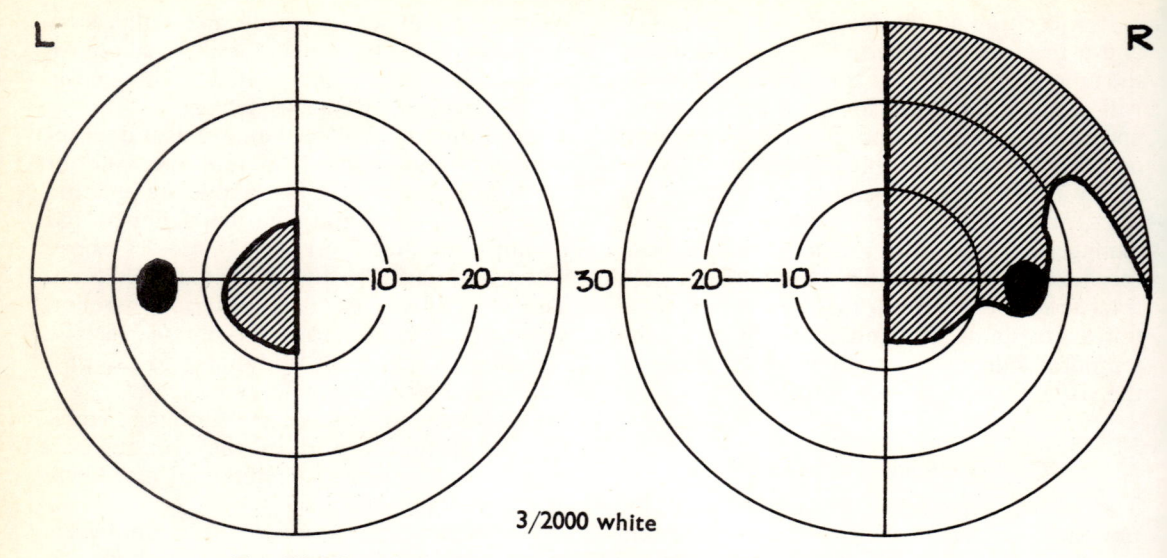

3/2000 white

FIG. 159. Bitemporal scotomata caused by a pituitary chromophobe adenoma.

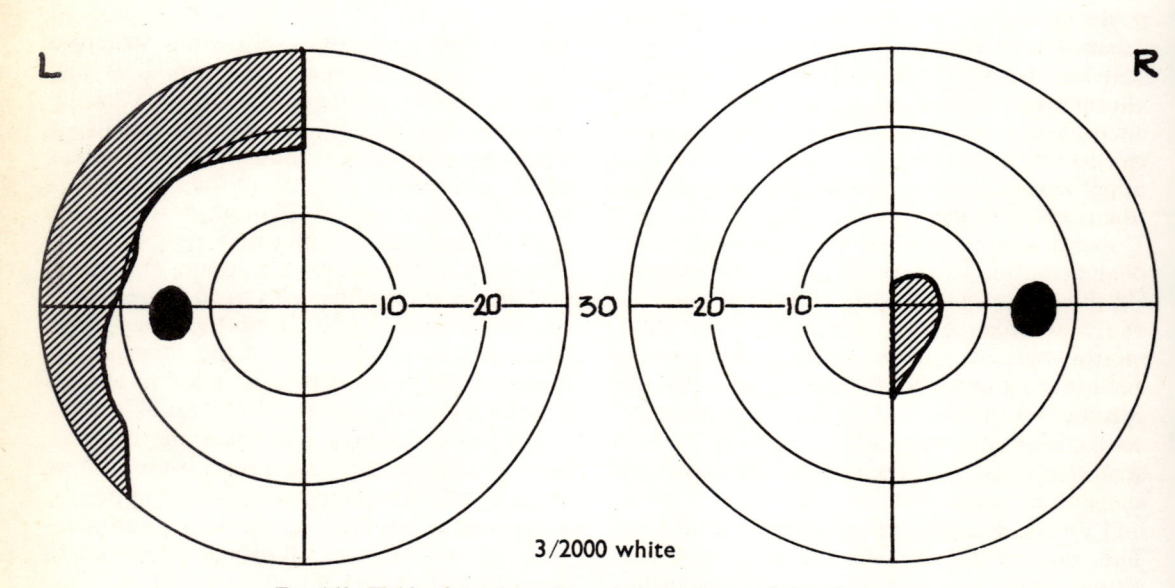

3/2000 white

FIG. 160. Fields of a patient with a pituitary chromophobe adenoma.

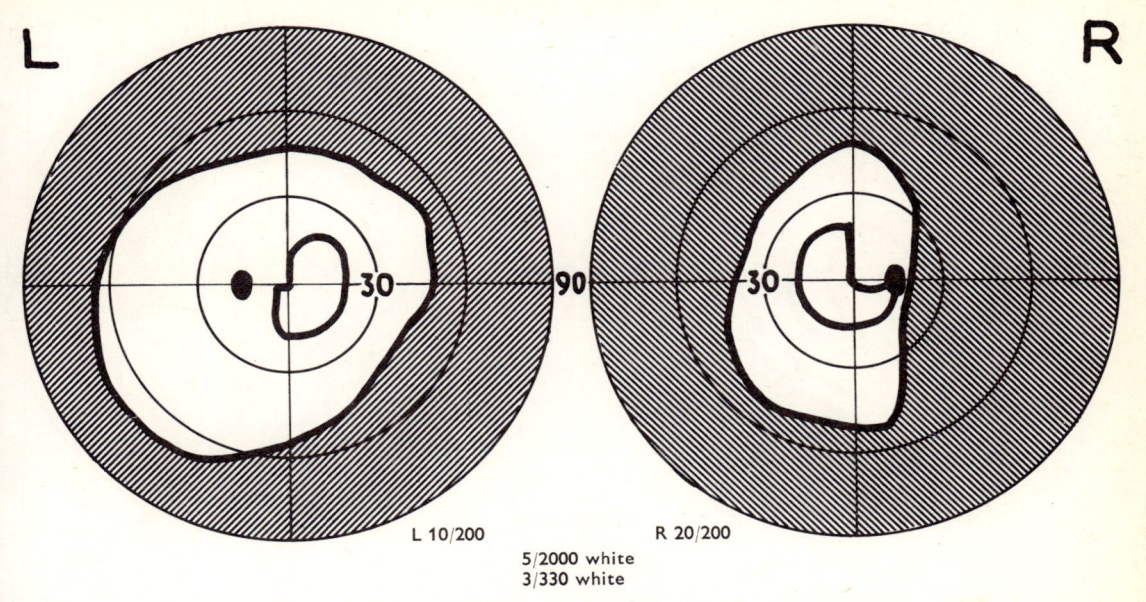

FIG. 161. Field changes in a patient with a suprasellar aneurysm.

is probable that interference with blood supply causes more visual failure than mere pressure on the nerve fibres and that stretching interferes with conduction in nerve fibres more than compression. Displacement of structures may result in nipping of a blood vessel which supplies an area distant from the tumour. The chiasma may be compressed against an artery. For example, Jefferson has suggested that bitemporal scotomata may result from a pituitary adenoma elevating the chiasma so that the posterior macular fibres are compressed by an anterior cerebral artery crossing behind its middle. Soft tumours occasionally grow and surround the chiasma and the optic nerve, and so cause generalized constriction of the visual fields which are of no localizing value.

The extent of the field defect gives little indication of the size of a tumour which may be compressing the chiasma. A slowly-growing tumour permits more adaptation to occur, and causes relatively less severe damage to the nerve fibres than a rapidly growing one. Tumours may, therefore, grow to a very large size before damaging the visual fibres. It has been stated that a pituitary adenoma must rise at least 2 cm. above the level of the clinoid processes before causing visual defects.

The advance of a field loss is not necessarily a steady one. It will be recalled that a sudden increase in the size of the field defects may result from haemorrhages into a tumour, ischaemic necrosis leading to cyst formation, and expansion of an aneurysm. Such a sudden increase is often followed by a period in which no change is observed. In pituitary adenomata a halt frequently occurs just before the invasion of the inferior nasal quadrant. This does not necessarily indicate that the tumour has ceased to grow. It may mean that it is expanding upwards between the uncrossed chiasmal fibres, which lie on either side of the tumour, relatively unharmed.

The tumour may extend forward to involve the optic nerve and cause a central scotoma on that side. If the neoplasm spreads backwards to involve a tract, the fields then combine in varying degrees the characters of a bitemporal hemianopia and a contralateral incongruous homonymous hemianopia [see FIGS. 156 and 158, pp. 131 and 132].

If the tumour spreads sideways and damages the uncrossed chiasmal fibres, the eye on the side suffering the greater damage will show the greater contraction of the nasal field.

Occasionally an arcuate defect may be found in the temporal field. Kearns and Rucker have

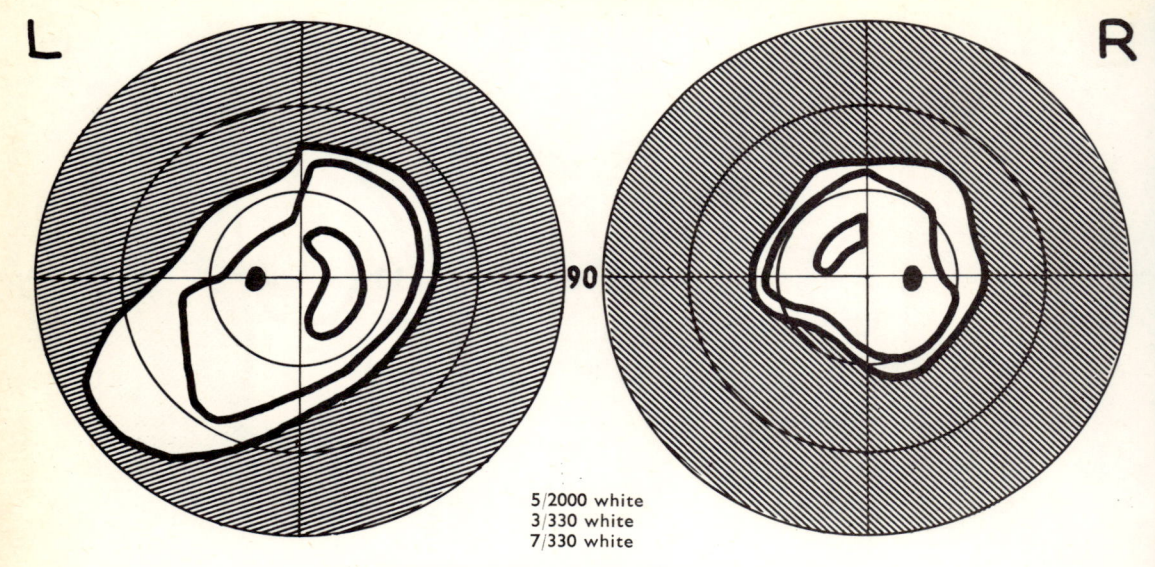

FIG. 162. Visual fields in optochiasmatic arachnoiditis.

5/2000 white
3/330 white
7/330 white

reported several patients with chromophobe adenomata exhibiting arcuate defects in the visual fields without any characteristic bitemporal changes. They were unable to explain the mechanism of production but suggested that the arcuate scotomata might be due to vascular changes in the optic nerve. Another explanation is that the arcuate fibres from the nasal halves of the retinae might cross the chiasma in bundles and be susceptible in some cases to damage by pressure.

OTHER CAUSES OF CHIASMAL LESIONS

Inflammations affect the chiasma rarely, but a few require special mention.

Disseminated Sclerosis

The field defects vary with the site of the demyelination. Bitemporal hemianopia, or a junction scotoma, may occur. Typically, bitemporal hemianopia develops rapidly with dense central defects. As in retrobulbar neuritis, the extent and shape of the field defects vary from day to day. The condition usually recovers almost completely in 2–3 months, leaving some pallor of both optic discs. The optic chiasma is affected much less commonly than the optic nerve in this disease.

Optochiasmatic Arachnoiditis

This is an ill-defined condition in which bands of arachnoid adhesions constrict the chiasma. Any cause of basal meningitis, such as syphilis, tuberculosis, blood in the subarachnoid space, and spread from inflammations of the paranasal sinuses, may cause this affection. But cases occur in which the pathogenesis cannot be satisfactorily explained.

It produces headaches and progressive loss of vision which may be slow or rapid. There may be nausea and dizziness. Exophthalmos occurs in about half the patients. Extra-ocular muscle palsies may occur. The optic disc may be normal, pale, or even oedematous. Bizarre field defects often accompany this condition. Bitemporal hemianopia may be found but irregular constriction of both visual fields in association with central scotomata is the most common finding [FIG. 162].

Occasionally arachnoid cysts may form, which act as space-occupying lesions.

Most authorities consider that a diagnosis of optochiasmatic arachnoiditis should be made only after an exploratory operation has revealed the condition. If exploration is omitted, operable tumours or cysts may be overlooked. Surgical removal of the adhesions surrounding the chiasma sometimes results in considerable

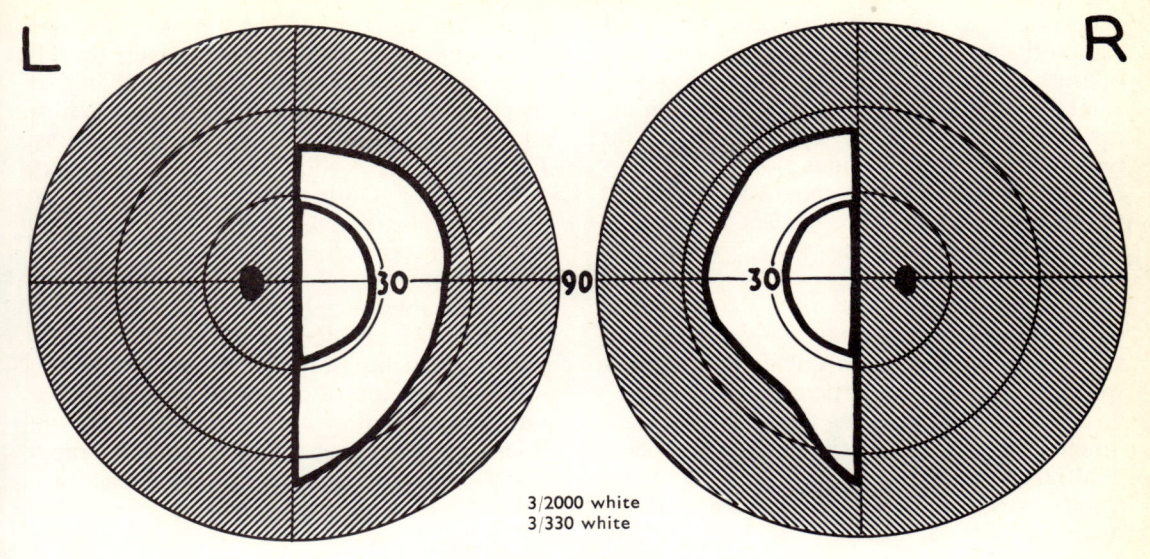

FIG. 163. Complete bitemporal hemianopia after a car accident.
(3/2000 white; 3/330 white)

visual improvement. At other times sight continues to deteriorate. Best results appear to result from early surgery followed by steroid therapy.

Syphilitic Basal Meningitis
This is seldom seen nowadays.

Severe Head Injuries
These, with or without fractures of the base of the skull, occasionally damage the chiasma. The chiasma may be torn by a bone fragment, or its blood supply may be impaired. Unfortunately these lesions are being seen more frequently with the increase in the number of car accidents. When it seems that only one eye is damaged the visual field of the other eye should always be examined because minimal changes may sometimes be found.

At first the patient is mentally confused as a result of cerebral contusion, so that examination of the visual fields may not be possible except by confrontation. The field defects resemble those found in chiasmal compression by a tumour but they have steep edges. They may increase during the few weeks following the injury because of cicatrization. Occasionally a complete bitemporal hemianopia with splitting of the macula occurs, presumably due to a midline tearing of the chiasma [FIG. 163]. Such field defects are almost never caused by a neoplasm.

INVESTIGATIONS
When the ocular and visual field examinations suggest that there is a chiasmal lesion, the following investigations are usually indicated:
1. A general medical and neurological examination.
2. X-ray of the skull and the optic foramina.

Pituitary adenomata expand and erode the walls of the pituitary fossa. The degree of erosion of the related bony structures depends on the direction in which the tumour expands. It may even encroach on the sphenoid sinus. The chromophobe adenoma grows large and balloons the fossa early so that lateral skull radiographs show some degree of enlargement in almost all cases. Erosion of the anterior clinoid processes, the posterior clinoid processes, and the dorsum sellae is also often seen. The eosinophil adenoma tends to be smaller, and the basophil adenoma is the smallest of the three.

Erosion of the dorsum sellae and the posterior clinoid processes is one of the earliest signs of an increase in intracranial pressure, whatever the cause. Erosion of an anterior clinoid process, or enlargement of an optic foramen, suggests the presence of a tumour such as an aneurysm, a meningioma, or a glioma of the optic nerve or chiasma.

Calcification may be seen in tumours such as craniopharyngiomata, gliomata, and sometimes meningiomata. It may occur as a late sign in the wall of an old aneurysm. The walls of atherosclerotic internal carotid arteries may sometimes show calcification. A meningioma may occasionally cause hyperostosis in the region of the sphenoid ridge.

3. Clinical studies for hormonal dysfunction if pituitary disease is suspected. The history and clinical examination usually supply more reliable information than laboratory and chemical studies.

4. Electroencephalography is sometimes of value, and has the great advantage of being without danger to the patient.

5. Brain scanning using radioactive compounds such as radioactive mercury is being used more frequently and will give a positive result in 80 per cent of cases. Superficial tumours such as meningiomas give positive results in almost all cases.

6. Ultrasonography is a newer technique which is proving of value in detecting the displacement of structures such as the falx cerebri.

7. Air encephalography, with special reference to the anterior end of the third ventricle and basal cisterns which may show distortion by a tumour.

8. Carotid arteriography. If optic atrophy is present, it usually indicates the side of the lesion, and the side which should, therefore, be injected for arteriography. Arteriography may demonstrate dilatation or displacement of the carotid artery, distortion or displacement of the vascular channels in the chiasmal area or increased vascularity in the region of the tumour.

PERIMETRY IN THE MANAGEMENT OF PITUITARY TUMOURS

There is a growing tendency to treat pituitary adenomata by radiotherapy, especially when the tumours are small or the patients are elderly and might not tolerate the operation. Where increasing field loss shows progressive visual failure despite radiotherapy, surgery is indicated. Very large or cystic tumours do not respond well to radiotherapy.

If visual field studies indicate progressive bitemporal field loss despite the lack of radiological or other confirmatory evidence, the neurosurgeon should be encouraged to undertake an exploratory craniotomy.

Chamlin has drawn attention to the value of repeated field studies, both during and after radiotherapy. He used the 1/2000 white and 2/330 white isopters almost exclusively for this purpose. The visual acuity and fields should be checked on alternate days during the therapy and then at monthly intervals for 6 months. Thereafter a check should be made about every 4–6 months. During the course of radiotherapy an extension of the field defects may occur, due to reactive oedema in the tumour. The radiotherapist should be informed, so that the dosage may be reduced, or the intervals between the doses prolonged. If the field loss continues to increase, surgery is usually indicated.

Rapid field loss suggests a haemorrhage or cystic degeneration within the tumour, but several cases have been reported in which rapid loss of central visual acuity followed excessive radiation therapy (above 3000 r). This visual loss was believed to be due to damage to the blood vessels supplying the visual pathway and to subsequent radiation necrosis.

In Chamlin's series visual improvement resulted in 60 per cent of patients, and in 30 per cent visual deterioration was halted by radiotherapy. Of those that improved, one half did so during the first year but in the other half improvement occurred as late as 2, 3, or even 4 years after treatment.

RECOVERY AFTER SURGERY

The degree of recovery depends upon the number of nerve fibres in the visual pathway which have atrophied. Recovery is less marked where tumours have grown slowly over a long period of time than in cases in which the visual failure has been rapid. Good visual recovery can be expected only if the visual symptoms have been present for less than 2 years [FIGS. 164 and 165].

Wilson and Falconer pointed out that almost all their patients who had had visual symptoms for 2 years or more had developed some optic atrophy, but the degree of pallor of the optic disc is not necessarily a reliable indication of the amount of recovery to be expected. Even when atrophy is fairly marked a considerable improvement in vision may occur. Wilson and Falconer reported that in their cases of chromophobe adenomas 94 per cent improved visually, one quarter regaining normal sight and one half regaining useful vision. The greatest improvement occurred in the scotomatous cases.

PERIMETRY IN THE MANAGEMENT OF PITUITARY TUMOURS 139

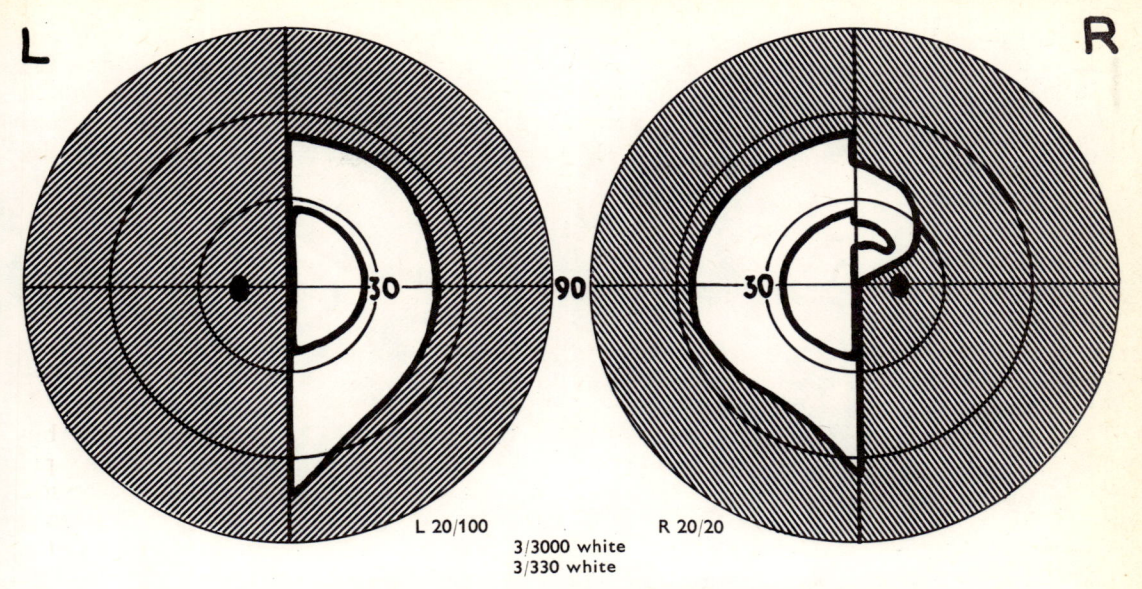

FIG. 164. Field changes in a patient with a chromophobe adenoma of the pituitary. The splitting of the macula which occurred in this case was unusual.

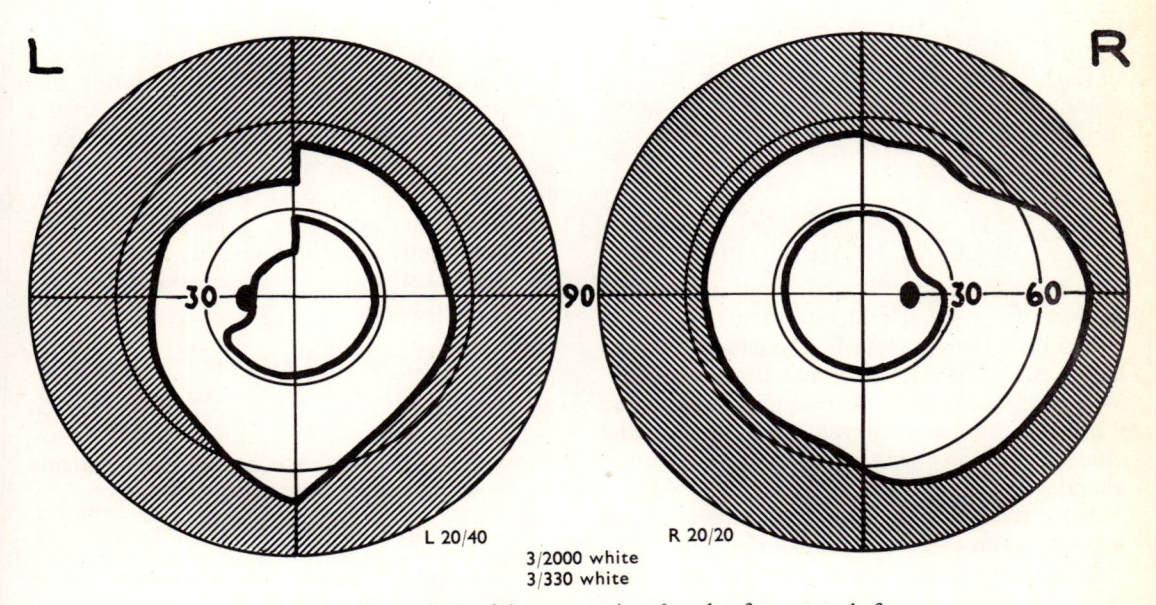

L 20/100   R 20/20
3/3000 white
3/330 white

FIG. 165. Visual fields of the same patient 6 weeks after removal of the tumour.

L 20/40   R 20/20
3/2000 white
3/330 white

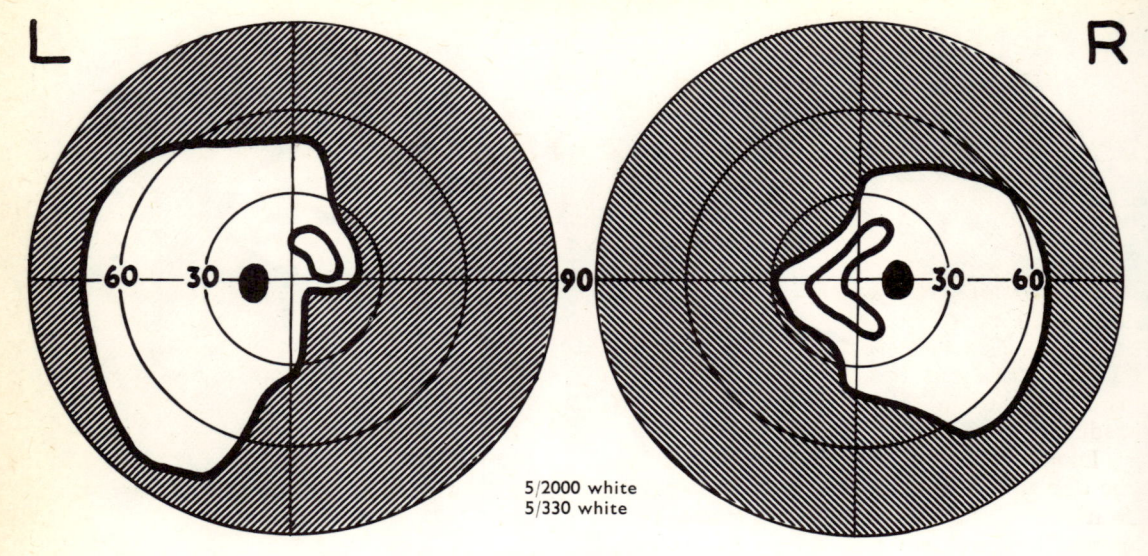

FIG. 166. Long-standing papilloedema with some contraction of the nasal fields.

5/2000 white
5/330 white

Improvement in vision occurs mainly during the first month after surgery and then little change can be expected. An interesting and important feature of the recovery is that regression of the defect retraces its development in reverse.

INTERNAL HYDROCEPHALUS AND BINASAL HEMIANOPIA

The effect of internal hydrocephalus upon the chiasma is not well understood. It will be recalled that the chiasma is situated at the anterior end of the floor of the third ventricle. When internal hydrocephalus occurs, the dilatation of the third ventricle stretches the chiasma and displaces it forwards and downwards.

Since the fibres from the nasal halves of the macular areas cross in the posterior part of the chiasma, one would expect to find bitemporal central scotomata. This sometimes occurs, but no characteristic defect is constantly associated with internal hydrocephalus.

Binasal hemianopia is sometimes found in these cases and much has been written in an attempt to explain the association. It was formerly believed that the dilated third ventricle displaced the chiasma anteriorly so that the internal carotid arteries compressed the uncrossed fibres from the temporal halves of the retina. This is no longer accepted. It is now considered that in most cases the binasal hemianopia results from post-neuritic atrophy, following long-standing papilloedema [FIG. 166]. It is not known, however, why the uncrossed fibres should be more vulnerable than the crossed fibres.

REFERENCES AND FURTHER READING

CHAMLIN, M. (1958) Visual field changes produced by X-ray treatment of pituitary tumours, *Brit. J. Ophthal.*, **42**, 193.

CHAMLIN, M., and DAVIDOFF, L. M. (1950) 1/2000 field in chiasmal interference, *Arch. Ophthal.*, **44**, 53.

JEFFERSON, G. (1955) *Clinical Neurosurgery*, Baltimore.

KEARNS, T. P., and RUCKER, C. W. (1958) Arcuate defects in the visual fields due to chromophobe adenoma of the pituitary gland, *Amer. J. Ophthal.*, **45**, 505.

MOONEY, A. J. (1964) Colour of optic disc and its relation to various field defects, *Trans. ophthal. Soc. U.K.*, **84**, 227.

WILSON, P., and FALCONER, M. A. (1968) Patterns of visual failure with pituitary tumours, *Brit. J. Ophthal.*, **52**, 94.

14
RETROCHIASMAL LESIONS

Retrochiasmal lesions may affect the optic tracts, the lateral geniculate bodies, the optic radiations, or the visual cortex. Interference with the tract and the lateral geniculate bodies is less common than damage to the optic radiations and visual cortex.

Damage to the retrochiasmal pathway may be due to inflammation, a vascular accident, trauma, or to a space-occupying lesion. In all cases, homonymous hemianopia or quadrantopia results.

In vascular accidents and in trauma the onset of the hemianopia is usually abrupt, but with space-occupying lesions it is slowly progressive. Since vascular accidents occur more frequently than space-occupying lesions, the onset of homonymous hemianopia is more often abrupt than gradual.

Hemiplegia may accompany the sudden development of hemianopia. If any hemiplegic signs are present, a lesion involving the posterior part of the internal capsule and the anterior end of the optic radiation should be suspected. The absence of hemiplegia suggests that the lesion is more posteriorly placed.

Lesions involving the optic tract alone are exceedingly rare. Far more commonly the tract is involved secondarily by a pituitary adenoma growing backwards. In this case the signs and symptoms of the chiasmal compression and local enlargement are more obvious than those of the involvement of the tract. Less frequently, a temporal lobe tumour will spread to involve a tract but again the effects of the involvement of the temporal lobe are usually more obvious than the signs of tract damage.

INFLAMMATORY LESIONS

Inflammatory disease, such as disseminated sclerosis and encephalitis, affect the retrochiasmal pathway rarely. When disseminated sclerosis attacks the retrochiasmal pathway it usually causes hemianopic homonymous scotomata, especially in young women. The onset is rapid and there is fairly prompt recovery [FIGS. 167 and 168], but unfortunately other manifestations of the disease usually supervene and the prognosis is poor. This contrasts with the prognosis of retrobulbar neuritis which in about 50 per cent of cases is good.

VASCULAR LESIONS

Cerebral arteriosclerosis may result in a great variety of clinical manifestations. These depend on the site of the occlusion, whether it is complete or partial, and on the vagaries of the collateral circulation. It is now realized that atherosclerotic narrowing of the main arteries, such as the internal carotid, basilar and vertebral, occurs more commonly than was previously thought. This narrowing results in a reduction in the rate and volume of blood flow. The cerebral tissue supplied by the artery suffers from ischaemia, and cerebral infarction of small or large areas may follow. These cause clinical manifestations which depend upon the site and extent of the infarction.

Since the narrowing develops gradually, the symptoms are often transient at first, due to ischaemic episodes in the affected cerebral tissue.

Atherosclerotic narrowing of the internal carotid or middle cerebral artery may result in a sudden onset of homonymous hemianopia, hemiplegia and numbness of the opposite side [FIG. 169]. But this end result is usually preceded by transient ischaemic attacks which may last from a few seconds to several hours. One to ten minutes is the usual duration. In about half of these cases amaurosis fugax may be experienced on the side of the narrowed internal carotid artery. Transient attacks occur if the arterial narrowing or a small embolus causes temporary cerebral ischaemia. Permanent

RETROCHIASMAL LESIONS

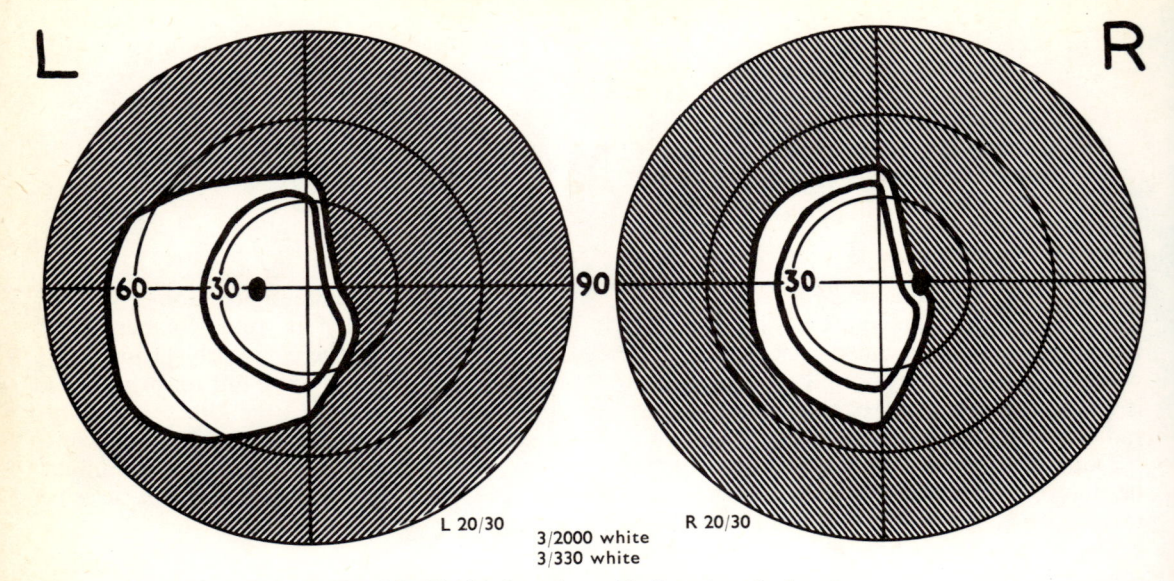

L 20/30   R 20/30
3/2000 white
3/330 white

Fig. 167. Fields of a patient with disseminated sclerosis.

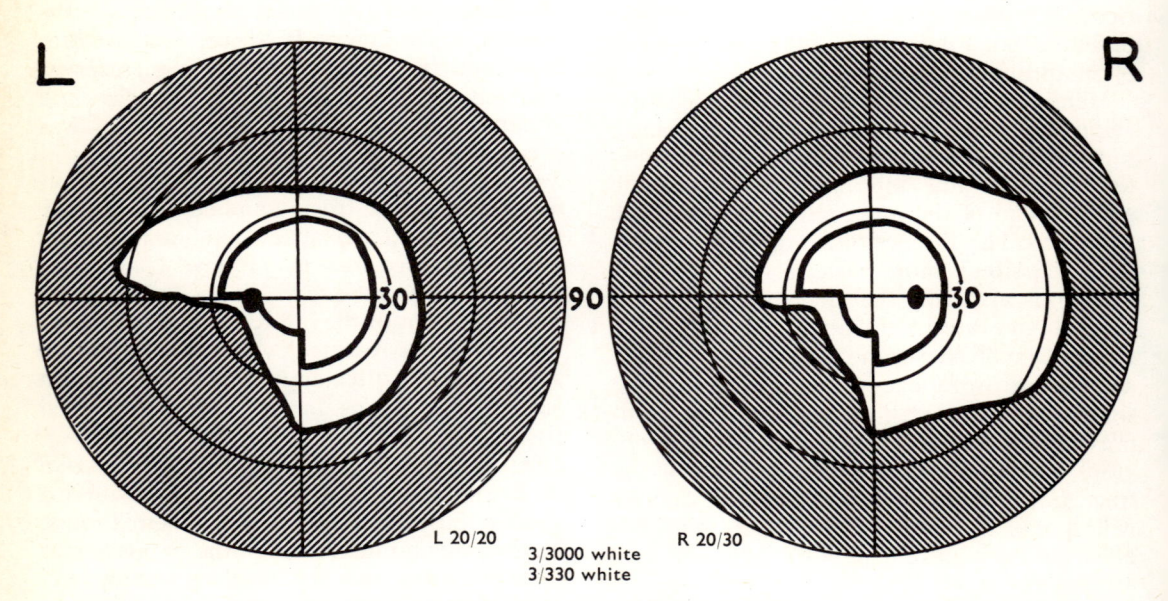

L 20/20   R 20/30
3/3000 white
3/330 white

Fig. 168. Fields of the same patient one month later.

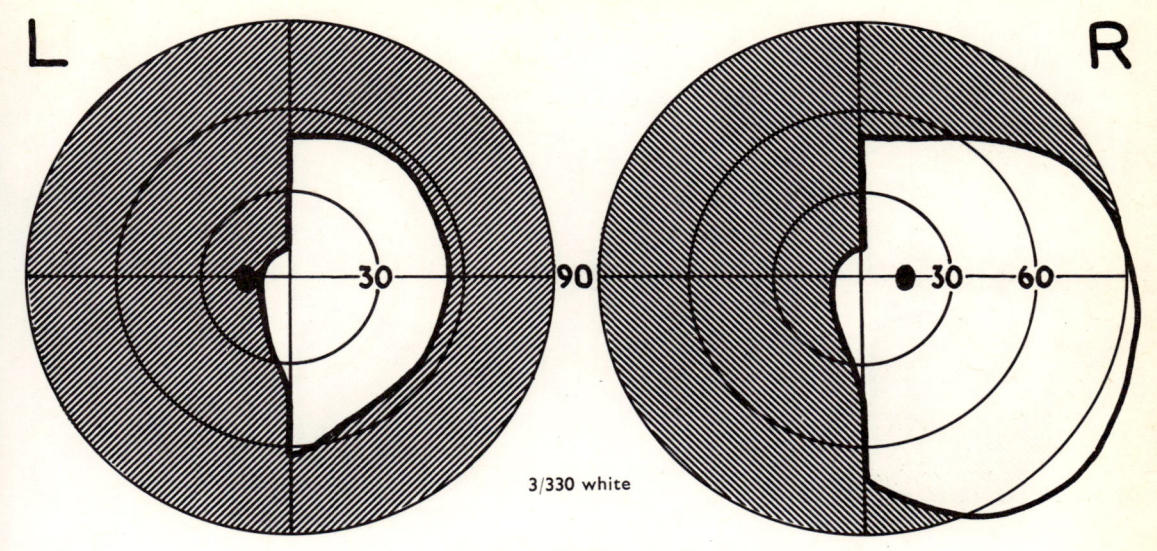

FIG. 169. Left congruous homonymous hemianopia with macular sparing in a patient with a sudden onset of left hemiplegia.

hemiplegia occurs if complete occlusion causes a cerebral infarction. When the infarction is widespread in the dominant hemisphere, aphasia often occurs, and, if the parietal area is involved, the patient may be strangely oblivious of his hemiplegic side.

Homonymous hemianopia is not uncommon in these patients. Very rarely the ophthalmic artery may be involved, so that monocular blindness occurs. The loss of vision in homonymous hemianopia due to atherosclerosis is not always permanent. There may sometimes be a considerable recovery but in almost all cases a quadrantic or partial hemianopic defect in the field of each eye is left.

The upper nerve fibres of the optic radiation are supplied solely by branches from the middle cerebral artery, but the lower fibres receive an additional supply from branches of the posterior cerebral artery. The upper fibres are therefore more commonly affected by ischaemic lesions than the lower fibres. This explains the relative frequency of homonymous inferior quadrantopia [FIG. 170].

Atherosclerotic stenosis of the basilar-vertebral arterial tree results in ischaemia of the midbrain. Transient ischaemic attacks may occur and give rise to a diverse symptomatology. The most common complaint is of dizziness either alone or in combination with other symptoms. Mental confusion, abducens and facial palsies, dysarthria, dysphagia, hemiparesis, and numbness, pallor, and sweating may occur. Ocular manifestations of midbrain involvement are nystagmus, internuclear ophthalmoplegia, corneal anaesthesia and orbicularis weakness.

Some cases of homonymous hemianopia may be due to a piece of thrombus breaking off a basilar or vertebral artery and lodging in the posterior cerebral or calcarine arteries. Homonymous scotomata may suddenly develop in elderly people, presumably due to a similar mechanism causing a small embolus in a terminal branch of a calcarine artery [FIG. 171].

Ophthalmologists should be familiar with these features of transient ischaemic attacks. In the majority of cases they precede the final occlusion. Thus if they are not recognized hemiplegia or death may result. Treatment with anticoagulants may be effective in preventing further ischaemic episodes and the threatened infarction.

Bilateral infarction of the occipital lobes may occur. One side is usually affected before the other. The interval between the two accidents may be weeks, months, or years. Its onset may be gradual but is usually sudden, often following sleep. There may be at first a complaint of

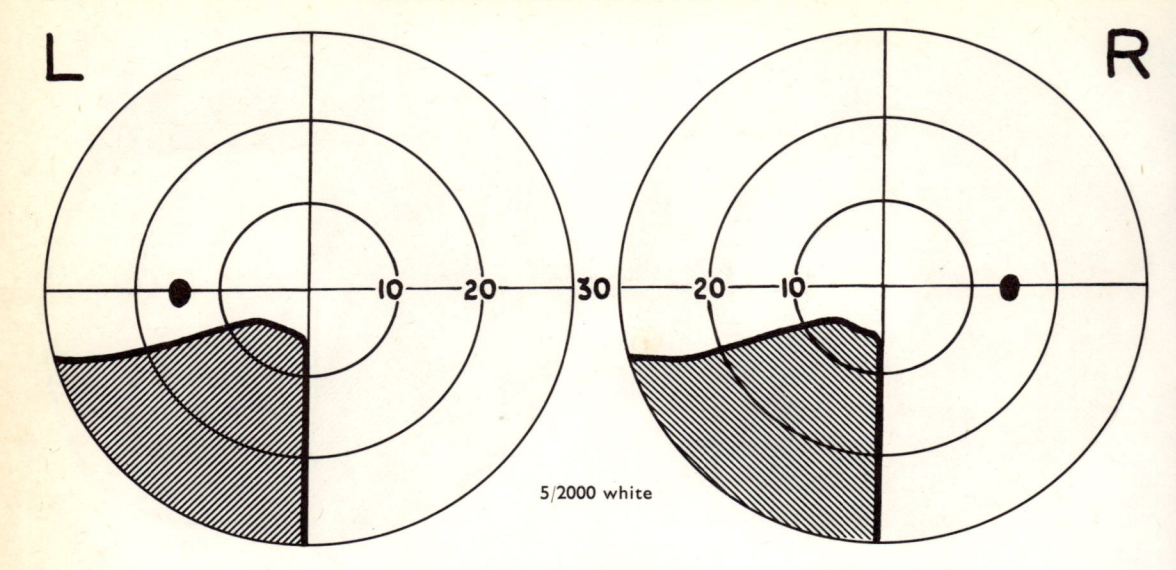

FIG. 170. Left inferior congruous homonymous hemianopia with macular sparing.

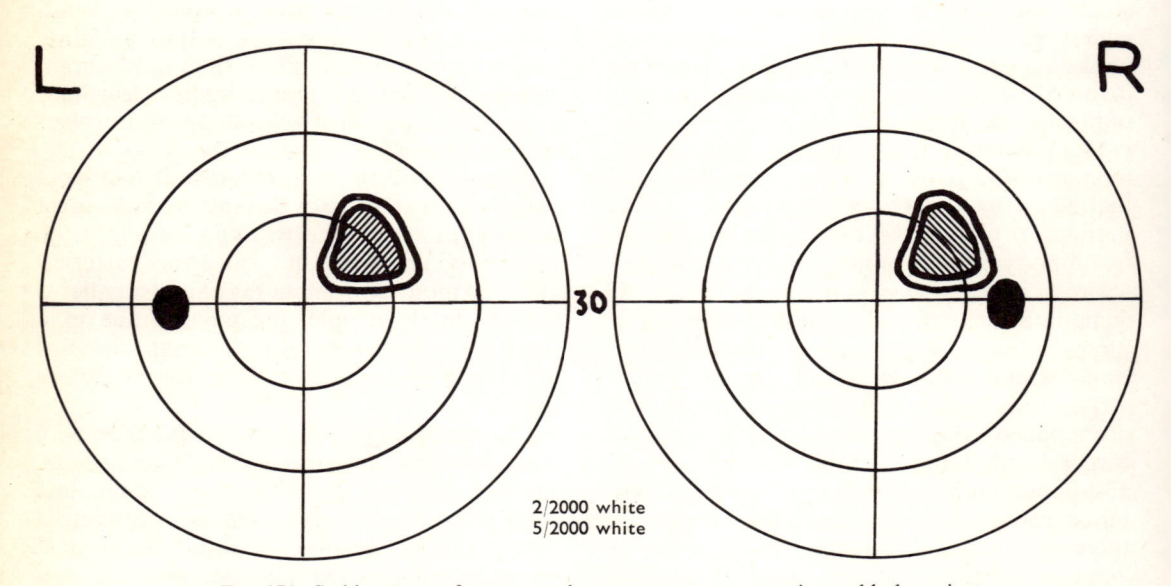

FIG. 171. Sudden onset of congruous homonymous scotomata in an elderly patient.

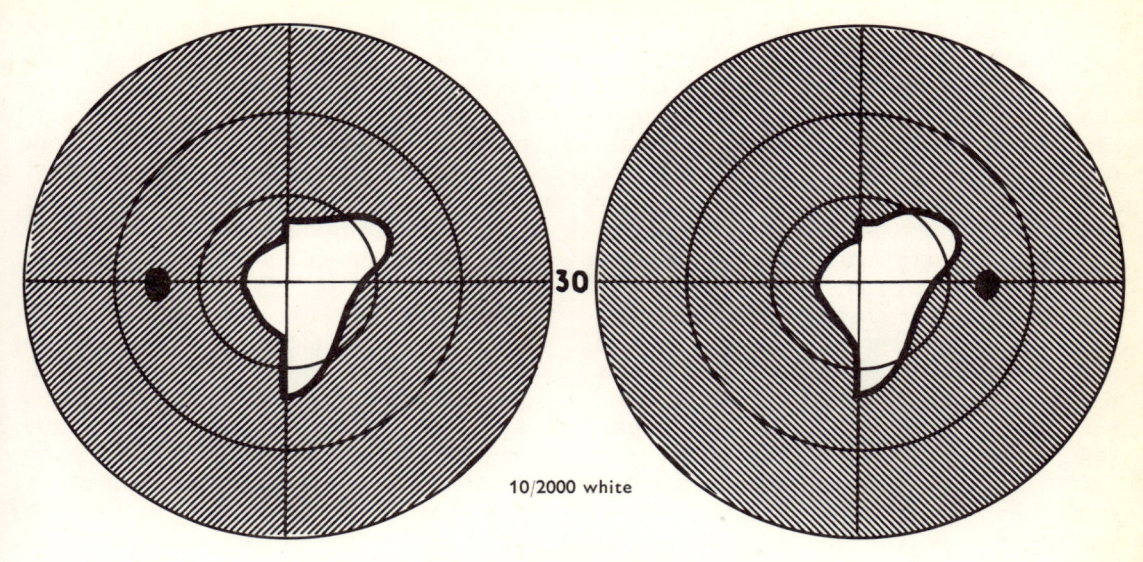

Fig. 172. Fields in bilateral infarction of the occipital lobes.

darkness followed by a gradual return of vision, first light, then movements and lastly colours. Complete recovery is unusual and homonymous field defects usually remain. In severe cases there is usually mental confusion, and the patients often deny that they are blind. The fact that they are unaware of visual failure may be due to destruction of the related visual association areas in the occipital lobes.

This condition is known as cortical blindness or Anton's syndrome and it has the following characteristics:
1. The patient does not know that he is blind.
2. The pupillary reactions are normal.
3. The fundi are normal.
4. The blinking protective reflex is absent.
5. The perception of light and the sense of light projection are absent.

This fully developed clinical picture is not commonly seen but incomplete manifestations in which the patient has only a clouded understanding of the severity of visual loss, some mental confusion, and a small residual central field are fairly common [FIG. 172].

In cases of *cerebral haemorrhage* the dramatic nature of the 'stroke' tends to confuse the clinical picture. The patient is often unconscious or stuporose when first seen, and a visual defect cannot be detected. Later, during convalescence, the patient may complain of loss of vision of one eye, or of bumping into objects on one side, and investigation may lead to the discovery of homonymous hemianopia.

Cerebral tumours which cause a rise in intracranial pressure may occasionally produce hippocampal herniation through the tentorium cerebelli. If this happens, the posterior cerebral artery may be compressed. Occlusion may follow and produce a sudden onset of homonymous hemianopia. The field defect in this case may be misleading, since it does not give a true indication of the site of the tumour.

TRAUMA

Injury to the retrochiasmal pathway is not often seen in civilian practice. A car accident may occasionally cause such an injury but these patients are more often seen by neurosurgeons than ophthalmologists. Wars produce many such injuries and there are several careful studies of visual field defects resulting from damage to the occipital lobes by shell fragments and bullets during the two world wars.

An injury to the head frequently causes partial or complete loss of consciousness. Accurate assessment of the damage to the visual pathway soon after the injury may therefore be very difficult. Since a sluggish or absent pupil reaction to direct light is dependent upon the visual pathway anterior to the lateral geniculate bodies, this sign is of little help in assessing damage to the retrochiasmal pathway.

When the patient is seen soon after the injury or upon regaining consciousness, it may not be possible to do more than assess the visual field by confrontation. Later, when the patient is stronger it may be possible to make a more thorough examination and to record the visual field changes. These patients are often unable to concentrate and this tends to make accurate and detailed assessment difficult or impossible.

If the patient's fixation tends to wander it is often helpful to put a white target 1–2 degrees in diameter in the centre of the blindspot on the screen. Any wandering of fixation causes this white target to be seen and both the patient and perimetrist are alerted.

Some workers have found the critical fusion frequency useful in assessing patients with injuries to the occipital cortex. They have recorded changes in the critical fusion frequency in abnormal areas of the field and have reported that this test is often more sensitive than the more usual methods of perimetry.

An hysterical component may often be added to the defect in traumatic cases so that it is difficult to make a true assessment of the severity of the lesion. However, there are two features which should always be remembered as characteristic of hysterical fields. First, the edge of the seeing area is usually smooth and steep. Secondly, if the defect is measured at three or four different distances from the screen the size of the defect on the screen will be found to vary little and will fail to change appropriately with the varying distances.

PATTERNS OF FIELD DEFECT

If a neoplasm begins at the occipital pole it will, at first, produce homonymous scotomata. As it spreads forward to affect more anterior parts of the visual cortex the scotomata will enlarge to involve more peripheral areas of the visual field. Similarly the nature of the field defect following injury depends upon the site of the trauma to the visual cortex. If a shell fragment destroys the occipital pole of one cortex, homonymous scotomata of the opposite halves of the two visual fields may result, their size depending upon the extent of the damage to the visual cortex [FIG. 173]. If both occipital poles are destroyed, bilateral homonymous scotomata result [FIG. 174]. But a missile passing through the visual cortex anterior to the posterior pole may result in a type of tubular field [FIG. 175].

Soon after an injury, variable or transient annular type scotomata may be found which may later either disappear or become permanent. With time *central or paracentral scotomata* may result in the development of 'false maculas' but the visual acuity of these extrafoveal areas does not increase significantly above the level to be expected in a similar extrafoveal area in a normal eye. Ocular torsion has occasionally been reported in the presence of large defects so that the vertical meridian is tilted. The use of an extrafoveal area and tilting of the vertical meridian may be confirmed by demonstrating a corresponding displacement of the blind spot. It should also be remembered that direct injury to an eye may occur at the same time as the occipital damage, causing traumatic oedema of the macula with an associated central scotoma.

Following the First World War, Holmes and Lister reported a number of cases of *altitudinal scotomata* resulting from gunshot wounds of the occiput. Other workers have reported similar cases which occurred in both world wars. These scotomata are caused by bullets or shell fragments passing horizontally through the occiput. If large, the defects may result in a vertical shift in fixation. This is readily demonstrated by plotting the blindspot. Inferior altitudinal defects [FIG. 176] are seen more frequently than superior altitudinal defects, probably because lesions below the occipital pole tend to involve venous sinuses or the brain stem and thus result in death.

Damage to the occipital lobes seen in civilian practice is usually the result of depressed fractures and contusion or destruction of brain tissue following car or motorcycle accidents. When first seen, the field defect may be extensive but healing may result in surprising recovery [FIGS. 177–180].

The destruction of the visual cortex of one lobe results in *homonymous hemianopia*. If the

TRAUMA

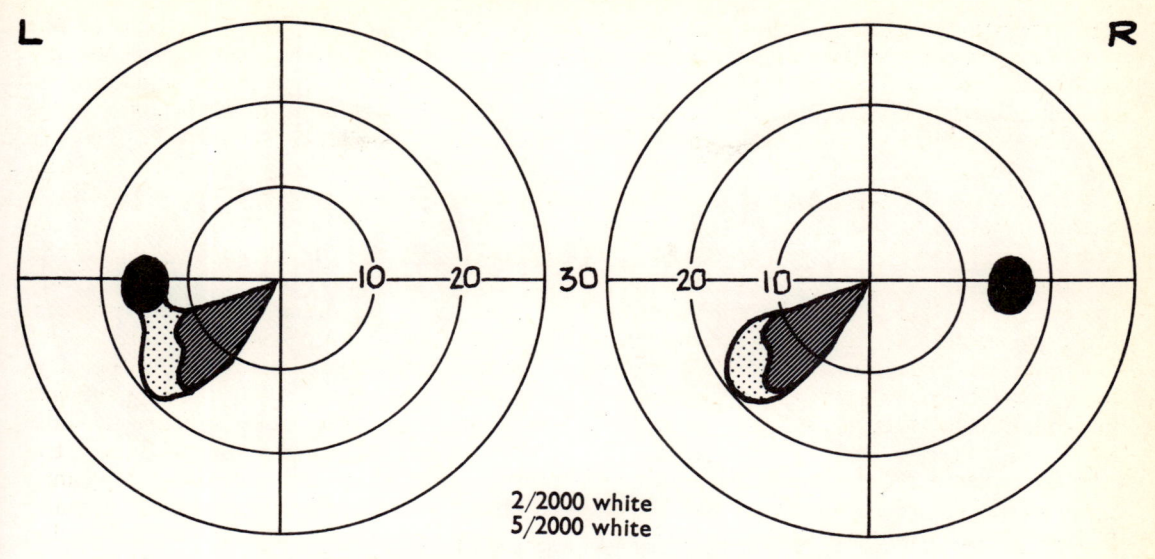

FIG. 173. Damage to occipital pole causing homonymous scotomata. 2/2000 white; 5/2000 white

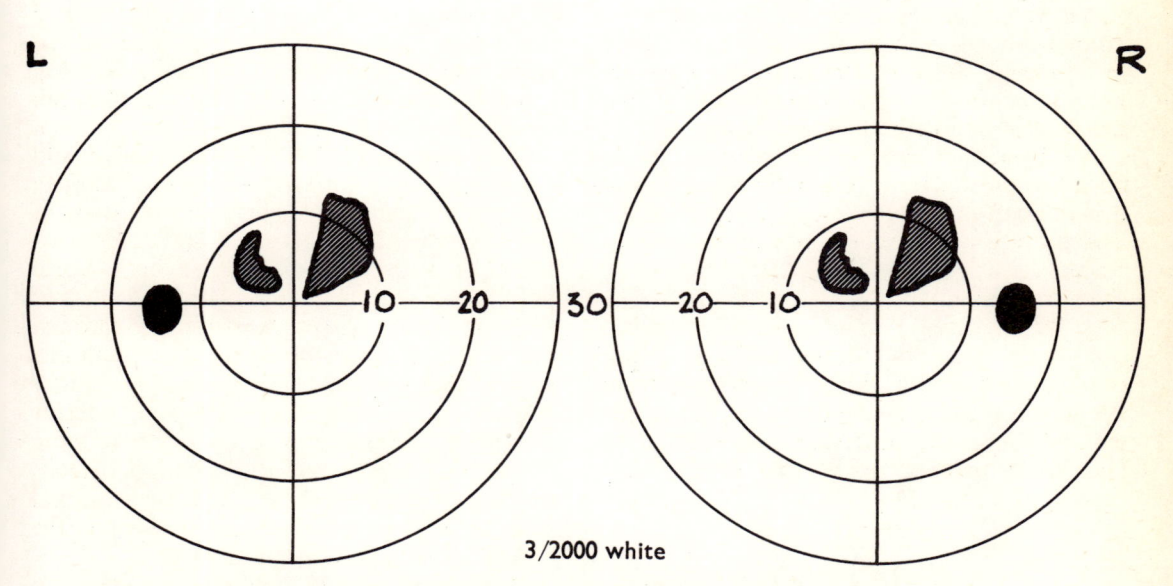

FIG. 174. Trauma to occipital lobe producing bilateral homonymous scotomata. 3/2000 white

148   RETROCHIASMAL LESIONS

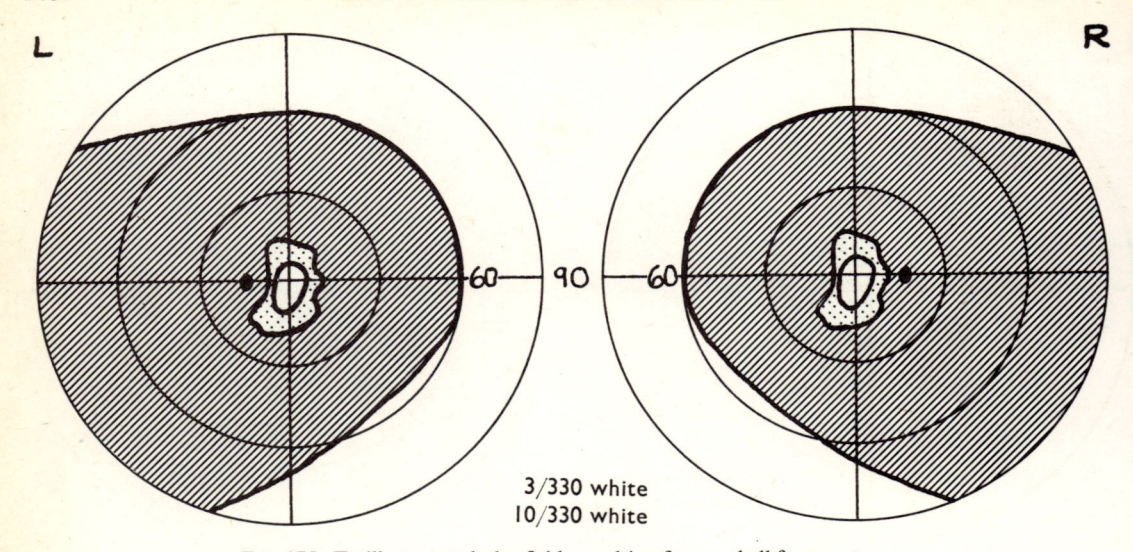

3/330 white
10/330 white

Fig. 175. To illustrate tubular fields resulting from a shell fragment damaging the anterior part of the visual cortex on each side.

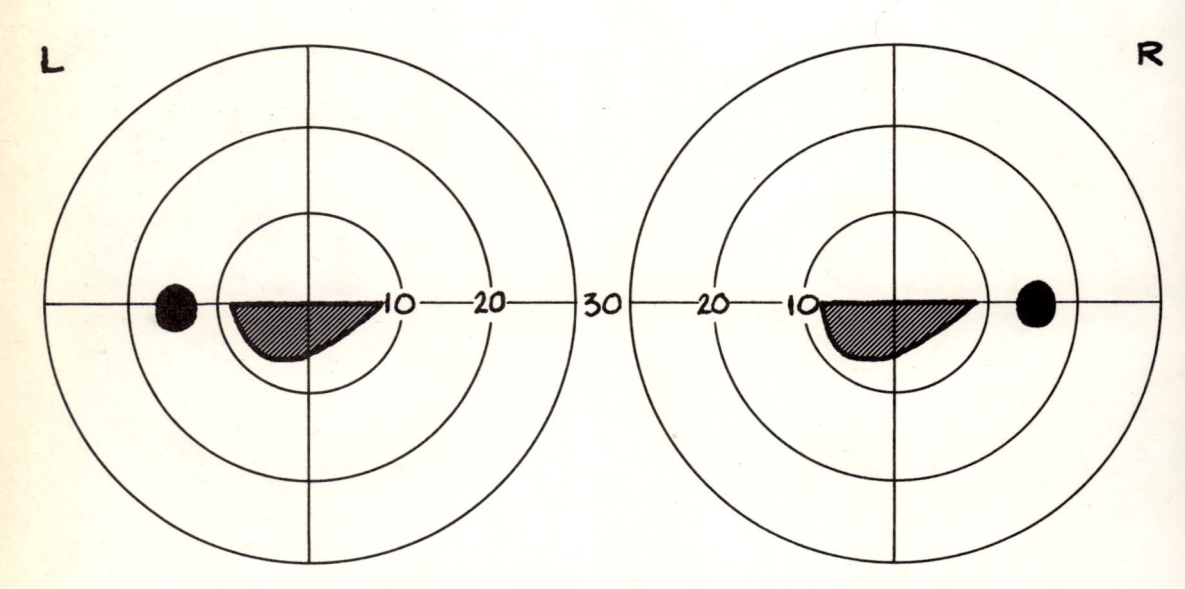

Fig. 176. To illustrate altitudinal defects caused by bullets passing horizontally through the occiput.

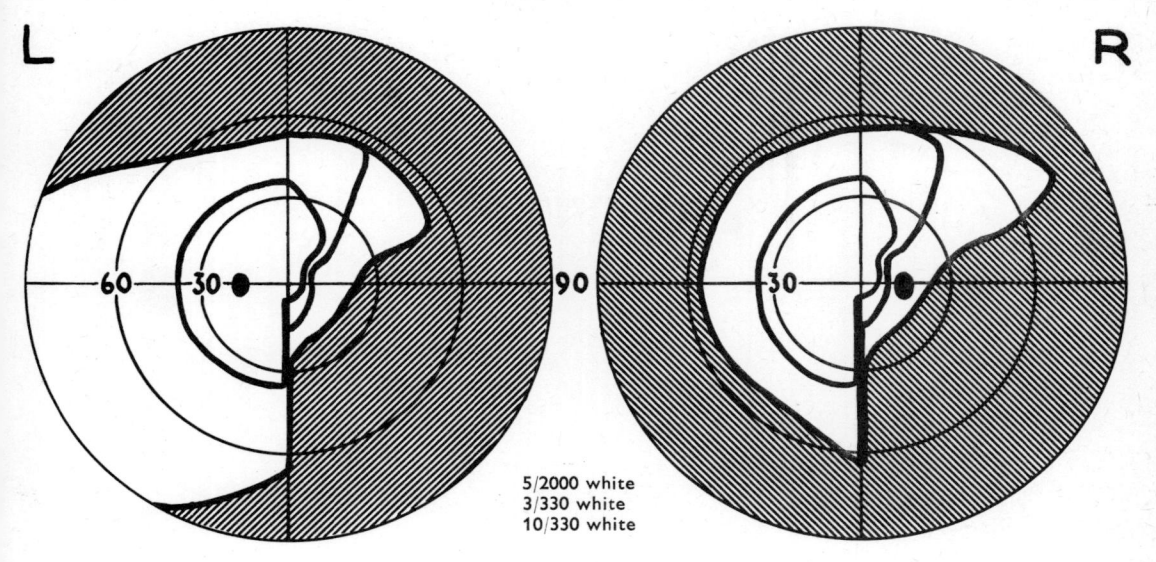

FIG. 177. Field defects one week after elevation of a depressed fracture of the skull in the left parieto-occipital region.

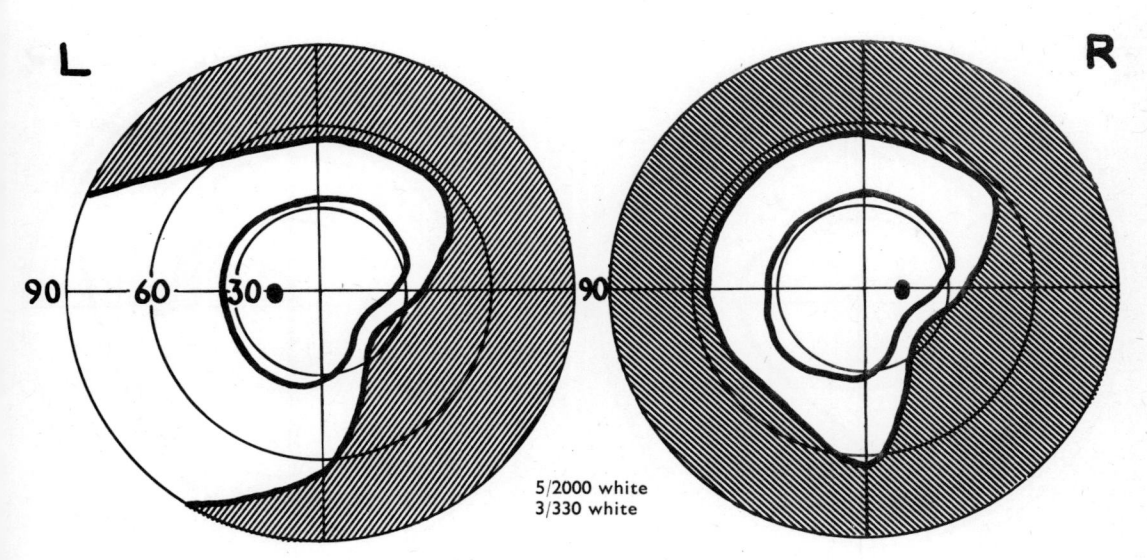

5/2000 white
3/330 white
10/330 white

FIG. 178. Six weeks after elevation of the depressed bone fragments.

5/2000 white
3/330 white

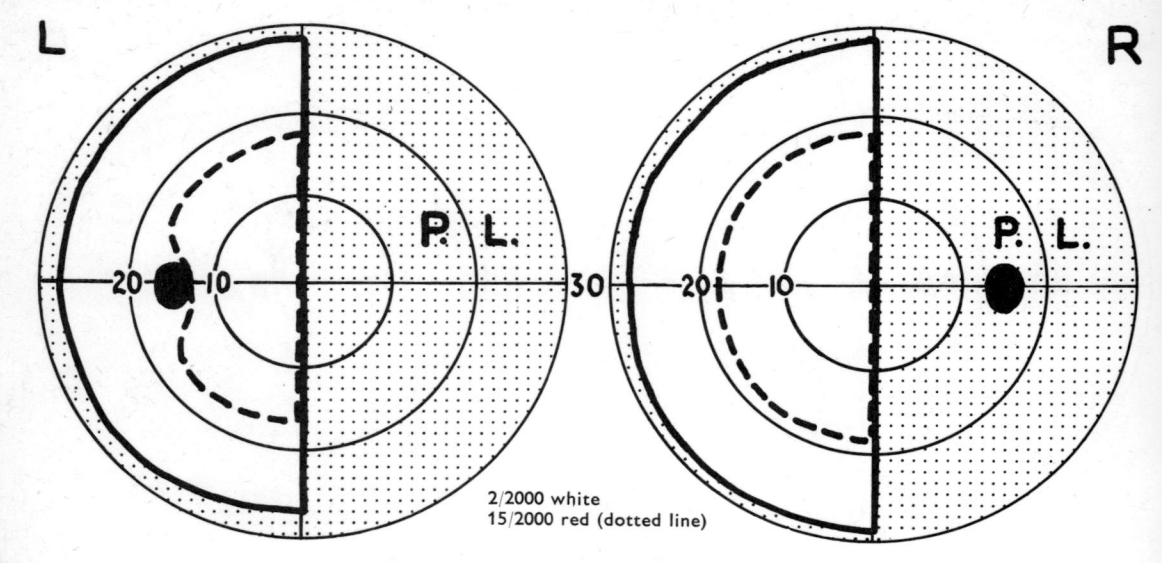

FIG. 179. Field defects 5 days after injury to the left occipital pole.

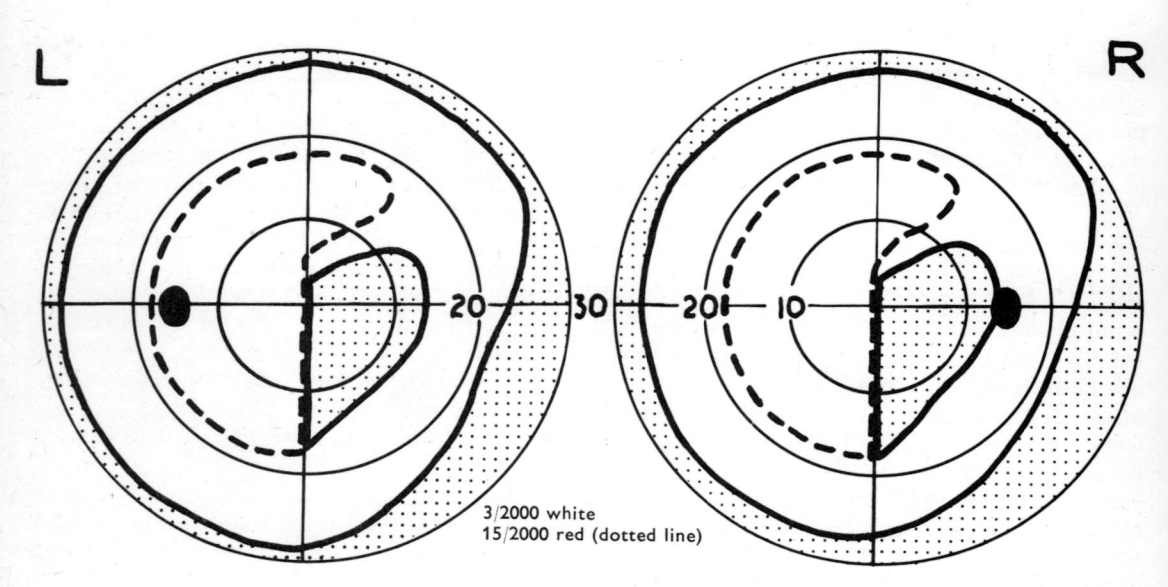

2/2000 white
15/2000 red (dotted line)

FIG. 180. Fields of the same patient 6 weeks after the injury.

3/2000 white
15/2000 red (dotted line)

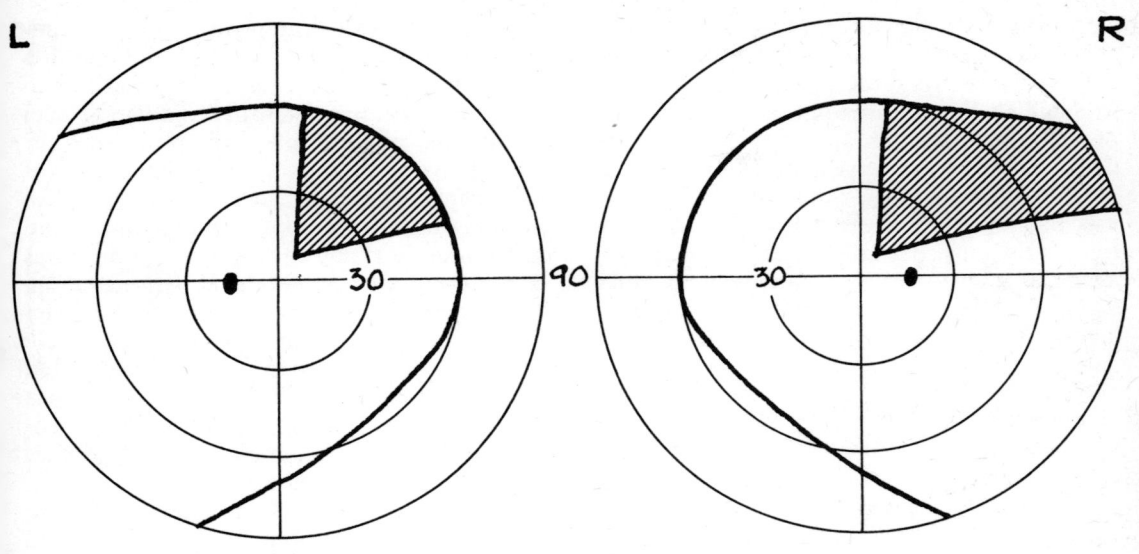

FIG. 181. Fields resulting from a gunshot wound damaging the anterior pole of the left temporal lobe.

destruction is the result of a gunshot wound, it is not uncommon to find a paracentral scotoma in the shape of an arc or claw in the opposite field. This may be transient or permanent. In such homonymous defects the patient complains of loss of vision in the eye with the temporal field defect. The loss of vision in the nasal field of the other eye is less obvious and is often overlooked.

Quadrantic defects may occur following gunshot wounds. They tend to be sector shaped, filling a triangular area within the quadrant with the apex pointing towards the fixation point [FIG. 181]. The horizontal meridian is usually spared. This type of quadrantic defect is usually due to damage to the anterior portion of the optic radiations and resembles the defects produced by amputation of the anterior pole of the temporal lobe [see p. 17]. Spalding suggested that in the anterior part of the optic radiations the fibres serving central vision are spread out over the lateral aspect of the radiation whilst the fibres serving peripheral vision are medial. Posteriorly the fibres are aggregated into three groups, the peripheral fibres being above and below and the central fibres intermediate in position.

Spalding was the first to point out that homonymous quadrantic defects due to injuries to the occipital pole seldom involve the horizontal meridian. This has been commented upon by others and the concensus is that it is due to the fact that the horizontal meridian is represented by cortical tissue in the depth of the calcarine fissure and is thus relatively protected.

It is interesting that the meticulous studies of several workers in this field have demonstrated that in homonymous quadrantopia or hemianopia due to injury, absolute *congruity* seldom occurs. In fact it may be said that the more careful the study the more frequently will small incongruities be found. It is usual for the fields to be similar but the finding of exact congruity is often the result of hasty or inaccurate plotting. It is probable that these incongruities are due to slight irregularities in the development of the nerve fibres. In some cases the incongruities may be due to vagaries of testing.

Macular sparing is very common in vascular accidents because of the anastomosis at the posterior pole of terminal branches of the middle and posterior cerebral arteries. It is much less common following injuries to the occipital region. In fact the macula may occasionally be completely 'split'. It is interesting that Allen reviewed a series of new growths affecting the occipital lobe and found that one third of the cases also showed macular splitting.

Another feature which the more careful

studies reveal is that the vertical line between seeing and blind portions of the hemianopic fields is rarely straight. Usually a slight curve is found. This feature, in addition to the finding of slight incongruities, supports the theory of irregular growth of nerve fibres.

Unlike patients who suffer visual loss from vascular lesions of the visual cortex, who are frequently only partially aware or even unaware of their visual loss, patients who suffer trauma to the visual cortex of one or both hemispheres are keenly aware of the visual defect.

SPACE-OCCUPYING LESIONS

Tumour tissue is itself inert. Tumours, therefore, cause symptoms by compressing nervous tissue, and interfering with function. They usually grow slowly. Thus, if any part of the retrochiasmal pathway is involved, a slowly progressive homonymous hemianopia occurs.

Patients may complain of gradual loss of vision on one side, or of increasing difficulty in reading, especially if the hemianopia is on the right side, due to difficulty in guiding the eyes along the line.

Compression or displacement of adjacent structures by a space-occupying lesion may lead to irritative phenomena which are akin to the symptoms of epilepsy. These occur much less frequently than simple visual failure, and vary with the site of the lesion. These irritative phenomena may take the form of visual hallucinations. They may be of two types. Unorganized hallucinations, such as flashes of light, colours, stars, and rainbows, result from lesions in the occipital lobe. Formed hallucinations, such as animals, human faces, or trees, are caused by tumours in the posterior areas of the temporal lobe.

Space-occupying lesions in the temporal lobe may cause epileptic phenomena, due to interference with other functions. If the uncinate region is involved, a complaint of appalling stinks, or of loathsome tastes may be made; or the patient may develop a habit of smacking his lips without apparent cause. If the auditory centre of the dominant hemisphere is affected, hallucinations of sound may occur in which the patient complains of hearing noises. He may also be unable to understand what people say to him.

Temporal lobe tumours occur fairly commonly. They cause homonymous upper quadrantopia with macular sparing of the opposite side of the visual field. Brain abscesses due to infection spreading from the middle ear may involve the related optic radiation, but they are relatively infrequent since the advent of antibiotics. They may give rise to perceptual illusions such as micropsia or macropsia, and sometimes they may cause peculiar symptoms of temporal and geographical disorientation. The patient may be unable to recall the order in time in which certain events took place. He may suddenly discover that he is unable to find his way home, or to describe the route to a familiar place, or to repeat well-known geographical facts, for example, that Canada lies to the north of the United States.

Parietal lobe tumours occasionally damage the upper bundle of optic radiation fibres and cause a congruous homonymous inferior quadrantopia with macular sparing of the opposite side. These tumours are liable to interfere with the body image, so that the patient becomes unaware of the side of his body which is controlled by the damaged hemisphere.

Cogan has demonstrated that temporoparietal lesions of the left hemisphere cause defective recognition of visual symbols as in alexia and agraphia, whilst lesions of the right temporoparietal region impair judgement of spatial relationships as in topographic agnosia and constructional apraxia.

Expanding supratentorial tumours may compress the posterior cerebral arteries against the tentorium thereby causing infarction of one or both occipital lobes. Increased supratentorial pressure from any cause, haemorrhage or tumour, may produce herniation of the hippocampal gyrus through the tentorial hiatus. Unless the increasing pressure is relieved it rapidly leads to death. The discovery of homonymous hemianopia in these cases is of no value as a localizing sign but it may indicate a state of emergency. Even if the tumour is removed and the pressure relieved, the hemianopia may remain.

In cases of retrochiasmal interference there is sometimes widespread cerebral damage, so that there is some clouding of consciousness and co-operation is poor. Field examination in these patients may be difficult, so that the confrontation test is the only method which

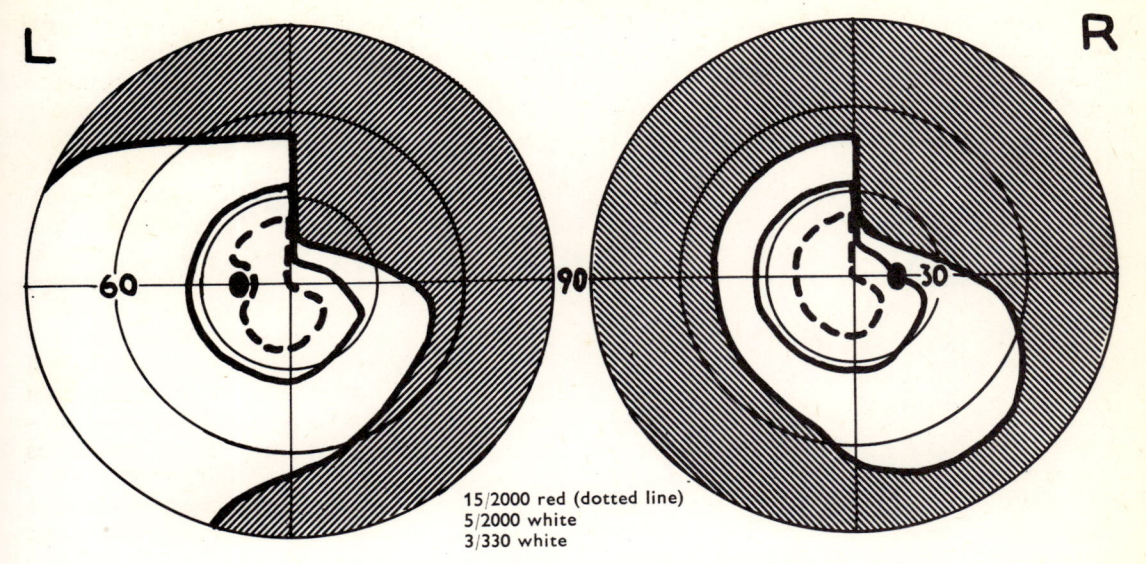

FIG. 182. Fields of patient with a glioma in the left temporo-occipital region.

15/2000 red (dotted line)
5/2000 white
3/330 white

reveals any information. This test is invaluable for detecting homonymous hemianopia. A congruous homonymous hemianopia with macular sparing can often be diagnosed with a white hatpin alone.

FIELD DEFECTS

It will be recalled that occlusions of branches of the middle cerebral and posterior cerebral arteries result in homonymous hemianopia or quadrantopia with macular sparing. In most cases the edges of the field defects are steep or vertical at their onset and they show little or no recovery.

Compression of an optic radiation by a tumour causes homonymous congruous defects with shelving edges. A tumour in the temporal lobe is likely to cause crossed homonymous congruous upper quadrantic defects by damaging the inferior fibres of the optic radiation [FIG. 182]. The more rapid the growth of the tumour the more gradual the slope of the margin of the defect. If the tumour is removed, some recovery usually occurs. The defect becomes smaller and its margin steeper. After about one month the field defect has usually adopted its permanent form and has a steep edge. The degree of recovery depends upon the extent of the destruction of the optic radiation.

Tumours in the occipital region usually involve the optic radiation and cause a typical radiation defect [FIGS. 183 and 184]. Much less commonly, the occipital pole is primarily involved and the macula is not spared. There may even be homonymous scotomata. Very rarely a meningioma may arise from the falx and damage both occipital poles. This results in bilateral homonymous scotomata, which are almost diagnostic of this condition.

Occasionally these patients seem to be quite unable to avoid looking towards the moving target. The method of examination used to demonstrate the extinction phenomenon or lack of awareness must then be tried. This will often unmask a hemianopia or quadrantopia. An aphasic patient is sometimes unable to give a clear indication vocally when a finger is moving. Asking him to blink when the finger moves may prove a better means of communication.

The extinction phenomenon may be demonstrated in cases in which a field defect is slight or absent. This occurs particularly in elderly arteriosclerotic patients in whom there is cortical damage involving the association areas. A complete hemianopic defect of attention may occur in lesions of the parietal area of the opposite side.

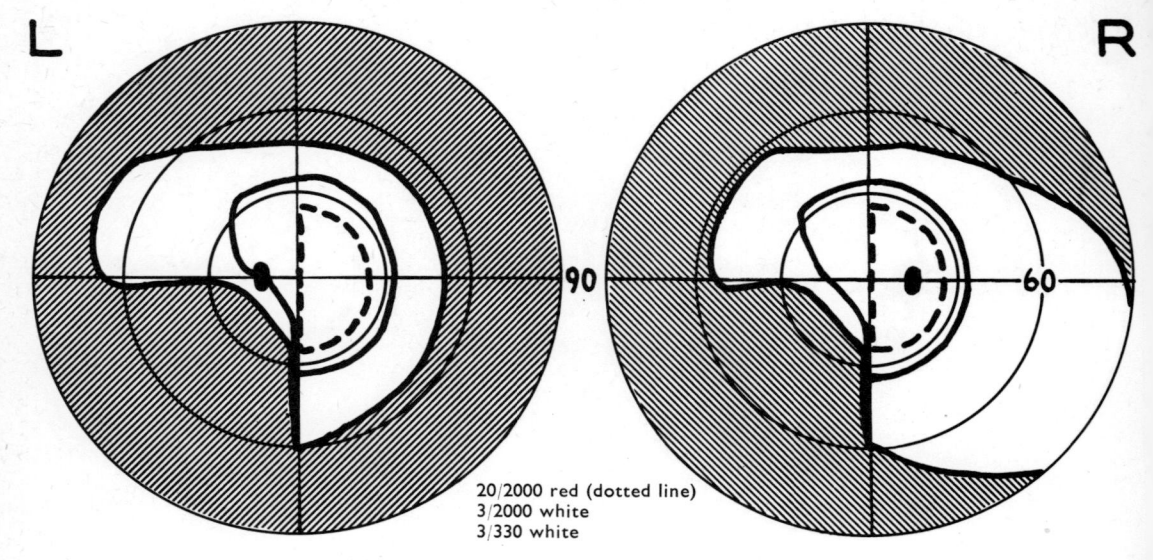

FIG. 183. Fields of a patient with a metastasis from a breast carcinoma involving the right geniculocalcarine pathway.

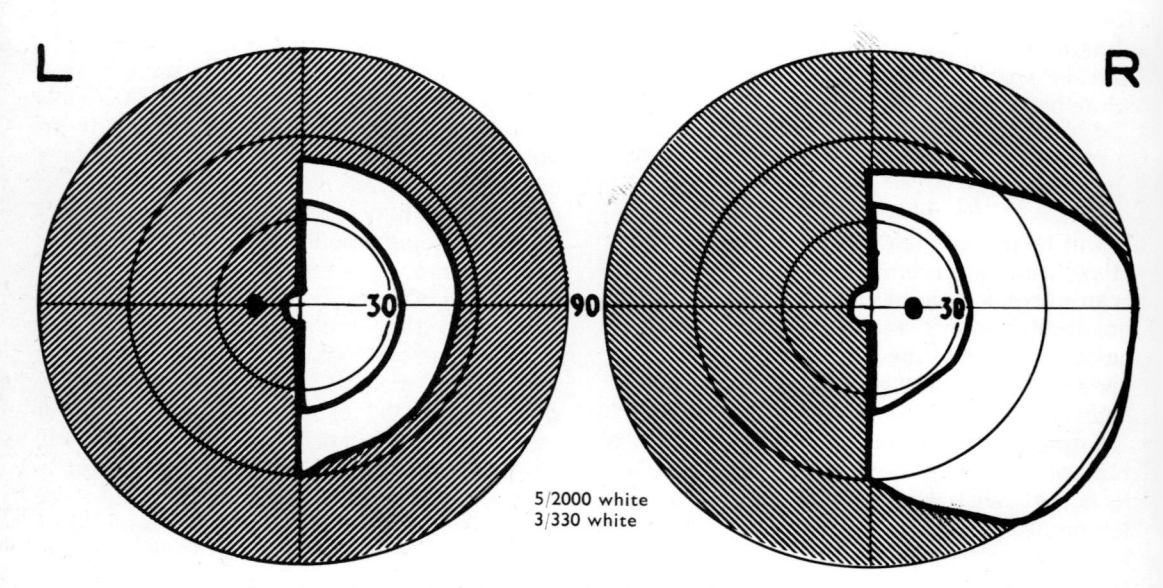

20/2000 red (dotted line)
3/2000 white
3/330 white

FIG. 184. Fields of the same patient 6 weeks later. She was developing a left hemiplegia at this time.

5/2000 white
3/330 white

FIELD DEFECTS

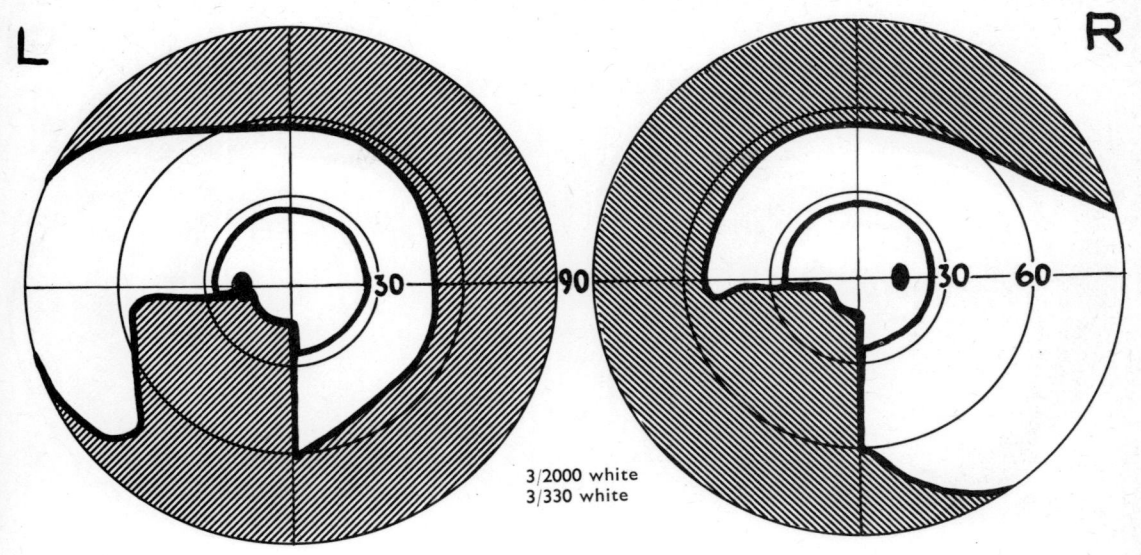

3/2000 white
3/330 white

FIG. 185. A vascular lesion leaving the left monocular crescent almost intact.

The perimeter is always required when a defect involving the monocular temporal crescentic portion of field is suspected [FIG. 185]. A lateral ventricle tumour, which is rare, would be likely to affect this part of the field of the opposite eye first. Bender and Strauss have suggested that the fibres of the optic radiation related to the monocular temporal crescent form a small compact bundle. Hence damage to this bundle is likely to affect all the fibres and cause total loss of the opposite temporal crescentic monocular field. In contrast, the macular nerve fibres are numerous and fan out widely in the optic radiation. Thus a lesion affecting a radiation rarely involves all the fibres, and macular sparing is a common feature.

LOCALIZING SIGNS

The exact site of a lesion in the retrochiasmal visual pathway if often difficult to determine on ocular findings alone, but there are some indications which are of value.

CONGRUITY

Congruity is said to be present when the edge of the field defect in each eye is identical in shape. Field changes due to lesions of the optic tract and lateral geniculate bodies are incongruous. Those due to interference with the optic radiations and visual cortex are congruous. Whilst these are sound working rules, certain comments should be made.

When assessing congruity care must be taken that the patient does not tilt his head to the left during the charting of the right eye, and to the right when the left eye is being examined. This is a common fault, and may give the impression of incongruity when the fields are in fact congruous.

It should also be borne in mind that the temporal field is larger than the nasal field. Occasionally only the uniocular temporal crescentic area disappears. This is caused by damage to the most medial group of optic radiation fibres, which pass to the anterior end of the visual cortex. Rarely the temporal crescent may remain intact in the presence of a homonymous congruous defect affecting the binocular field [FIG. 185].

A tumour which is basically a chiasmal lesion, e.g. a pituitary adenoma, may grow posterolaterally to involve a tract [FIG. 186]. Sometimes a tumour in the anterior part of the temporal lobe which is damaging the optic radiations may spread to involve the adjacent tract or lateral geniculate body. Incongruity in

156   RETROCHIASMAL LESIONS

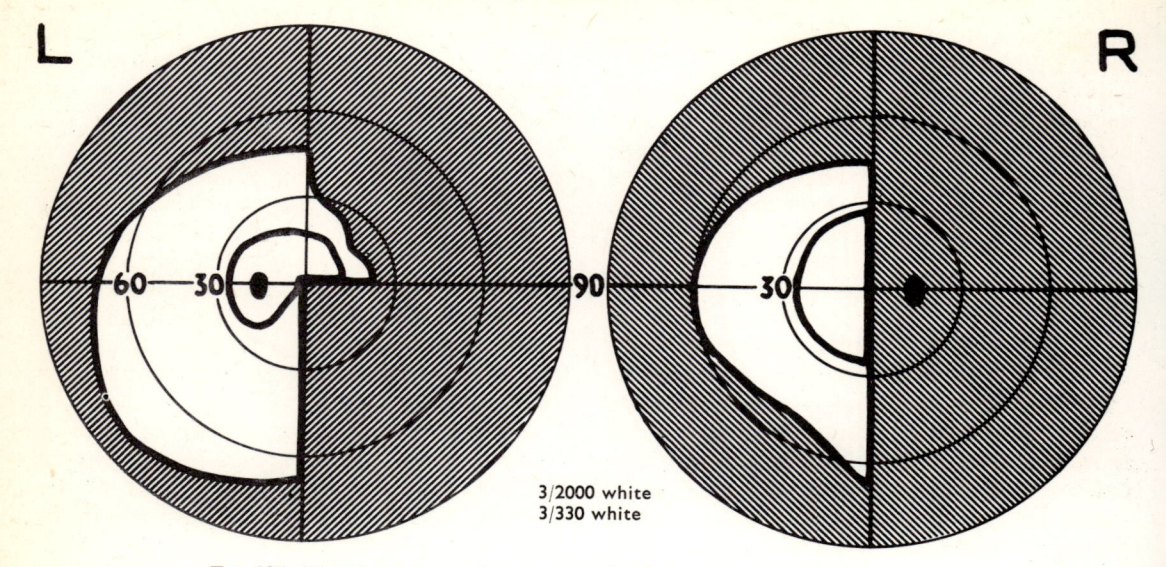

3/2000 white
3/330 white

Fig. 186. Right incongruous homonymous hemianopia in a patient with a chromophobe adenoma which at operation was found to compress the left optic tract.

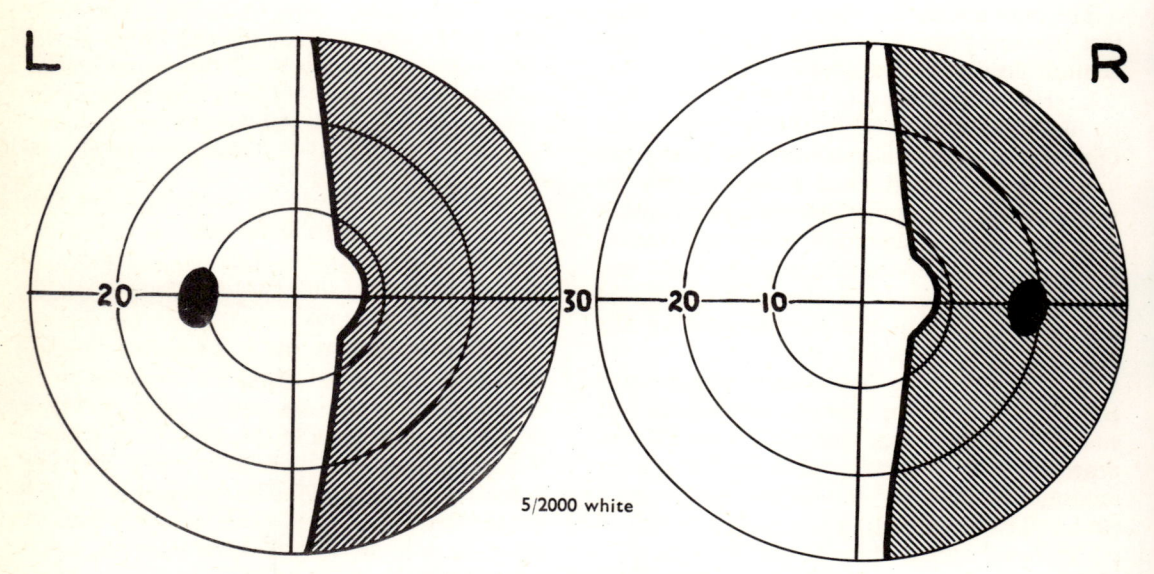

5/2000 white

Fig. 187. The patient's fixation was wandering to the hemianopic side. The blind spots have also moved to the right.

these cases would not indicate primary damage to the optic tract.

Involvement of the optic tract and lateral geniculate body is much less common than damage to the optic radiation. Thus, incongruous homonymous field defects are seen less frequently than congruous ones. When the optic tract is involved by a space-occupying lesion, there are usually accompanying clinical signs which clearly indicate damage to related structures such as the brain stem and basal ganglia.

Authorities differ in their opinions regarding the frequency of incongruity in lesions of the radiations and visual cortex, but during recent years it has become obvious that the more meticulous the analysis of homonymous defects, the more frequently incongruity is found. Incongruity can often be discovered in lesions of the anterior parts of the optic radiations and in injuries of the visual cortex. This finding of incongruity, which is seldom marked, suggests that at least in the anterior parts of the optic radiations, the nerve fibres carrying impulses from corresponding retinal points may not be together. It is also possible that in some people anomalies in the development of nerve fibre bundles may occur.

MACULAR SPARING

Damage to the visual pathway by lesions behind the lateral geniculate bodies usually results in field defects in which the central area is intact for about 5 degrees from the fixation point. Exceptions to this general rule may occur, particularly in injuries to the occipital pole and lesions of the anterior half of the optic radiation.

In the past there was some controversy about the reason for this macular sparing. It was at first believed that each macula was represented in both occipital lobes. There is no anatomical basis for this belief. Anatomical studies have pointed to a complete crossing of all the nasal retinal fibres at the chiasma.

One suggestion for the cause of macular sparing is that the patient learns to fix eccentrically [FIG. 187]. There is no doubt that patients do learn to look towards the blind field, but it is doubtful whether true eccentric fixation ever develops. If the patient's fixation is wandering towards the blind side, it may be demonstrated by the fact that the vertical edge of the half-field in which vision is intact will move into the hemianopic area. Moreover, if the blind spot in the 'seeing' half-field is plotted, it will be found to be closer to the fixation point than normal.

The macular sparing which occurs in vascular occlusions of the occipital lobe is due to an anastomosis of the middle and posterior cerebral arteries in the region of the posterior pole of the occipital lobe, the area which represents the macula. Thus, when the branches of the posterior cerebral artery are occluded, the middle cerebral artery continues to supply the posterior pole, and the macula is spared.

This explains macular sparing in vascular lesions, but it does not account for its frequent occurrence in injuries and tumours of the occipital lobe. It has even been known to occur after occipital lobectomy.

Its occurrence in these cases may be due to the fact that the macular bundle consists of about one half of the total number of fibres in each optic radiation, and the macular representation occupies about one half of the total area of the visual cortex. A lesion is therefore likely to leave undamaged some fibres of the optic radiation and part of the visual cortex associated with macular function because of this abundant representation. There may also be minor anatomical variations in the site of visual representation.

OPTIC ATROPHY

Optic atrophy occurs in tract lesions because the nerve fibres comprising the tracts arise in retinal ganglion cells and pass to the lateral geniculate body without interruption. It does not occur in lesions behind the lateral geniculate bodies, because the optic radiation fibres arise from cells in the lateral geniculate bodies. If optic atrophy is present in cases showing homonymous hemianopia, it suggests a tract lesion. Since, however, optic atrophy usually takes some months to develop when an optic tract is damaged, at an early stage the optic discs may appear to be normal.

It should be noted that the optic atrophy will be bilateral because each tract receives fibres from both optic nerves. This makes the comparison of the two optic discs valueless and assessment of the optic atrophy difficult. The absence of obvious optic atrophy does not, therefore, rule out a tract lesion.

WERNICKE'S PUPIL REACTION

The afferent fibres connected with the light reflex leave the anterior two-thirds of the optic tracts and pass to the third nerve nuclei. Lesions of the anterior two-thirds of an optic tract will therefore damage these fibres and affect the light reflex.

Wernicke's pupil reaction is said to be present when the direct pupil reaction resulting from light shone from the hemianopic field onto the defective area of the retina is sluggish compared with that elicited by light shone from the normal field. Its presence indicates damage to the anterior two-thirds of an optic tract.

It is difficult to demonstrate this reaction because internal reflection and spherical aberration cause some light to reach the normal half of the retina. Moreover, it is not easy to estimate changes in the size of so mobile a structure as the pupil, when it is illuminated from each side. Some observers use the ophthalmoscope beam in a semi-darkened room to demonstrate this phenomenon. Others prefer the slit lamp beam. But a cinematographic recording of the pupil, when each side of the retina is illuminated under constant conditions, is the best method of all.

VISUAL AWARENESS

The majority of patients with a homonymous defect complain only of loss of vision of the eye on the side of the hemianopia. Few are aware that both are involved.

Interference with the posterior part of the optic radiation is rarely localized to a small area. Adjacent areas which subserve the associational and interpretive functions are sometimes affected too. This does not happen in lesions of the tracts or of the anterior parts of the optic radiations. On the whole, the more posterior the lesion, the more marked is the lack of insight into the bilateral nature of the visual defect.

Whilst this principle is basically true, many other factors are involved. The native intelligence of the patient must always be considered when assessing the significance of lack of awareness.

The value of this sign is sometimes diminished by the nature of the lesion. Since lesions of the optic tract, lateral geniculate bodies and the anterior part of the optic radiations are often due to tumours, the development of the field defect is gradual and does not attract attention. Moreover, if there is raised intracranial pressure, the associated confusion and drowsiness render these patients less likely to notice the field loss. On the other hand, interference with the optic radiations and visual cortex is usually vascular in origin. The onset is, therefore, abrupt and more likely to attract attention, unless the infarct is widespread and involves associational areas.

The patient is usually well aware of visual loss due to injury. No matter what the cause, in homonymous hemianopic or quadrantic defects, he is more conscious of the loss in the eye with the temporal defect than the loss in the eye with the nasal defect.

It is possible that the macular sparing found in retrochiasmal lesions may often be the reason for the patient's inability to realize the presence of a field defect. A similar phenomenon occurs in diseases such as simple glaucoma and tobacco amblyopia, which affect the visual pathway anterior to the lateral geniculate bodies. In these conditions, patients may lose a large part of their visual field, and be totally unaware of the loss until it encroaches on the fixation area.

Occasionally, when there is widespread cerebral damage, patients may fail to understand that each eye is hemianopic, even when it is demonstrated to them. This is characteristic of cortical blindness which has already been mentioned.

THE INVESTIGATION OF HOMONYMOUS HEMIANOPIA

It is the task of the ophthalmologist to report on the ocular signs and symptoms in cases of homonymous hemianopia to assist in the localization of the lesion. The history and results of a complete ophthalmological examination should be recorded. The visual fields should be charted, using both the perimeter and Bjerrum screen. In most cases two or three isopters give sufficient information, e.g. 3/330 white, 2/2000 white, and 15/2000 red, but more isopters may be required in cases showing disproportion. The five localizing signs should be assessed, namely:

1. Congruity

2. Macular sparing
3. Optic atrophy
4. Wernicke's pupil reaction
5. Visual awareness

From a consideration of these signs, and from the results of the general physical examination, an attempt should be made to suggest the site and nature of the lesion. Other investigations which should be considered are:

1. Radiographic examination of the skull
2. Electroencephalography
3. Brain scanning using radioisotopes
4. Ultrasonography
5. Air encephalography
6. Carotid arteriography

REFERENCES AND FURTHER READING

ALLEN, I. M. (1930) A clinical study of tumours involving the occipital lobe, *Brain*, **53**, 194.

BENDER, M. B., and STRAUSS, I. (1937) Defects in visual field of one eye only in patients with a lesion of one optic radiation, *Arch. Ophthal.*, **17**, 765.

COGAN, D. G. (1965) Ophthalmic manifestations of bilateral non-occipital cerebral lesions, *Brit. J. Ophthal.*, **49**, 281.

HARRINGTON, D. O. (1961) Visual field character in temporal and occipital lobe lesions, *Arch. Ophthal.*, **66**, 778.

SPALDING, J. K. K. (1952) Wounds of the visual pathway, *J. Neurol. Neurosurg. Psychiat.*, **15**, 99 and 169.

SYMONDS, C., and MACKENZIE, I. (1957) Bilateral loss of vision from cerebral infarction, *Brain*, **80**, 415.

TEUBER, H. L., BATTERSBY, W. S., and BENDER, M. (1960) *Visual Field Defects after Penetrating Missile Wounds of the Brain*, Cambridge, Mass.

15

OTHER LESIONS CAUSING FIELD DEFECTS

The diagnosis of many ocular lesions may be made by the ophthalmoscopic appearance alone. Although these lesions often cause characteristic field defects, the ophthalmoscopic features are so unmistakable that perimetry is seldom called for. Occasions sometimes arise, however, when a knowledge of the field defects produced by these conditions is of importance. This group of ocular affections is discussed in this chapter.

AFFECTIONS OF CHOROID AND RETINA

CHOROIDITIS

It will be remembered that the two inner neurones of the retina are supplied by the retinal circulation, whilst the outer neurone is dependent upon the choriocapillaris for its nutrition. Thus when the choroid is inflamed, the adjacent retina seldom escapes damage. The extent to which the toxic process spreads through the retina depends upon the severity of the inflammation.

In *disseminated choroiditis* the outer neurone only is affected in most cases. Thus the field defects should correspond exactly to the atrophic areas left from the inflammation [FIG. 188]. This is seldom found, and the visual defects are usually smaller than the fundal appearances suggest. The diagnosis, however, is rarely in doubt in this condition. As one would expect, it causes scattered scotomatous defects corresponding to the situation of the retinal lesions, but there is less functional damage than the ophthalmoscopic picture would indicate.

In *exudative choroiditis* the toxic process often extends through the three neurones of the retina and damages the nerve fibre layer, so that sector defects may occur which correspond to the course of the nerve fibres [FIG. 189]. In the active phase of the disease, vitreous opacities often make it difficult or impossible to demonstrate a sector field defect, but it becomes easier to do so when the inflammation subsides.

The shape of the field loss depends upon the site of the inflammation. A patch of juxtapapillary choroiditis close to the lower margin of the optic disc may damage the inferior arcuate fibres and cause a superior arcuate defect [FIG. 189]. If the inflammation involves the nasal retinal fibres, a sector-shaped area in the temporal field will be produced [FIG. 190].

Rarely the inflammatory reaction may affect the outer layer of peripheral fibres in the nerve fibre layer of the retina and leave the inner layer intact. In this case, there will be a peripheral field defect, separated from the scotoma caused by the patch of choroiditis by a small area of decreased or normal perception [FIG. 191]. This fact has been used by Wolff and Penman as evidence for their belief that in the nerve fibre layer the fibres from peripheral retinal ganglia are external to those arising more centrally.

COMMOTIO RETINAE

The recognition of macular oedema following a blow on the eye gives rise to no difficulty. Perimetry is unnecessary as an aid to diagnosis, but it may be of value in prognosis. If a central scotoma can be demonstrated with the blue target only, the oedema usually clears in a few days and leaves no visual defect. A central defect demonstrable with red and white targets suggests that the scotoma will be permanent.

It is interesting that a crescentic rupture of the choroid gives rise to no characteristic defect. A central scotoma due to the commotio retinae is all that is usually found.

AFFECTIONS OF CHOROID AND RETINA

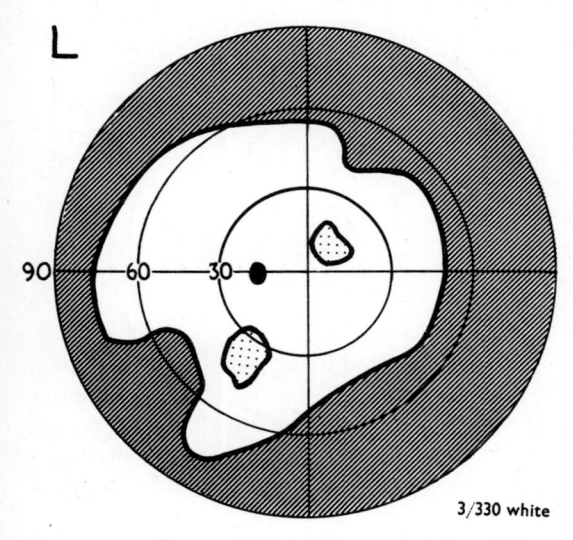

FIG. 188. Left visual field in disseminated choroiditis.

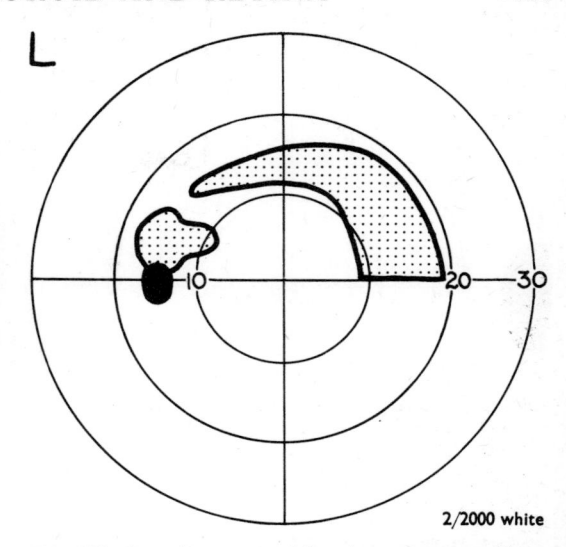

FIG. 189. Superior arcuate defect due to juxta-papillary choroiditis adjacent to the lower margin of the optic disc.

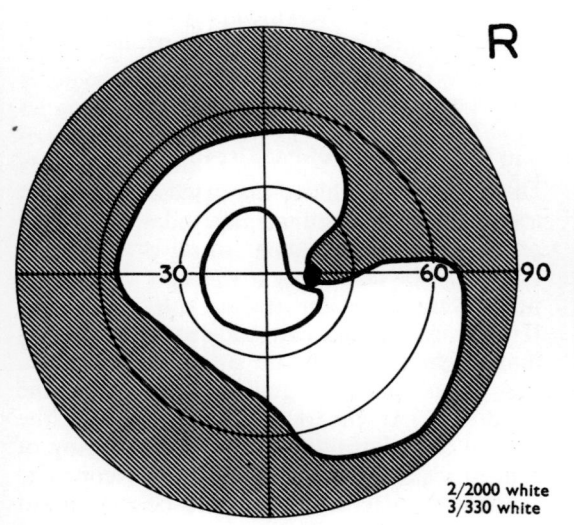

FIG. 190. Sector defect in the temporal field due to a patch of choroiditis on the nasal side of the optic disc.

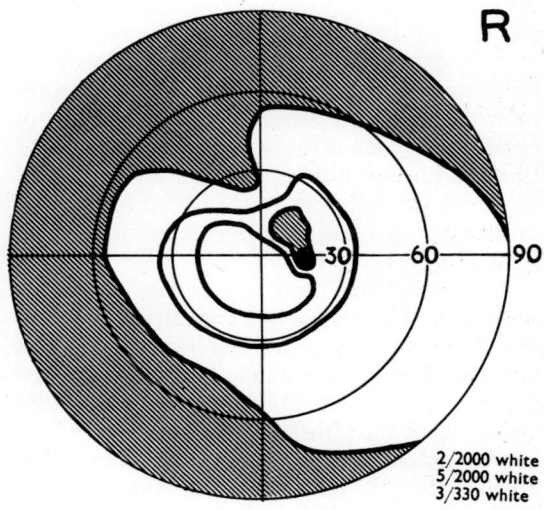

FIG. 191. A peripheral defect separated from a scotoma due to choroiditis.

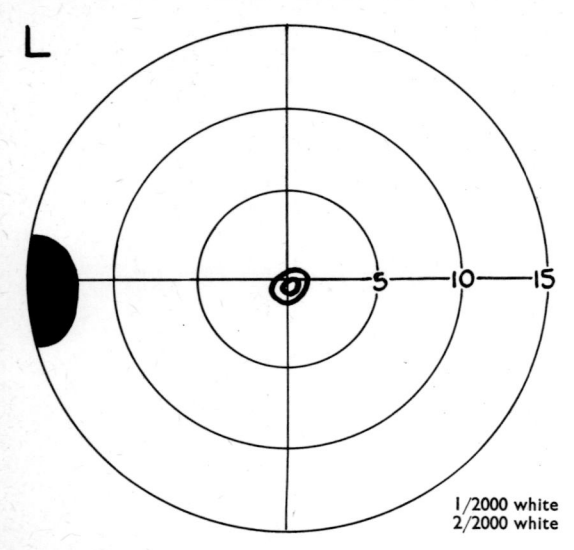

FIG. 192. An eclipse scotoma of the left eye.

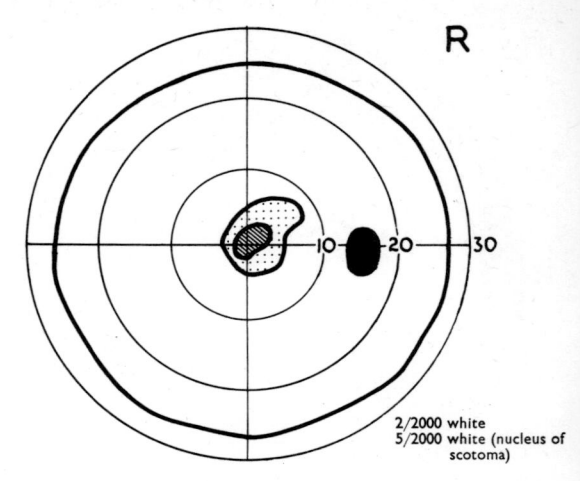

FIG. 193. Field defect due to central serous retinopathy.

ECLIPSE SCOTOMA

This condition results from looking at the sun without protection for the eyes. The eclipse of the sun of 1912 was followed by reports of thousands of cases from many European countries. In primitive countries it is still common. In educated communities the danger of gazing at the sun is more fully appreciated and this condition is not so common. In about half the cases the right eye only is affected, the left in about a quarter, and both eyes in about a quarter.

The symptoms and signs vary with the severity and duration of exposure. A positive central scotoma usually results and obscures central vision. If the damage is slight the distortion of the central area may be demonstrated with the Amsler chart.

The vision is reduced and may vary from 20/60 to 20/200. Examination of the fundi immediately after the injury may reveal no abnormality, but, after a few hours, macular oedema usually appears. The oedema gradually subsides. Several weeks later a small circular cyst-like area of reddish hue surrounded by slight pigmentation is all that can be seen.

The patient is left with a permanent central scotoma, often slightly eccentric, ½–3 degrees in diameter [FIG. 192]. The margins are steep and well defined and the peripheral field is unaffected.

The retinal burns in eclipse scotoma are caused by visible radiation. Meyer-Schwickerath made use of this fact to develop the field of photocoagulation which plays so important a role in the treatment of various retinal diseases.

CENTRAL SEROUS RETINOPATHY
(CENTRAL ANGIOSPASTIC RETINOPATHY)

This condition, which was originally thought to be due to spasm of choroidal or retinal arterioles in the macular area, is now considered to be caused by a vascular defect permitting transudation of fluid into the retina. If such a leakage can be demonstrated by fluorescein studies to be situated away from the fovea, photocoagulation may cure the condition. At the onset of the disease the patient complains of distortion or blurring of central vision. With the ophthalmoscope the central macular area is seen to be raised and oedematous. It is often surmounted by a few yellow dots. Vision is reduced to between 20/60 and 20/200. The distortion is best demonstrated with the Amsler chart. A circular central scotoma of 3, 5 or more degrees in diameter may be plotted on the Bjerrum screen [FIG. 193].

Static perimetry in a typical case shows the characteristic defect associated with oedema of the macula. There is diminished foveal sensi-

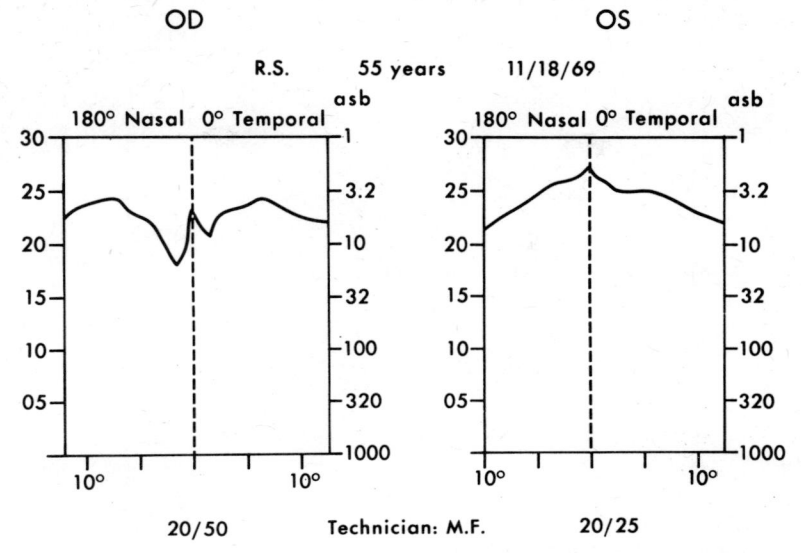

FIG. 194. Static profile of central serous retinopathy of the right eye, showing a diminished foveal sensitivity surrounded by a depression within 2 degrees of fixation. The other eye shows normal function.

tivity surrounded by a depression which is more pronounced [FIG. 194].

In most cases the oedema is absorbed after some weeks or months. The retina may then appear normal, or a cyst-like formation or pigment may be seen at the macula. There may be no remaining field defect, but sometimes a small central or paracentral scotoma may persist, which requires minute targets and reduced illumination for its detection.

SOME CONGENITAL AND DEVELOPMENTAL ANOMALIES

Among the various congenital and developmental abnormalities of the optic discs which are associated with anomalies in the visual field, there are some that might be considered as either congenital or developmental. Nasally directed scleral canals, medullated nerve fibres, and inferior conus, should probably be considered as developmental in origin rather than congenital.

A *coloboma* of the optic disc may be diagnosed on its ophthalmoscopic appearance alone. Even in cases with normal visual acuity, an arcuate field defect resembling that found in glaucoma is often present. In more severe cases, enlargement of the blind spot, and gross sector defects involving the central area may cause considerable reduction in vision.

A *crater-like hole or pit* is usually situated in the inferior temporal quadrant although any area of the disc may be involved. It is most commonly considered to be a minimal form of coloboma but others believe these 'holes' to be glial cysts. The distribution of the vessels at the disc is usually anomalous, with a shift to the side of the disc away from the pit. Cilioretinal vessels are frequently present. In about one third of the cases there is an associated macular lesion. Some present with pigmentary macular changes. Others at first resemble central serous retinopathy. Most are accompanied by nerve fibre bundle defects, i.e. arcuate scotomata, in the upper temporal field corresponding to the pit in the inferior temporal sector of the optic disc.

A *nasally directed scleral canal* or tilting of the optic disc may cause a field defect resembling that found in glaucoma. When present in both eyes, bitemporal defects may result which mimic those produced by a pituitary tumour [FIG. 195]. Rucker has pointed out that when the field defect is due to a disturbance at the nerve head, the contracted 2/2000 white isopter passes without a break from the temporal to the nasal field. This enables it to be

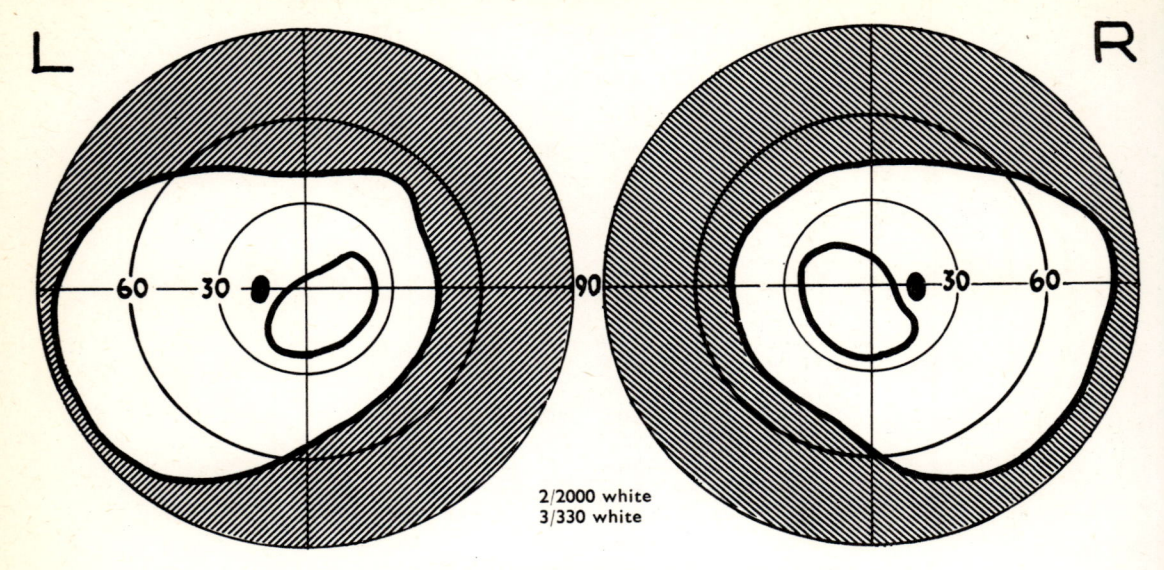

FIG. 195. Visual fields of a patient with nasally directed scleral canals.

2/2000 white
3/330 white

distinguished from a true bitemporal hemianopia due to a chiasmal lesion, in which there is a step up from the temporal to the nasal field [FIGS. 154 and 195].

Medullated nerve fibres cause enlargement of the blind spot corresponding to their site and extent. But their ophthalmoscopic appearance is so striking that they are unlikely to be mistaken for any other condition.

An *inferior conus* is often associated with a superior arcuate scotoma and baring of the blind spot. It may be bilateral, so that the field defects resemble those of an early chiasmal lesion [FIG. 196]. But the ophthalmoscopic appearance is characteristic, the field defects are connected with the blind spot, and the radiological appearance of the pituitary fossa is normal. Thus, it is not difficult to make the diagnosis.

MYOPIA

The central fields of a myopic patient are best examined with the patient wearing his glasses. If the patient has bifocals, they should not be worn. The visual field of the fully corrected myope shows no contraction but many myopes have an enlarged blind spot, particularly in the horizontal diameter, due to the temporal crescent of choroidal atrophy. Myopia is often accompanied by a partial ectasia particularly of the areas below the papilla. This can be seen by a pallor of the choroid below when compared with areas above the disc. In the visual field this manifests itself as a superior temporal depression [FIG. 197 and PLATE 1B, p. 78], which when bilateral may resemble chiasmal involvement or arcuate defects. With the addition of concave lenses (as much as 5–7D may be necessary) the 'defective' areas disappear. The addition of concave lenses will, of course, blur the rest of the visual field so that the fields have to be interpreted as a whole, composed of parts tested with different refraction.

The presence of degenerative changes in myopia is accompanied by bizarre, localized field defects and central scotomata resulting from macular haemorrhages or central areas of chorioretinal atrophy [FIG. 198]. Peripheral defects suggest retinal separation.

DRUSEN
(SEE PSEUDOPAPILLOEDEMA)

Drusen or hyaline bodies appear as glistening, more or less spherical bodies in the optic disc. Microscopically they can be seen to be anterior to the lamina cribrosa and the greater concentration is usually on the nasal side of the disc. They may occur sporadically or as a hereditary phenomenon. Some authors consider the inheritance to be irregular dominant

L   R

2/2000 white

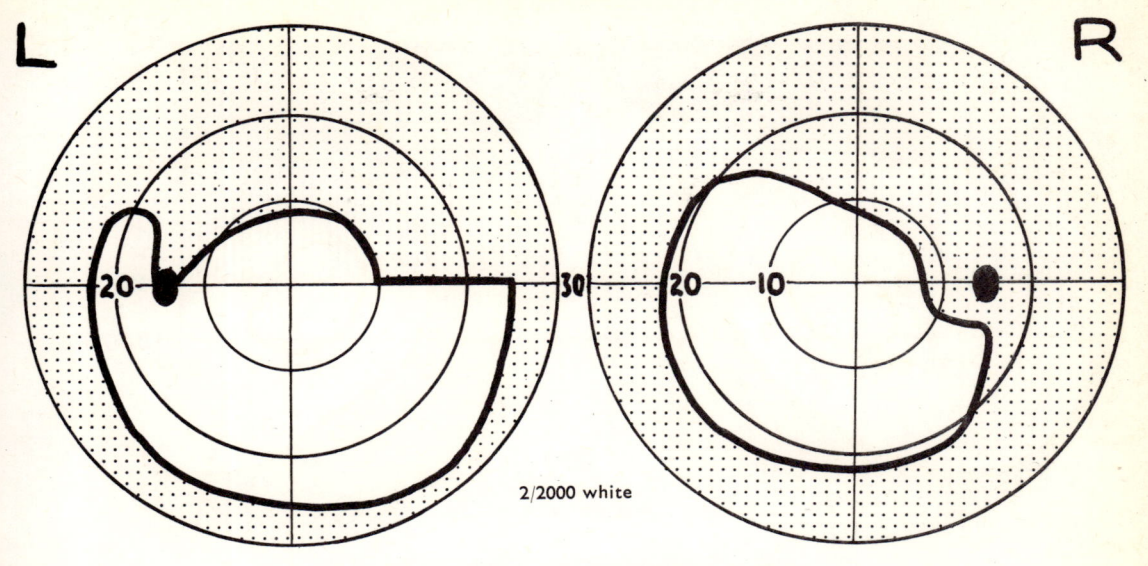

Fig. 196. Visual fields of a patient with bilateral inferior conus.

with variable expressivity. Others believe sporadic drusen may represent *formes frustes* of Bourneville's disease. Histologically drusen are similar to the tumours of Bourneville's disease and are commonly found in families with this condition. Sometimes drusen are found in association with neurofibromatosis. They may also be secondary to optic neuritis and to some affections of the retina such as retinitis pigmentosa, angioid streaks, and macular dystrophy.

In some cases the visual fields are normal, but defects are usually found if a careful search is made. No one type of defect is characteristic. Enlargement of the blind spot, arcuate and pericentral scotomata, sector defects, and irregular contraction of the fields have all been described [Fig. 199]. In most cases the changes are stationary, but slow progression sometimes occurs, though never so far as to cause blindness. Drusen increase in number and size particularly in retinitis pigmentosa.

This condition has been mistaken for papilloedema, and the associated field defects have been taken as evidence of interference with the visual pathway. Thus, patients have been subjected to unnecessary intracranial investigations. It will be appreciated, therefore, that the recognition of the drusen glistening in the nerve head is of the utmost importance.

PSEUDONEURITIS OR PSEUDOPAPILLOEDEMA

This condition, in which the optic disc is heaped in such a way as to resemble papillitis or papilloedema, is not uncommon. It is sometimes very difficult to distinguish between the benign developmental anomaly and the pathological entities. Gross dilatation of veins, haemorrhages and exudates are never found in pseudopapilloedema. Loss of vision and inflammatory cells in the posterior vitreous indicate the presence of papillitis. It is with early minimal papilloedema that confusion arises.

In early papilloedema a small central physiological cup usually persists. The oedematous nerve fibres arching into the optic disc may surround and blur the main retinal blood vessels emerging from the disc. The disc margin is blurred by the oedematous nerve fibres which form a smooth elevation and tend to spread onto the peripapillary retina. The veins are tortuous and dilated and pulsation cannot be provoked by slight digital pressure on the globe through the lid. Field studies will show a slight enlargement of the blind spot. Examination with the binocular indirect ophthalmoscope or the binocular microscope fundus contact lens and Hruby lens is often valuable in these cases by providing stereopsis.

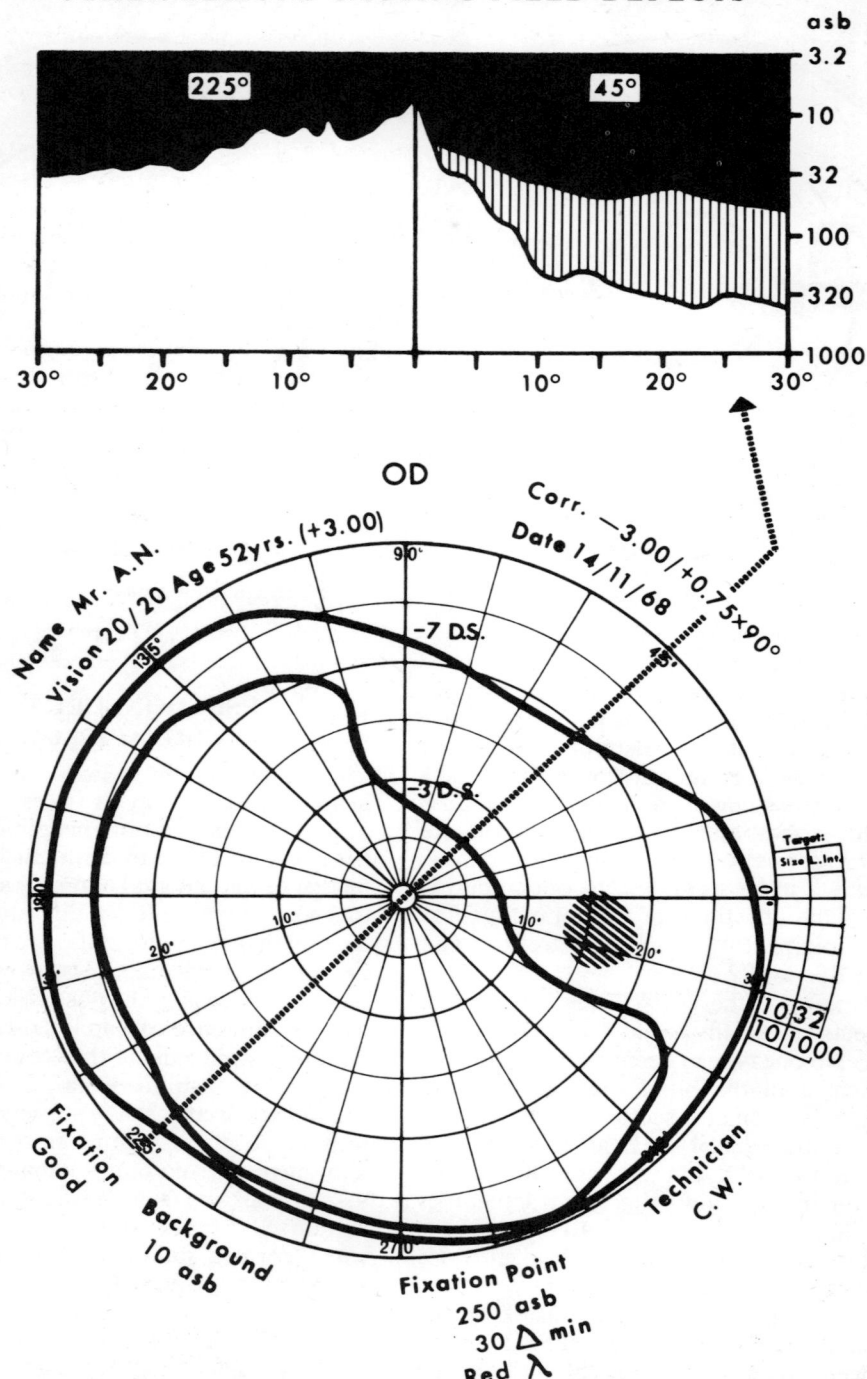

FIG. 197. Visual field of a patient with —3D myopia. A baring of blind spot and contraction in the upper temporal quadrant is present with the patient's own correction. There is some ectasia of the sclera below the optic disc and more concave lenses are necessary to expand these isopters. Similar changes can be seen on the static profiles along the 45 degree meridian.

PSEUDONEURITIS

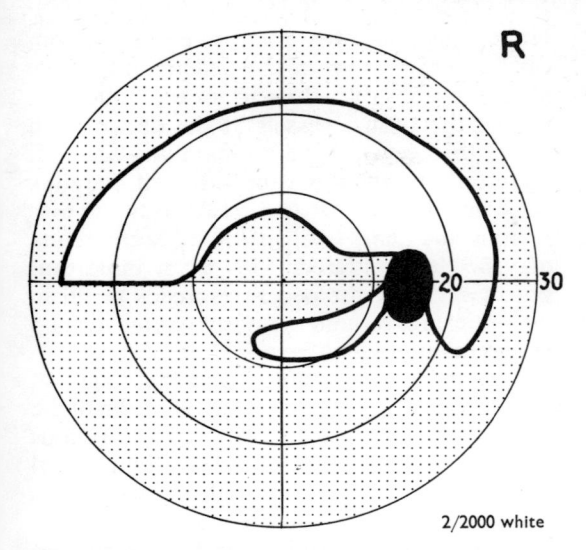

FIG. 198. Visual field in myopia with macular degeneration.

In pseudopapilloedema the central cup is obliterated by glial tissue. The retinal blood vessels are usually clearly seen anterior to the central elevation of the disc but occasionally flecks of glial tissue obscure segments of the blood vessels. The elevation, unlike that in papilloedema, is confined to the disc and does not spread onto the surrounding retina. If hyaline bodies are present the elevation and margins are likely to be irregular and if a slit lamp beam is cast upon the disc the hyaline material may be seen to glow beneath the overlying nerve fibres. The retinal veins are often tortuous but never markedly dilated. The optic disc may be tilted with the scleral canal piercing the globe at an unusual angle. If the pseudopapilloedema is due to drusen the blind spot may be enlarged and arcuate scotomata may be present. There may also be associated refractive errors such as astigmatism, hypermetropia or myopia.

If there is any doubt about the diagnosis there is seldom any harm in waiting a few weeks. In papillitis, severe visual failure develops rapidly and in papilloedema the swelling of the disc usually increases with the swelling of the tumour so that the diagnosis becomes obvious. But in pseudopapilloedema the vision and the appearance of the disc remain unchanged.

Pseudopapilloedema is sometimes hereditary and in doubtful cases it is often of value to examine other members of the family. The finding of a similar condition in the eyes of one of the parents or of siblings is suggestive evidence of pseudopapilloedema.

PAPILLOEDEMA

It is becoming the rule to confine the term papilloedema to plerocephalic oedema. This is

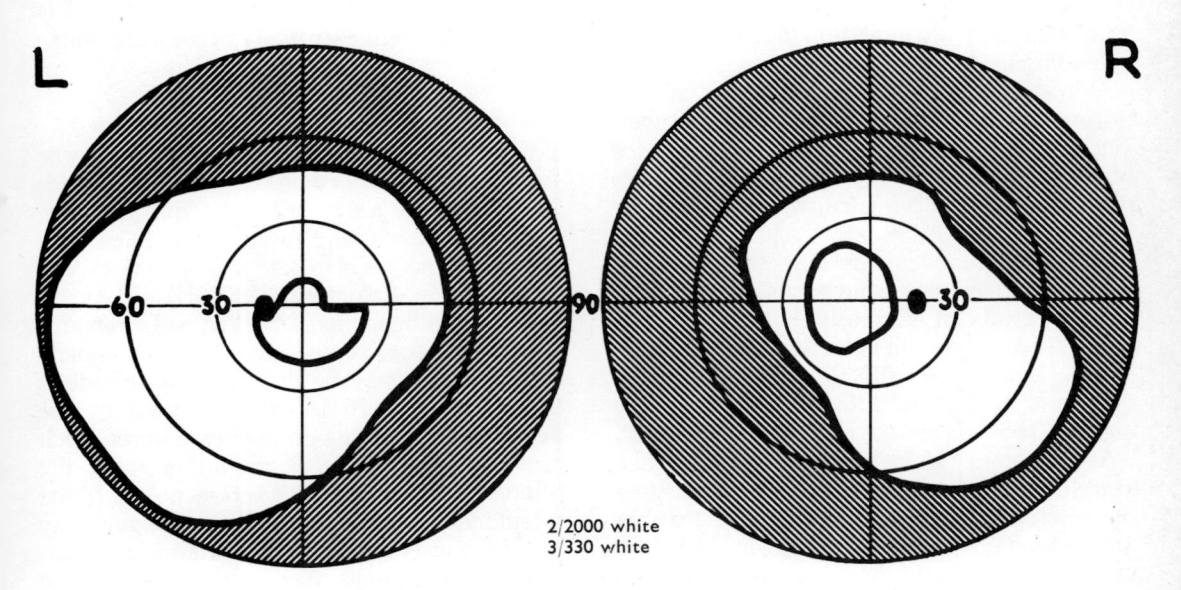

FIG. 199. Visual fields of a patient with drusen of the optic disc.

a passive oedema of the nerve head due to raised intracranial pressure.

The meninges of the optic nerve are continuous with those of the brain. Increased intracranial pressure is therefore transmitted to the subarachnoid space surrounding the optic nerve. Just behind the eyeball the central retinal vein crosses this space, and if the intracranial pressure rises above the pressure in the central retinal vein, the venous drainage from the eye is impeded and papilloedema occurs.

Oedema of the optic disc may be caused by cerebral tumours, particularly when they are situated in the posterior fossa, because they obstruct the drainage of the cerebrospinal fluid. It may also occur in the last stages of various blood dyscrasias, in lead and uraemic encephalopathy, in malignant hypertension, meningitis, subarachnoid haemorrhage, and conditions causing venous back pressure, such as dural venous sinus thrombosis, emphysema, and pulmonary insufficiency.

Plerocephalic oedema does not cause loss of central vision until a late stage. This is an important diagnostic feature in distinguishing papilloedema from papillitis and thrombosis of the central retinal vein. In addition to the swelling of the optic disc, these last two conditions cause marked loss of vision and a central scotoma. A few haemorrhages sometimes occur close to the optic disc in papillitis, but in central venous occlusion haemorrhages can be seen scattered throughout the fundus and extending to the periphery.

Whilst the eye with papilloedema retains normal vision until secondary atrophy supervenes, a characteristic complaint is of sudden blurring of vision. This is often particularly marked when the patient lowers the head by bending down.

When papilloedema is marked and is associated with exudates and haemorrhages there is no difficulty in diagnosis. It is in the early cases, where there are no exudates or haemorrhages, that it is so difficult to be sure of the diagnosis. It is these difficult early cases that are so often referred to the ophthalmologist.

Hyperaemia and blurring of the disc margins are usually said to be the earliest signs of developing papilloedema. These features are undoubtedly always present but the colour of the optic disc and the degree of blurring of the disc margins vary so widely in normal individuals that their assessment is seldom easy. A heaping up of the oedematous nerve fibres develops over the edge of the optic disc, raising the retinal vessels at the disc margin above their level in the peripapillary area. If, therefore, the pupil is widely dilated, parallax between the arch of the vessels over the disc margin and their level in the adjacent retina may be demonstrated. This is an important sign. Gradually the oedema spreads to fill in the optic cup, though in an early stage the cup may remain obvious.

The most important diagnostic sign of papilloedema is tortuosity and dilatation of the retinal veins. If these are observed and venous pulsation cannot be produced by slight digital pressure on the globe through the lid, this is strong evidence for the presence of papilloedema. Later, when exudates and haemorrhages appear around the disc, the diagnosis becomes obvious.

The use of the indirect binocular ophthalmoscope permits a better assessment of the protrusion of the disc by providing stereopsis. A binocular microscope and slit lamp with a Hruby lens or contact lens is also of value on occasions when the diagnosis is in doubt.

Sometimes even the experienced ophthalmologist is unable to be sure of the presence or absence of papilloedema. In these doubtful cases all one can do is to wait and re-examine every week or two weeks. If papilloedema is developing it will eventually become obvious.

FIELD CHANGES IN PAPILLOEDEMA

Early in this condition no field changes may be found, but as the oedema increases it extends beyond the edges of the optic disc and displaces the retinal end organs. The blind spot gradually increases in size and it may exceed 10 degrees in diameter [FIG. 200].

If the papilloedema is marked and it remains unrelieved for some time, an incomplete 'macular star' may develop on the nasal side of the fovea [FIG. 201]. This is caused by the action of the oedema on the nerve fibres. Such cases show a 'tongue' extending from the blind spot towards the fixation point. If the papilloedema is not relieved, the 'tongue' may creep towards the fixation area and finally include it. These field changes are characteristic of long-standing papilloedema [FIG. 202].

PAPILLOEDEMA

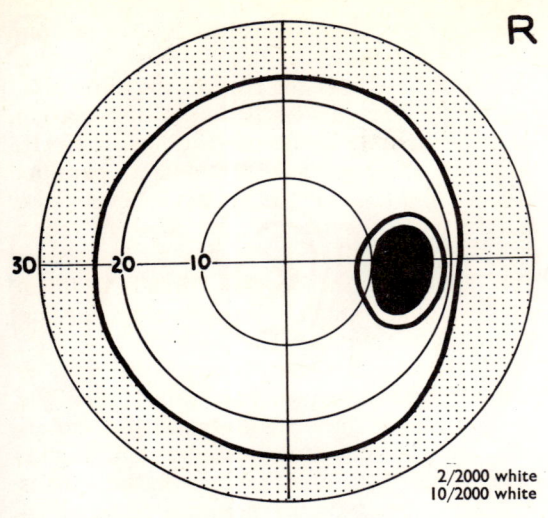

FIG. 200. Enlargement of the blind spot in papilloedema.
2/2000 white
10/2000 white

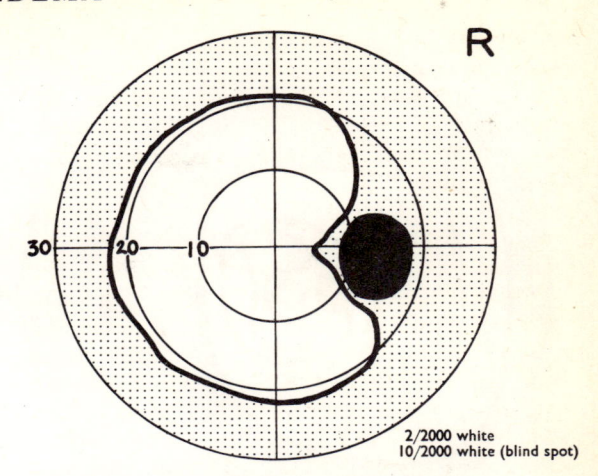

FIG. 201. Long-standing papilloedema developing a 'tongue' towards the central area.
2/2000 white
10/2000 white (blind spot)

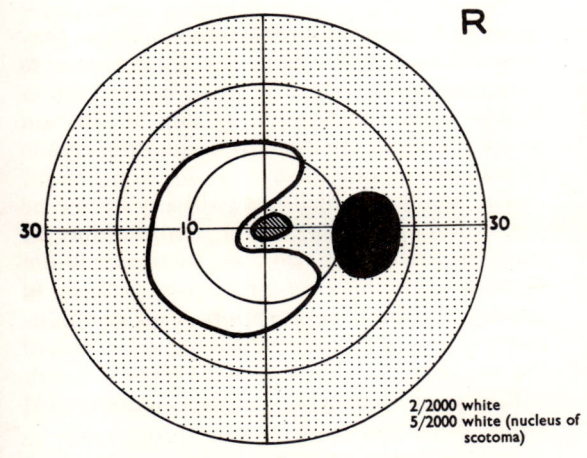

FIG. 202. Field defect in long-standing papilloedema, with a 'macular star' causing a central scotoma.
2/2000 white
5/2000 white (nucleus of scotoma)

POST-NEURITIC ATROPHY (SECONDARY OPTIC ATROPHY)

As has been previously mentioned, oedema of the optic disc may arise from a variety of causes. When this oedema subsides, it is replaced by fibrous tissue. The optic disc pales and the related blood vessels become attenuated. This ophthalmoscopic appearance is known as post-neuritic or secondary optic atrophy.

The field changes in post-neuritic atrophy are similar to those found in syphilitic optic atrophy in that there is a gradual irregular contraction of all isopters. These changes are, of course, added to any that may have occurred as a result of the original condition.

At the onset of post-neuritic atrophy, the visual fields begin to contract. At this stage the removal of the intracranial tumour causing the raised intracranial tension may not prevent further visual deterioration.

The loss is usually more marked nasally than temporally and in the final stages of atrophy following papilloedema due to raised intracranial pressure, the shrunken fields may suggest binasal hemianopia [FIG. 203]. This was formerly thought to be due to dilatation of the third ventricle pushing the optic chiasma against the internal carotid arteries, but this theory is not generally accepted [see binasal hemianopia, p. 140].

All cases of papilloedema should be examined, using the Bjerrum screen and perimeter, because any changes other than those due to this condition are most probably due to interference with the visual pathway by the lesion responsible for the raised intracranial pressure. These additional field changes may give much information about the site of the primary lesion.

2/2000 white
5/2000 white
3/330 white

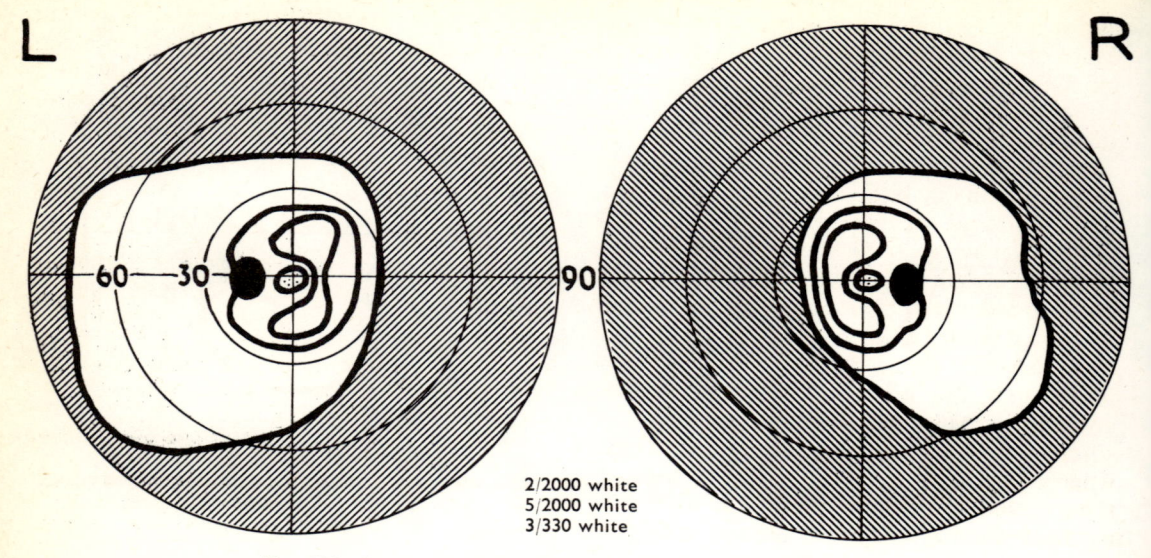

FIG. 203. Commencing optic atrophy in long-standing papilloedema.

DECOMPRESSION OPERATIONS

In times past, ophthalmic surgeons were occasionally asked to advise neurosurgeons of the onset of post-neuritic atrophy, so that patients with inoperable intracranial tumours might be saved from blindness by a decompression operation. Nowadays, neurosurgeons often prefer to do their own visual field examination, the advance of neurosurgery has rendered more tumours operable, and radiotherapy is often capable of reducing the size of a tumour, at least temporarily. If, however, an opinion should be called for, the signs of secondary atrophy are best sought by using the 1 mm. or 3 mm. white targets with the perimeter. A constriction of these isopters suggests the onset of post-neuritic atrophy.

SUPPRESSION SCOTOMA IN STRABISMUS

A child with strabismus learns to suppress the deviating eye in order to overcome diplopia. If the strabismus remains uncorrected, the suppression becomes dense and a scotomata develops. The physiological mechanism underlying this phenomenon is not fully understood.

These suppression scotomata are difficult to plot and they vary in size and density. Since they result from a desire to avoid diplopia, they are more readily demonstrated when both eyes are in use at one time. The two eyes must therefore be open during the test, and the position of the squinting eye must be maintained by the fixation of the other eye.

The methods which have already been described for plotting a central scotoma may be used. The red and green glass method and the stereocampimeter are the most useful in clinical practice. Travers adopted an ingenious method in which a mirror was arranged before the fixing eye so that it saw a Bjerrum screen with a small light at its centre, superimposed on the one observed by the squinting eye.

In alternating strabismus each eye develops two suppression scotomata. One is a central scotoma and the other corresponds to the macula of the other eye. They can be plotted, however, only when the other eye is fixing. If the squinting eye is covered, no scotomata can be demonstrated in the fixing eye. In esotropia, the extramacular scotoma is in the temporal field, and its distance from fixation varies with the angle of squint. In exotropia, the scotoma is in the nasal field.

In constant strabismus, the suppression scotoma of the macular area of the squinting eye is denser. As a general rule, the poorer the vision the more obvious the scotoma. If the fixing eye is covered, the scotoma is relative, and it may be difficult to define, not only because of poor fixation but because its edge is indefinite. It is an area of depressed sensitivity rather than a hole in the visual field. If a stereoscopic device is used so that the dominant eye is able to fix, the scotoma becomes obvious and may be plotted more readily.

In moderate degrees of suppression, the scotoma may be relative and its edges impossible to define with certainty. When suppression is dense, the edges of the scotoma may be plotted fairly exactly with a 1 or 2 mm. white target on the 2 metre Bjerrum screen. Travers found that the more closely the angle of anomaly approached the objective angle of squint, the denser and larger the scotoma. Thus when normal retinal correspondence is present, the scotoma, if demonstrable, will be small, and not more than 3–5 degrees in diameter.

The more marked the abnormal retinal correspondence, the denser and larger the scotoma will be. In severe cases it may be as much as 20 degrees in diameter. If the abnormal retinal correspondence can be reduced by straightening the eyes by surgery, the scotomata become smaller and less dense.

REFERENCES AND FURTHER READING

Lansche, R. K., and Rucker, C. W. (1957) Progression of defects in visual fields produced by hyaline bodies in optic disks, *Arch. Ophthal.*, **58**, 115.

Rucker, C. W. (1946) Bitemporal defects in visual fields resulting from developmental anomalies of optic disks, *Arch. Ophthal.*, **35**, 546.

Schmidt, T. (1955) Perimetric relative scotomata, *Ophthalmologica (Basel)*, **129**, 303.

Travers, T. à B. (1938) Suppression of vision in squint and its association with retinal correspondence and amblyopia, *Brit. J. Ophthal.*, **22**, 577.

INDEX

Absolute field, 26
Absolute scotoma, 31
Acromegaly, 124
Adenoma of pituitary, 124
   X-ray findings in, 137
Alcohol, ethyl, 98
   methyl, 99
Altitudinal hemianopia, 114, 146
Amblyopia, 95
   nutritional, 109
   toxic, 54, 60
Amsler's charts, 40
Analysis of field defects, 46
Anatomy of retina, 3
   optic chiasma, 9
   optic radiations, 16
   visual cortex, 20
Aneurysms of circle of Willis, 118, 124
Angioscotometry, 48
Aniline, 107
Anterior knee of Wilbrand, 9, 112, 118, 133
Anton's syndrome, 145
Aphakia, effect of, 49, 89
Apparatus, 33, 40
   charts, 38, 46
   Friedmann analyser, 40
   perimeter, hand, 35
      Goldmann, 36
      Oculus, 36
      standard, 35
      Tubingen, 36
   stereocampimeter, 37
   tangent screen, 34
Arachnoiditis, 66
Arcuate defects or scotomata, 4, 61, 64, 66, 72
   in colloid bodies at disc, 164
   in coloboma of disc, 163
   in inferior conus, 164
   in myopia, 164
Arcuate fibres, 4
Arsenic poisoning, 105
Arterial occlusion in retina, 61, 91
Arteries, basilar, 143
   central retinal occlusion, 91
   cilioretinal, 92
   internal carotid, 66, 141
   middle cerebral, 141
   superior temporal occlusion, 92
   thrombosis of cerebral, 141
Aspidium, 105
Atherosclerosis of cerebral arteries, 141
Atrophy of optic disc, 4, 111, 119, 122, 126, 157
Avulsion of optic nerve, 121

Awareness, 48, 158
   lack of, 48

Baring of blind spot, 66, 164
Basilar artery stenosis, 143
Binasal hemianopia, 140
Binocular field, 26
   cerebral representation of, 21
   examination of, by confrontation, 33
Bitemporal hemianopia, 11, 62, 64, 127
   scotomata, 133
Bjerrum screen, 34, 40
   examination with, 44
Bjerrum's scotoma, 71
Blindness, cortical, 145
   in poisoning (see Toxic amblyopia)
Blind spot, 25
   baring of, 66, 164
   enlargement of, 51, 66
   in glaucoma, 66
   in papilloedema, 168
   size of, 25
Blood pressure in glaucoma, 74
Blood supply,
   optic chiasma, 11
   optic nerve, 7
   optic radiations, 19
   optic tracts, 14
   retina, 5
   visual cortex, 20, 157
Blood vessel(s) basilar artery, 143
   central retinal artery, 91
   central retinal vein, 92
   cilioretinal artery, 92
   internal carotid, 141
   middle cerebral, 141
   posterior cerebral, 143
   superior temporal artery, 92
Brain, calcarine fissure in, 20
   frontal lobe tumour, 119
   occipital lobe, 20, 21, 143, 146
   occipital visual cortex in, 21, 143, 146
   parietal lobe, 152
   post-calcarine fissure, 20, 21
   temporal lobe, 152

Calcarine fissure, 20
Calcification in tumours, 43
Carbon bisulphide, 107
Carotid, internal thrombosis, 66, 141
Cataracts, effect on visual field, 49
Central angiospastic retinopathy, 40, 60, 162
Central retinal artery, 7, 91
   occlusion, 66, 91

INDEX

Central retinal vein, 91
  thrombosis of, 91
Central scotoma, analysis of, 53, 117
  in hereditary optic atrophy, 108
  in nutritional amblyopia, 109
  in retrobulbar neuritis, 110
  in toxic amblyopia, 95
Central serous retinopathy, 40, 60, 162
Central vision, examination of, 40, 45, 53
Centrocaecal scotoma, 96
Cerebral arterial thrombosis, 141
Cerebral haemorrhage, 145
Cerebral representation, 20
Cerebral tumours, 152
Charts, 25, 46
  Amsler's, 40
  Bjerrum screen, 46
  Crick's, 46
  Harrington and Flock's test, 39
  multiple pattern test, 39
  for perimeter, 47
  for stereocampimeter, 38
  for tangent screen, 46
  Walker's, 47
Chiasma (see Optic chiasma), 9
Chloramphenicol, 106
Chloroquine, 100
Choroid:
  choroiditis, 160
  disseminated choroiditis, 160
  exudative choroiditis, 160
  juxtapapillary choroiditis, 66, 160
  neoplasms of, 94
  rupture, 160
  trauma, 160
Cilioretinal artery, 92
Circle of Willis, 10
Colloid bodies of the optic disc, 66, 164
Coloboma of optic disc, 66, 163
Colour targets, 28
  diagnostic value of, 28, 29
  disproportion, 28
Commotio retinae, 160
Compression,
  of chiasma, 124
  of optic nerve, 116
Conduction defects, 3
Confrontation test, 33, 44
  extinction phenomenon or inattention, 48
  with a light as a test object, 49
  with a sheet of white paper, 44
Congruity, 14, 15, 62, 64, 155
Congruous homonymous hemianopia, 20, 62, 64, 155
Contraction of field,
  in hysteria, 50
  in malingering, 50
  in post-neuritic atrophy, 169
  in syphilitic optic atrophy, 114
Conus, inferior, 164
Corneal opacities, effect on the visual field, 49
Correspondence, between field defect and lesion, 118, 133, 152
  between retina and visual cortex, 21
Cortex visual (see Visual cortex), 20
  vascular occlusions, 141

Cortical blindness, 145
Cortical representation, 20, 152
Cranial arteritis, 123
Craniopharyngioma, 124, 129
Crater-like hole of disc, 163
Crick's chart, 48
Critical fusion frequency, 38
Cushing's syndrome, 125

Decussation in optic chiasma, 9
Detachment of retina, 93
Devic's disease, 112
Digitalis poisoning, 103
Dimercaprol (B.A.L.), 105
Disproportion, 28
  in chiasmal compression, 29
  in retrobulbar neuritis, 111
  in syphilitic optic atrophy, 114
Disseminated choroiditis, 160
Disseminated sclerosis, 114, 136, 141
  retrochiasmal pathway, 141
Drusen, 66, 164

Eclipse scotoma, 162
Enlarged blind spot, 51
Ergot, 107
Ethambutol, 106
Evans' studies on angioscotomata, 48
Examination,
  analysis of defect, 46
  Bjerrum screen, 34, 44
  by confrontation, 33, 44
  dull patient, 50
  of field, 42, 43
  of malingerer, 50
  with perimeter, 35, 46
  in poor fixation, 52, 53
  with stereocampimeter, 37
  with tangent screen, 34, 44
  with test objects, coloured, 28
  unreliable patient, 45
Exophthalmic ophthalmoplegia, 66, 118
Exophthalmos, endocrine or pituitary, 66, 118
Exsanguination optic atrophy, 121
Extinction phenomenon, 48, 158

Field defect,
  analysis of, 32, 46
  in aphakia, 49
  baring of blind spot, 66
  in central area, 12, 14, 40, 61, 64
  centrocaecal scotoma, 96
  in chiasmal lesions, 11, 62, 64
  congruity, 18, 62, 63, 64
  contraction, 28
  depression, 28
  factors affecting, 133
  in glaucoma, 61
  due to head tilting, 51
  hemianopia,
    altitudinal, 115, 148
    bitemporal, 12, 62, 64
    congruous, 18, 20, 62, 63, 64
    heteronymous, 62, 64
    homonymous, 13, 62, 63, 64

Field defect—*contd.*
  in hysteria, 50
  incongruity, 64
  interpretation of, 133
  in lead poisoning, 106
  macular sparing, 18, 64
  in malingering or simulation, 50
  from medullated nerve fibres, 164
  nasal step, 72
  occipital cortex lesion, 22
  opacities of media, 49, 54, 58
  in optic radiation lesion, 22
  in optic tract lesion, 22, 157
  due to ptosis, 51
  quadrantopia, 17, 18
  in quinine poisoning, 104
  in retinal lesions, 61, 64
  in retrochiasmal lesions, 62, 63, 64
  in toxic amblyopia, 95
Filix mas, 105
Fixation in cases of central scotoma, 53, 146
Flicker fusion perimetry, 38
Foster Kennedy syndrome, 119
Friedmann analyser, 40

Glaucoma,
  angioscotometry in, 66
  angle-closure, 89
  aphakic, 89
  arcuate scotoma in, 61, 66
  baring of blind spot in, 66, 67
  Bjerrum's scotoma, 66, 67, 79
  blood pressure in, 74
  cause of field defects, 74
  closed-angle, 89
  detection of, 73
  double arcuate defect in, 73
  low tension, 123
  management, 87
  nasal step in, 72
  nerve fibre bundle defects in, 71
  paracentral defects, 72
  pathogenesis of, 74
  progress, 77
  secondary, 89
  static perimetry in, 54, 67
  temporal island of vision in, 87
Glioma of temporal lobe, 15
  of optic chiasma, 118
  of optic nerve, 118

Harrington and Flock's test, 39
Harrington's method using ultra-violet light, 45
Head injuries, 121, 137, 145
Head tilting, effect of, 51
Hemianopia, altitudinal, 114, 146
  binasal, 140
Hemianopia, bitemporal, 11, 64, 124
  heteronymous, 64, 124
  homonymous, 12, 17, 62, 63, 64, 141
    congruous, 18, 20, 64, 155
    incongruous, 14, 151, 155
    investigation, 158
    in subgeniculate lesions, 155
    in suprageniculate lesions, 155

Hemiplegia associated with hemianopia, 141
Hill of vision, Traquair's, 28, 55
Hippocampal herniation in cerebral tumours, 145
History, 42
  amenorrhoea, 124
  hirsuties, 124
  impotence, 124
  lactation, 114
  pregnancy, 114
  symptoms and signs of importance, 42
Homonymous hemianopia (see also Hemianopia), 12, 17, 62, 63, 64, 141
  investigation of, 158
  scotomata, 143, 146
Hughes' quadrants of central scotoma, 117
Hydrocephalus, 140
Hydroxychloroquine, 100
Hysteria, 50
  field defects in, 50
    concentric contraction, 50
    reversal, 50
    spiral field, 50

Illumination of Bjerrum screen, 35
  reduced, use of, 52
  ultra-violet light, 45
  variations in, for detection of field defects, 45
Inattention, 48, 158
Incongruity, 14, 15, 64, 151, 158
Instruments, choice of, 40
Internal capsule, 16
  relation of, to optic radiations, 16
    to optic tract, 12
Intracranial pressure, increased, effect on field defects, 50, 167
  X-ray indications, 43
Iodoform, 104
Isopters, 28
  contraction of, 28
  definition, 28
  disproportion, 28

Junction scotoma, 12, 118, 132

Knee of Wilbrand, 9, 12, 118, 132

Lactation and retrobulbar neuritis, 114
Lateral geniculate body, 14
  blood supply of, 15
Laurence-Moon-Biedl syndrome, 91
Lead poisoning, 106
Leber's optic atrophy, 108
Localizing signs in retrochiasmal pathway, 155
  of X-ray examination, 43

Macula,
  fibres of, 3
  lesions of, 40, 160
  sparing of, 18, 64, 157
  splitting of macula, 14, 137
Macular degeneration, examination of, 40, 52
Macular fibres, 3
  in lateral geniculate body, 5
  in occipital cortex, 21
  in optic chiasma, 5

INDEX

Macular fibres—contd.
  in optic nerve, 5
  in optic radiation, 16
  in optic tract, 5, 9
Macular sparing, 18, 20, 64, 157
Maculopapillary fibres, 4, 5
Malingering, 50
Medial opacities, 28, 49, 54, 58
Medullated nerve fibres, 164
Melanoma of choroid, 94
Meningioma,
  compressing chiasma, 124
  olfactory groove, 119
  of optic nerve, 118
  of sphenoid ridge, 66, 118
Menopause and retrobulbar neuritis, 114
Methods of examination, 33
  Bjerrum screen, 34, 44
  confrontation, 33, 44
  perimeter, 35, 46
  stereocampimeter, 37
Methyl alcohol, 99
Meyer's loop, 17, 152
Miles' method of flicker fusion perimetry, 38
Miosis, effect of, 54, 58
Monocular field, 26
  cerebral representation of, 21, 155
Multiple pattern test, 39
Multiple sclerosis,
  of chiasma, 136
  of optic nerve, 112
  retrobulbar neuritis in, 112
  suprageniculate pathway, 141
Myopia, 58, 66, 164

Nasal step in glaucoma, 72
Nasally directed scleral canal, 163
Nerve fibre bundle defects, 4, 64, 66, 71
Nerve fibres,
  crossed, 9
  in lateral geniculate body, 14
  macular, 3
  in occipital visual cortex, 21, 146, 157
  in optic chiasma, 9
  in optic nerve, 5, 9
  in optic radiation, 16, 155
  in optic tract, 5, 9
  in retina, 3
Neuromyelitis optica, 112
Nutritional amblyopia, 109

Occipital cortex, 20
  field defects in lesions of, 141
  post-calcarine fissure in, 21, 143
Occipital lobe tumours, 153
Occlusion of central retinal artery, 66, 91
  central retinal vein, 92
  cilioretinal artery, 92
  superior temporal artery, 92
  superior temporal vein, 93
Opacities of the media, 28, 49, 54, 58

Optic atrophy,
  arteriosclerotic, 123
  exsanguination, 121
  hereditary, 108
  post-neuritic, 169
  secondary, 169
  syphilitic, 28, 114
Optic chiasma,
  anatomy of, 9
  anterior and posterior knees of Wilbrand, 9
  blood supply, 11
  compression of, 10, 29, 124
  factors affecting field changes, 118, 133, 152
  lesions at, 11, 29
    arachnoiditis, 136
    disseminated sclerosis, 136
    inflammation, 136
    syphilis, 28, 137
    trauma, 137
    tumours, 124
  loop of knee of Wilbrand, 9, 12, 118, 132
  pre- and post-fixation, 10, 133
  relationship to other structures, 9, 10
Optic disc,
  anatomy at, 4
  atrophy of, 43, 111, 119, 126, 138, 157
  coloboma of, 66, 163
  crater-like hole, 163
  cupping of, 43, 74
  nerve fibres of, 4
  neuritis of, 110
  oedema of, 119, 167
  pallor of, 3, 4, 43, 111, 119, 126, 138, 157
Optic nerve,
  anatomical relations of, 6
  arrangement of fibres in, 5
  atrophy, 3, 4, 43, 111, 119, 126, 138, 157
  avulsion of, 121
  blood supply of, 7
  cavernous, 123
  compression, 116
  exsanguination, 121
  due to haemorrhage, 121
  inflammation of, 110
  lesions of, 66, 108
  multiple sclerosis, 114
  neuritis (see Retrobulbar neuritis), 110
  papillitis, 110
  post-neuritic, 169
  retrobulbar neuritis, 110
    bilateral forms of, 112
    pain in, 6, 111
  syphilitic optic neuritis, 114
  toxic amblyopia, 95
    bilateral central scotoma in, 95
    bilateral peripheral contraction, 114
    centrocaecal scotoma in, 95
  trauma, 120
  tumours of, 117
  vascular lesions of, 121
Optic radiation,
  abscesses, 152
  anatomy of, 16
  blood supply, 19
  congruous homonymous hemianopia in, 20, 64, 155

INDEX

Optic radiation—*contd.*
  lesions of, 141
    associated symptoms in, 141
    congruity, 20, 64, 155
    field defects in, 20, 64, 141, 153
    pupil in, 157
    sparing of macula in, 157
    trauma, 145
    vascular, 141
  macular fibres in, 16, 146, 157
  Meyer's loop in, 17, 152
  relationship to internal capsule, 16, 141
  vascular supply to, 19
Optic tract,
  anatomy of, 12
  blood supply, 14
  lesions of, 14, 141, 152
    incongruity in, 14, 62, 155
  nerve fibres in, 6, 14
  relationship to basis pedunculi, 12
  splitting of macula in, 14
  vascular supply, 14
Optochiasmatic arachnoiditis, 66
Orbital tumours, 117

Papillitis, 66, 110
Papilloedema, 66, 167
Parietal lobe tumours, 152
Perimeter, 35
  charts for recording findings, 38, 46
  correspondence to retina, 25
  examination with, 46
  Goldmann, 36, 40
  hand, 35
  hemispherical, 36
  Oculus, 36, 40
  relationship to tangent screen, 30
  standard, 35
  test objects used, 36, 37
  Tubingen, 36, 40
  ultra-violet light, 45
Perimetry, aspects of,
  Bjerrum tangent screen, 34, 40
  confrontation tests, 33, 44
  flicker fusion, 38
  instruments, choice of, 40
  kinetic, 37, 54
  perimeter, 35, 46
  profile, 37, 54
  static, 37, 54
  stereocampimeter, 37, 38
  tangent screen, 34, 40
  threshold, 37, 54
Peripheral neuritis due to toxins, 95
Pernicious anaemia, 109
Phenothiazine, 106
Pituitary gland
  basophil tumour, 125
  chromophobe tumour, 66, 126
  eosinophil tumour, 125
  tumours, 124
    acromegaly in, 126
    management of, 138
Plerocephalic oedema, 167
Poor fixation, examination of fields in, 53

Post-neuritic optic atrophy, 169
Pre- and post-fixation of chiasma, 10, 133
Pregnancy and chiasmal tumours, 125
Pregnancy and retrobulbar neuritis, 114
Proptosis, unilateral, 43, 117
Pseudoneuritis, 165
Pseudopapilloedema, 165
Ptosis, effect on visual field, 51
Puberty and retrobulbar neuritis, 114
Pupil,
  in pregeniculate lesions, 111, 121
  reactions of, in cortical blindness, 145, 146
  Wernicke's reaction, 158

Quadrantopia, 17
  lower, 63, 143, 151
  upper, 17, 151, 152
Quinine amblyopia, 104
Quinoline, 106

Radiation (see Optic radiation), 16
Records, 29
Refractive errors, 58
Regeneration, absence of, in visual pathway, 3
Relative field, 26
Retina, affections of, 61, 90
    blood supply, 5
    central serous retinopathy, 40, 60, 162
    commotio retinae, 160
    detachment, 93
    eclipse scotoma, 162
    retinitis pigmentosa, 31, 90
    separation of retina, 93
    trauma, 160
    vascular, 91
  anatomy of, 3
    arcuate fibres in, 4
    arrangement of nerve fibres in, 3
    blood supply of, 5
    central artery of, 91
    central vein of, thrombosis of, 92
    cerebral representation of, 21, 146, 157
    corresponding points, 21
    detachment of, 93
    horizontal raphe of, 4
      vascular supply, 5
    maculopapillary fibres, 4, 5
    nerve fibre layer, 3, 71
Retinitis pigmentosa, 31, 90
Retinopathy, central serous, 40, 60, 162
Retrobulbar lesions, 64, 110
Retrobulbar neuritis, 66, 110
  examination of central area of field, 40, 53
  sinusitis, 114
Retrochiasmal lesions, 64, 160
Roenne's nasal step, 4, 72
Rupture of choroid, 160

Salicylate poisoning, 105
Scleral canal, nasally directed, 163
Scotomata, 30, 53, 60
  absolute, 31
  analysis, 32, 53
  angio-, 48

INDEX

Scotomata—*contd.*
  arcuate, 61, 66, 72, 73
    double, 77
  bitemporal, 133
  Bjerrum, 73
  central, 53, 95, 108
    pathogenesis of, 7
    plotting, 53
    use of polarized light, 53
    use of red-green goggles, 53
    in retrobulbar neuritis, 61, 110
    use of stereoscopic devices, 53
  centrocaecal, 95
  congruous homonymous, 146
  homonymous, 146
  junction, 12, 118, 132
  negative, 30
  nuclei of density in, 96, 112, 146
  paracentral, 60, 72
  positive, 30
  relative, 30
  retrobulbar neuritis in, 110
  ring, 31, 77
  suppression in strabismus, 170
  visual acuity, relation to, 31
Screen, Bjerrum, tangent, 34, 40
Secondary optic atrophy, 169
Sellar and extrasellar lesions, 124
Sinusitis, 114
Size, of blind spot, 25
  of monocular field, 25
Slope, gradual, 31, 32, 54
  in retinitis pigmentosa, 31, 32
  in retinal detachment, 93
  steep, 31, 32, 54
Space-occupying lesions, 124, 152
Sparing of macula, 18, 20, 64, 157
Sphenoidal ridge, tumour of, 118
Spiral field in hysteria, 50
Splitting of macula, 14, 137, 146
Stereocampimeter, examination with, 37
Strabismus, scotoma in, 170
Striate area in visual cortex, 20, 145
Sulphonamide intoxication, 103
Suppression scotoma in strabismus, 170
Suprageniculate lesions,
  absence of optic atrophy in, 157
  field defect in (see Hemianopia), 13, 141
Syndrome,
  cortical blindness, 145
  Foster Kennedy, 119
  Laurence-Moon-Biedl, 91
Syphilitic optic atrophy, 28, 114

Tangent screen (Bjerrum), 34, 40
Targets, 33, 35
  coloured, 28
  size in mm. compared to degrees, 30
  value of, 28
Temporal arteritis, 123
Temporal crescent, 21, 26, 155
Temporal lobe lesion field defects, 18, 152
Temporal lobe tumours, 152

Test objects, 33, 35
  coloured, 28
  conversion of size of, from mm. to degrees, 30
  value of, 28
Thallium scotomata, 103
Thrombosis (see Atherosclerosis),
  central retinal artery, 91
  central retinal vein, 92
Thyroid exophthalmos, 66, 118
Tobacco amblyopia, 95
Toxic amblyopia, 95
  aniline, 107
  arsenic, 105
  aspidium, 105
  carbon bisulphide, 107
  chloroquine, 100
  chloramphenicol, 106
  digitalis, 103
  ergot, 107
  ethambutol, 106
  ethyl alcohol, 98
  filix mas, 105
  iodoform, 104
  lead, 106
  methyl alcohol, 99
  phenothiazine, 106
  quinine, 104
  quinoline, 106
  rare causes of, 107
  salicylates, 105
  sulphonamides, 103
  thallium, 103
  tobacco, 95
Traquair's hill of vision, 27, 28, 54
Trauma avulsion of optic nerve, 121
  of occipital cortex, 145
  to optic chiasma, 137
  to optic nerve, 120
Tryparsamide, 105
Tubular field,
  glaucoma, 87
  hysteria, 30
  quinine, 104
  retinitis pigmentosa, 31

Ultra-violet light in perimetry, 45
Uniocular field, 21, 26, 155

Vascular lesions of cortex, 141
Vascular occlusion of retinal blood vessels, 91
Vein, central of retina, 92
  superior temporal vein occlusion, 93
Vertebral-basilar insufficiency, 143
Vision,
  acuity of, 28, 31
  field of,
    binocular, 26
    monocular, 25
  importance of, 28
  medial opacities, effect of, 28, 49
  refractive error, 28, 49
  relation to visual field, 28, 31, 49, 58
Visual awareness, 48, 158
Visual cortex,
  adjacent structures, relation to, 16

Visual cortex—*contd.*
  anatomy of, 20
  blood supply, 20
  calcarine fissure in, 20
  cortical representation, 21
  lesions of, 143, 145
    characteristics of, 155
    congruous hemianopia in, 151, 155
    homonymous hemianopic scotoma in, 146
    macular sparing, 151, 157
    representation of retina in, 21
  sparing of macula, 151, 157
  striate area in, 21
  temporal crescent in, 21, 26, 155
  trauma, 145
  tumour of, 152

Visual cortex—*contd.*
  types of field defects in lesions of, 64, 141
  vascular lesions, 141
  vascular supply to, 20, 157
Visual field, 25
Vitamin deficiency, 109

Walker's chart, 47
Wernicke's pupil reaction, 158
White line of Gennari, 20
Wilbrand's knee, 9, 12, 118, 132
Wolff and Penman, 4
Wood alcohol poisoning, 99

X-ray examination, 43, 119, 137
X-ray findings in chiasmal compression, 137